TRADITIONAL THAI YOGA

TRADITIONAL THAI YOGA

The Postures and Healing Practices of Ruesri Dat Ton

Enrico Corsi and Elena Fanfani

Photographs by Enrico Magri

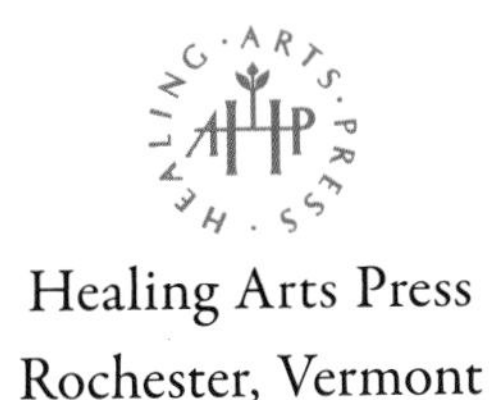

Healing Arts Press
Rochester, Vermont

Healing Arts Press
One Park Street
Rochester, Vermont 05767
www.HealingArtsPress.com

Healing Arts Press is a division of Inner Traditions International

Note to the reader: *This book is intended as an informational guide. The remedies, approaches, and techniques described herein are meant to supplement, and not to be a substitute for, professional medical care or treatment. They should not be used to treat a serious ailment without prior consultation with a qualified health care professional.*

Library of Congress Cataloging-in-Publication Data
Corsi, Enrico.
Traditional Thai yoga : the postures and healing practices of Ruesri dat ton / Enrico Corsi and Elena Fanfani.
p. cm.
Includes index.
ISBN: 978-1-59477-205-4 (pbk.)
1. Hatha yoga—Therapeutic use. 2. Medicine, Thai. I. Fanfani, Elena. II. Title.
RA781.7.C677 2008
613.7'046—dc22

2007049473

Printed and bound in India by Replika Press Pvt Ltd.

10 9 8 7 6 5 4 3 2 1

Text design and layout by Jon Desautels
This book was typeset in Garamond Premier Pro with Phaistos and Franklin Gothic used as the display typefaces

To send correspondence to the authors of this book, mail a first-class letter to the authors c/o Inner Traditions • Bear & Company, One Park Street, Rochester, VT 05767, and we will forward the communication.

To Prem Rawat

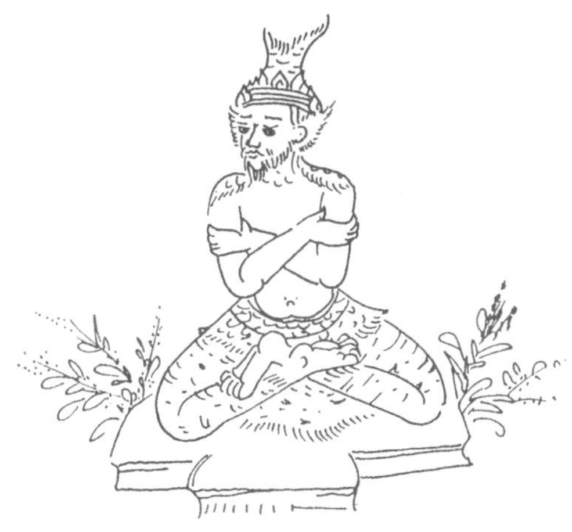

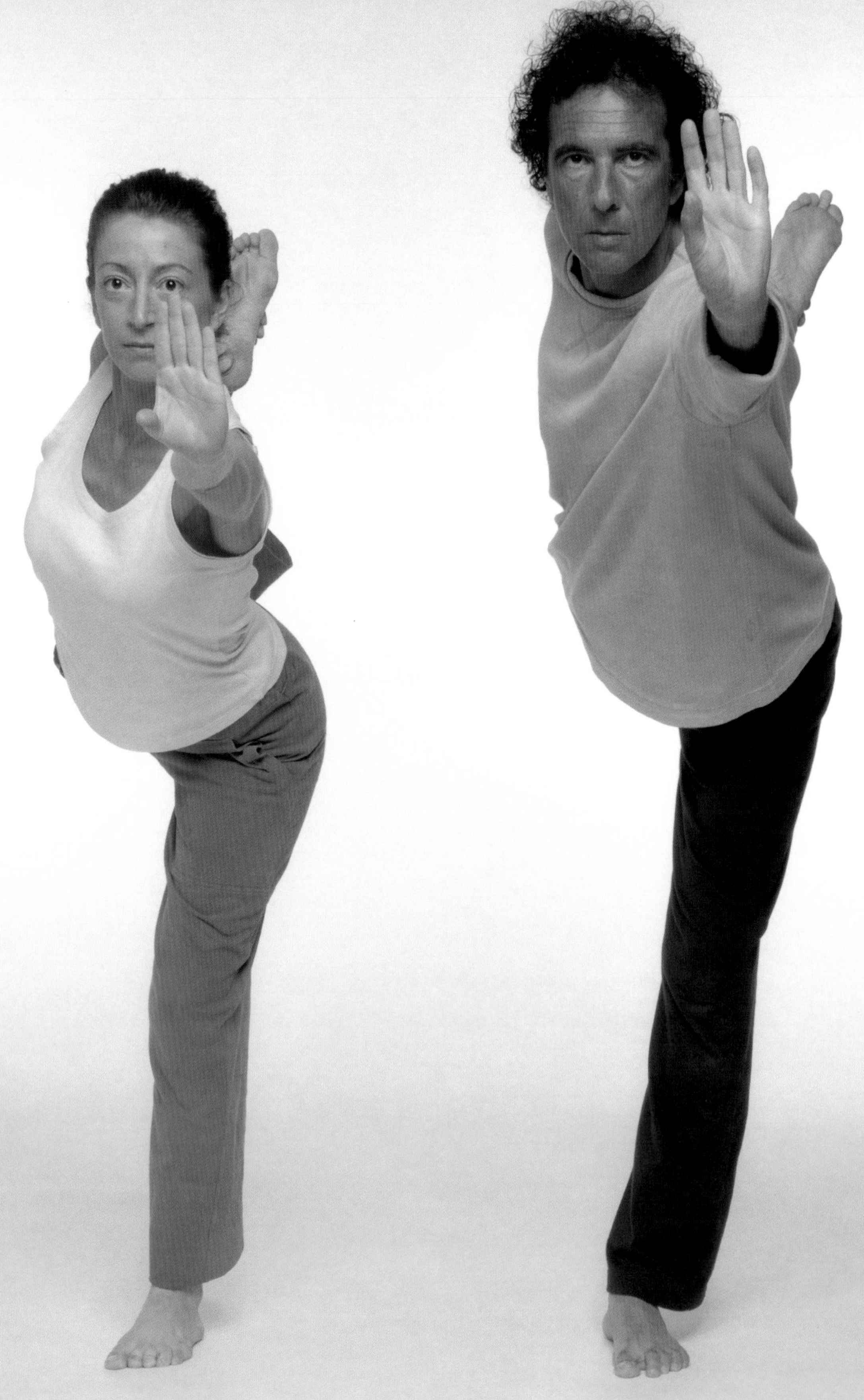

Contents

Acknowledgments

We truly thank our Thai teachers Tung and Sonh Pohn for sharing their skill in and enthusiasm for this priceless treasure, Andrea Macario for translating from Thai, Nerio Brugna for the location, our parents Rosa and Antonio Fanfani and Elena and Mario Corsi, Cristiano Cori, Vittorio Maiullari, Bruna Gabrielli, Silvio Satta, Susan Athol, Linda Murray, and all our students who helped us grow with their feedback. We also thank the editorial and production staff at Healing Arts Press for producing this beautiful book.

Preface

We first had the opportunity to experience Ruesri Dat Ton—traditional Thai yoga—after we had been visiting Thailand for many years in order to deepen our knowledge of Thai medicine. We almost immediately understood that we had discovered a priceless jewel that nobody had yet tried to unveil. But only by regularly practicing its techniques have we come to understand how deep are the qualities of this discipline.

We sincerely hope that our readers will be able to perceive in this text at least one sparkle of the enthusiasm that accompanied its composition. During every stage of this project we felt both privilege and responsibility in exposing a discipline formed by absolute qualities.

We also hope, with all our heart, that many of you will be able to draw benefit from the brilliant intuition that someone, more than 2,500 years ago, placed at mankind's disposal. And it is to this person, to Jivaka, physician and Buddha's personal friend, that we dedicate the memory of this book.

We don't know whether Jivaka, when he developed these techniques, could ever have imagined that one day his work would be spread so widely. And we don't know whether he is able, in some transcendental shape alien to our understanding, to observe his work enduring through time and expanding into space.

Still, sometimes, practicing Ruesri Dat Ton and the other disciplines that Jivaka created, we imagine him to be next to us.

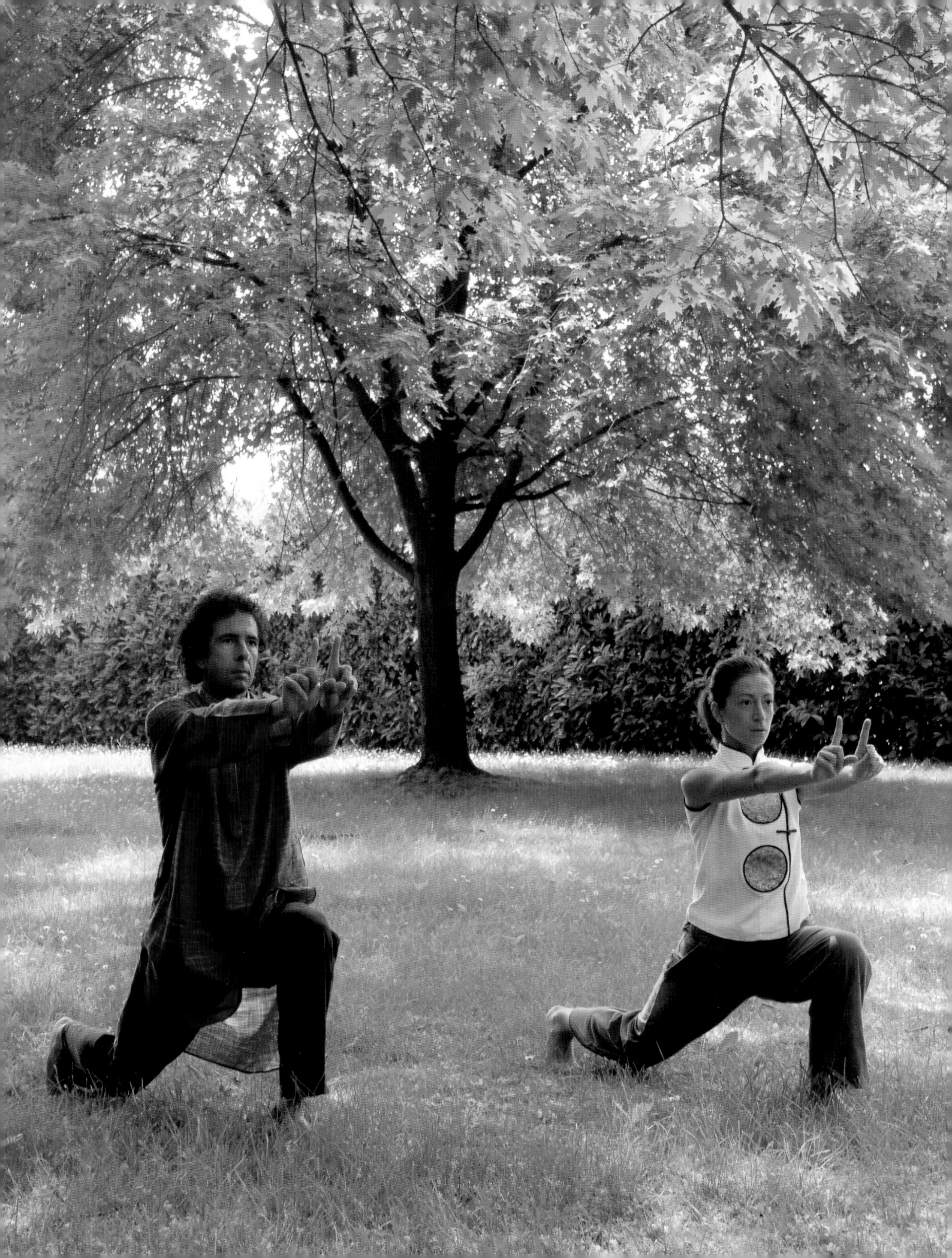

PART ONE

About the Practice of Ruesri Dat Ton

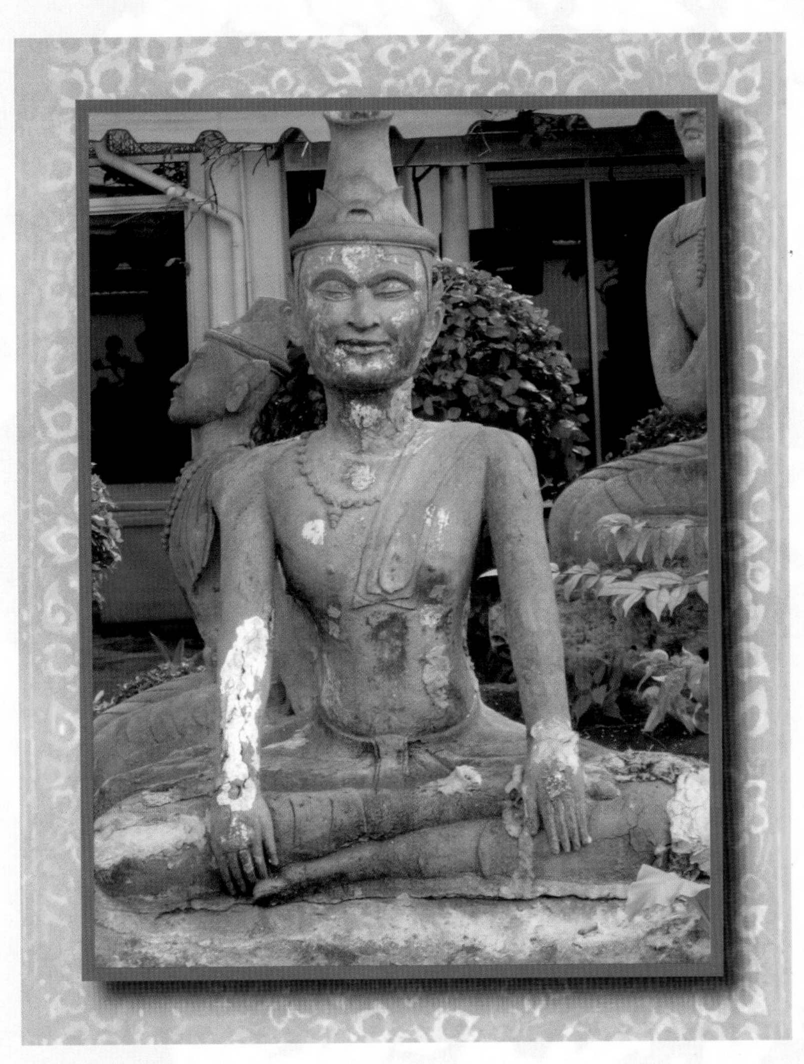

ONE

The History of Ruesri Dat Ton

The origins of ancient Siamese medicine are still today the object of research and debate. In the past the kingdom of Siam (in what is present-day Thailand) enjoyed long periods of splendor, and we must assume that independent therapeutic arts were developed during that fertile age. Furthermore, Thailand represents a natural borderline and meeting point between two great civilizations: India and China. Consequently the practice of Thai medicine received the benevolent influence of both Ayurvedic medicine and traditional Chinese medicine.

TRADITIONAL THAI MEDICINE

Traditional Thai medicine includes three main branches: traditional Thai massage (Nuad Bo Rarn), traditional Thai yoga (Ruesri Dat Ton), and Thai herbal medicine. Like traditional Chinese medicine and Ayurvedic medicine, traditional Thai medicine is a holistic system that heals by facilitating the free flow of energy throughout the body. All of the Thai healing practices seek to balance the flow of energy in the *sen* energy channels, a network of energy pathways in the body in which life energy circulates.

Many Westerners are most familiar with traditional Thai massage, in which a Thai massage practitioner helps the massage recipient into

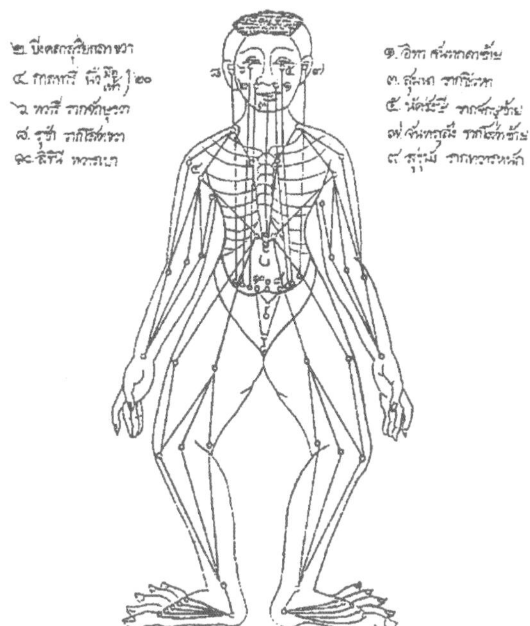

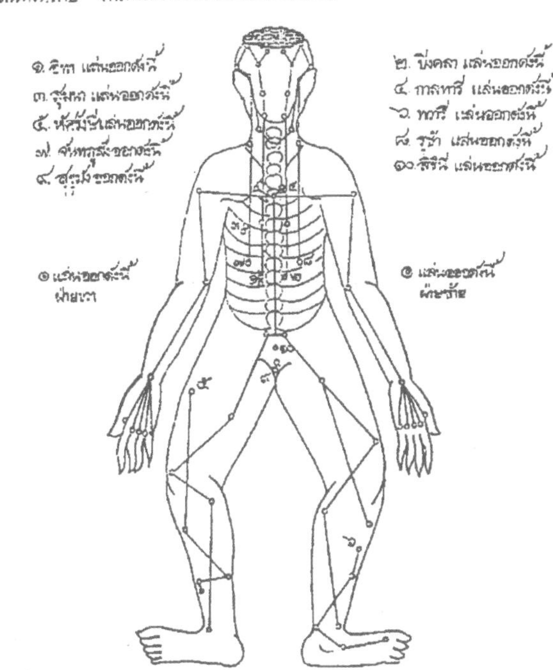

An ancient Thai temple drawing of the sen energy system, showing the energy pathways on the front and back of the body.

beneficial postures, stretches various parts of the body, and applies pressure to trigger points along the sen pathways. Ruesri Dat Ton—which translates literally as "the hermit's autocure"—is different from Thai massage in that it is a solo yoga practice. Practitioners can perform the healing postures on their own without the assistance of a trained massage professional. Though some of the postures may seem challenging at first, and it is important to follow the directions precisely for the best results, the system is, overall, a simple one. With diligent practice, an individual can significantly improve his or her own health.

In fact, one of the main characteristics of Thai medicine is its simplicity. All its therapeutic instruments are made up of essential conceptual virtues. In fact, emphasis is placed on the ability to "feel," to "perceive," and, with practice, to "grow" toward these virtues in order to improve the result of the medicine. This is why it may be defined as "popular medicine": because it may be used by anyone, regardless of his or her education. The practice of the various therapeutic instruments of Thai medicine, particularly massage and herbal medicine, is widespread among the Thai population, in which techniques and secrets are usually handed down from one generation to the next.

One characteristic of Thai medicine that, along with the healing techniques, has been handed down over the centuries is the Buddhist concept of *metta*. The most appropriate translation of this term is "loving-kindness." In other words, the techniques of traditional Thai medicine are often taught and practiced in Thailand in a spirit of loving care, with the goal of providing comfort.

THE FATHER OF THAI MEDICINE: JIVAKA KUMARABHACCA

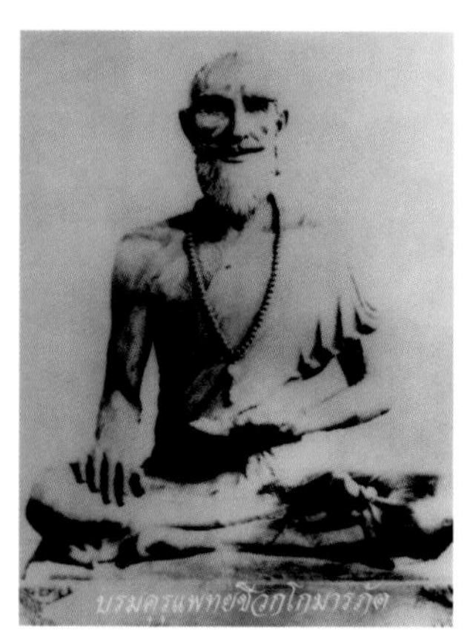

Jivaka Kumarabhacca

Tradition holds that Thai medicine derives from the teachings of Jivaka Kumarabhacca, who lived in approximately 500 BC and was not only a personal friend of Buddha but also the physician of the master's community. Jivaka, also known as Khun Shivago or Shivago Komparpaì, was a rishi before joining Buddha's community.

According to ancient sacred Hindu scriptures, in particular the Ramayana, the rishis were hermits who lived in the remote valleys of the Himalayas and practiced very particular internal exercises that enabled them to meditate for extremely long periods. The practice of such contemplation allowed them to develop a perceptive sensitivity of their bodies on a very high level. When the rishis interrupted this state of immobility, it was essential that they use some therapeutic techniques to restart their bodily functions within a relatively short time. Most of the active and passive ancient Asian disciplines that are used today probably derive from the exercises performed by these extraordinary people.

Jivaka's therapeutic techniques arrived in Thailand thanks to a Buddhist community that, over the course of centuries, driven by historical events and hostility toward its religious beliefs, migrated from the Indian subcontinent. From India this community moved to Ceylon and then on to Cambodia, where it found hospitality with the Khmer civilization in the Angkor empire. In 1238 the Thai kingdom conquered Sukhothai and absorbed the Khmer culture. The Thais converted to Buddhism and developed their own language, which derived from Pali and Sanskrit, and they began to study the ancient scriptures

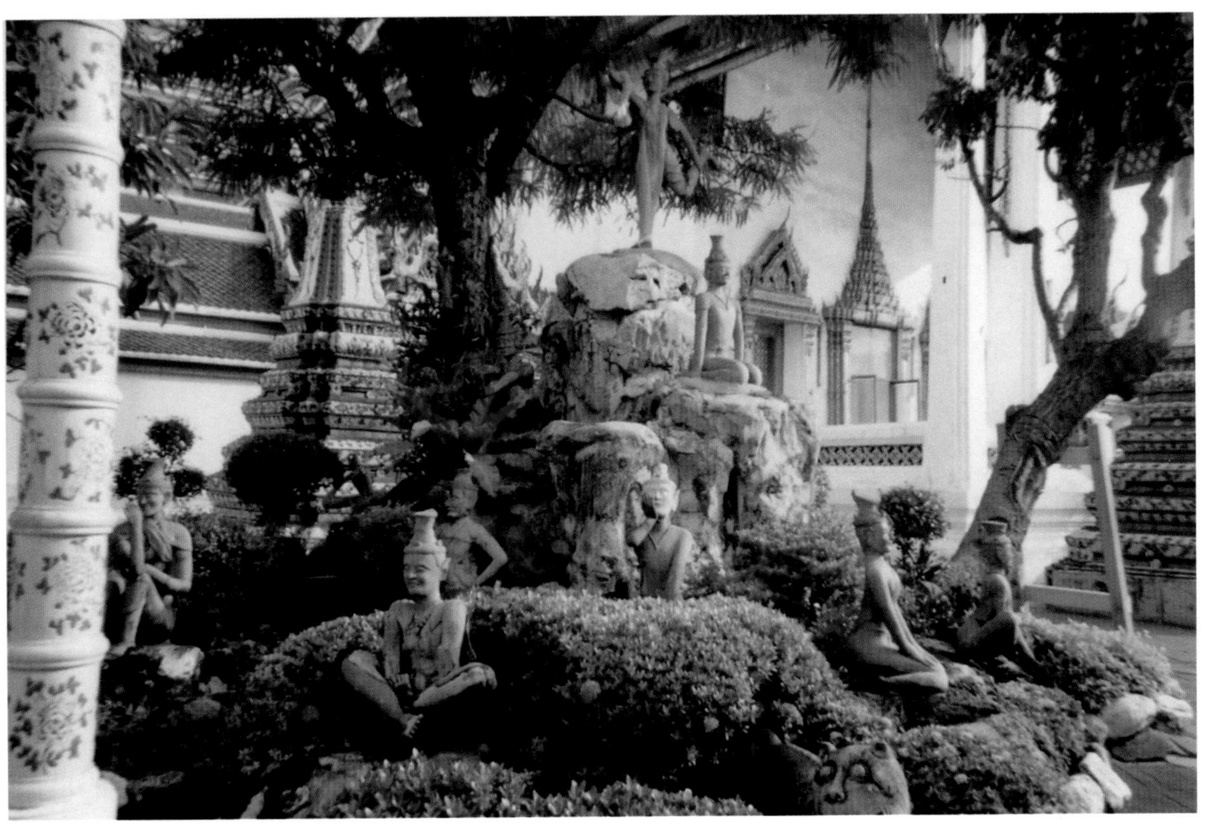

Garden at the temple of Wat Pho in Bangkok, showing some of the remaining statues of Jivaka performing traditional Thai yoga postures.

of this culture. They evidently began to practice yoga and other disciplines handed down by Jikava's teachings. These disciplines were practiced and evolved over the centuries, thanks mainly to the exercise and teachings of the monks inside the temple walls.

Following the 1787 Burmese conquest of Ayutthaya, which was then the capital of Thailand, many Thai medical texts were lost. At the beginning of nineteenth century King Rama III ordered the collection of all the remaining ancient medical texts throughout the Thai kingdom in order to catalog, compare, and preserve them. Some of these pieces are still preserved in the temple of Wat Pho in Bangkok. Among these is the representation of the sen energy system conceived by Jivaka, the oldest existing historical representation of the body's energy systems.

The Wat Pho temple also contains what remains of the original 120 statues of Jivaka performing traditional Thai yoga techniques and eighty drawings of the actual statues. King Rama I began the construction of the statues, which were based on an examination of the texts,

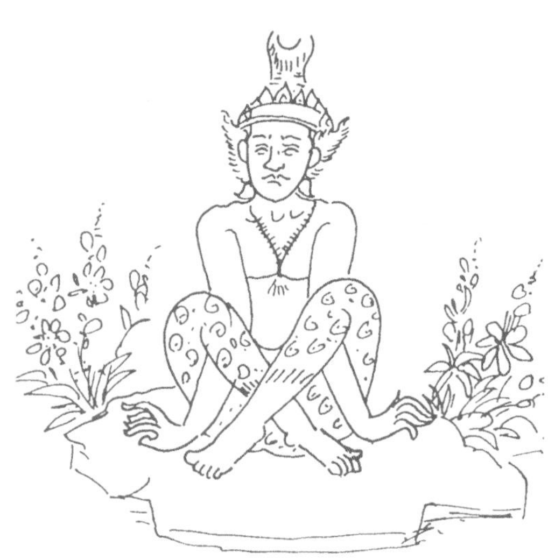

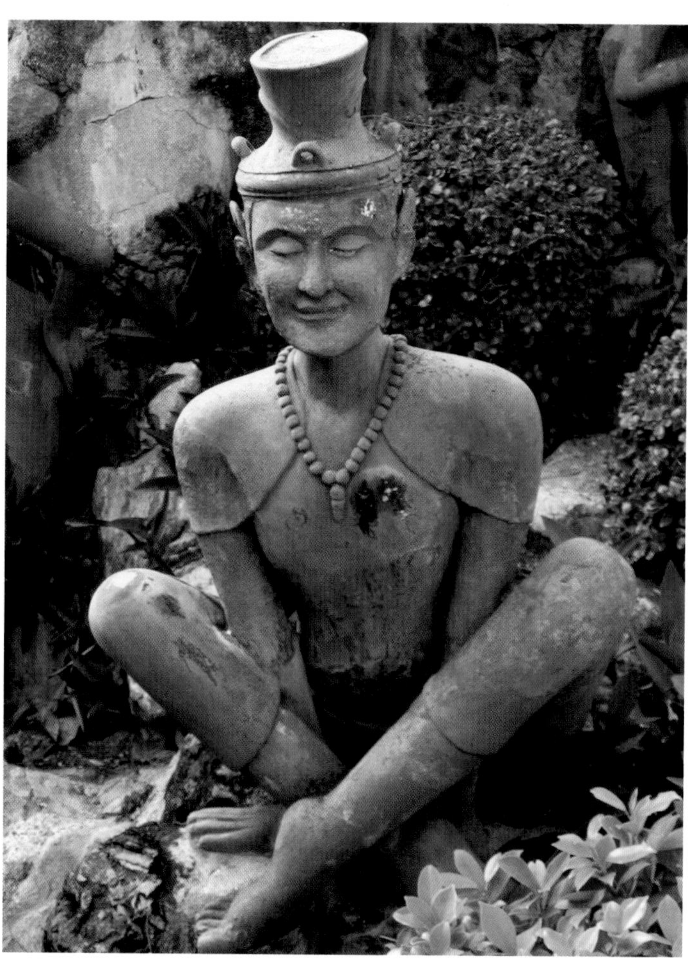

Above: An archival drawing of the statue shown on the right

Right: A statue of Jivaka performing a posture to remedy stiff knees

and they were completed by Rama III. The drawings, which were commissioned to famous artists of that time, were executed to preserve likenesses of the statues, which have inevitably suffered degradation. Each drawing is accompanied by a description, written in verse by a famous poet, of the performance and therapeutic benefit of the exercise it depicts.

As you can see, the history of Thai medicine has its origins in mythological times and characters. Nevertheless, even today, Thai medicine is practiced according to the principles and practices defined centuries ago. The effectiveness of the knowledge and the techniques leads one to feel that the scientific inheritance handed down from Jivaka is a true gift. This is why Jivaka is still a very popular and respected figure throughout the kingdom. The Thais call him the Father of Medicine or, more affectionately, Daddy Doctor.

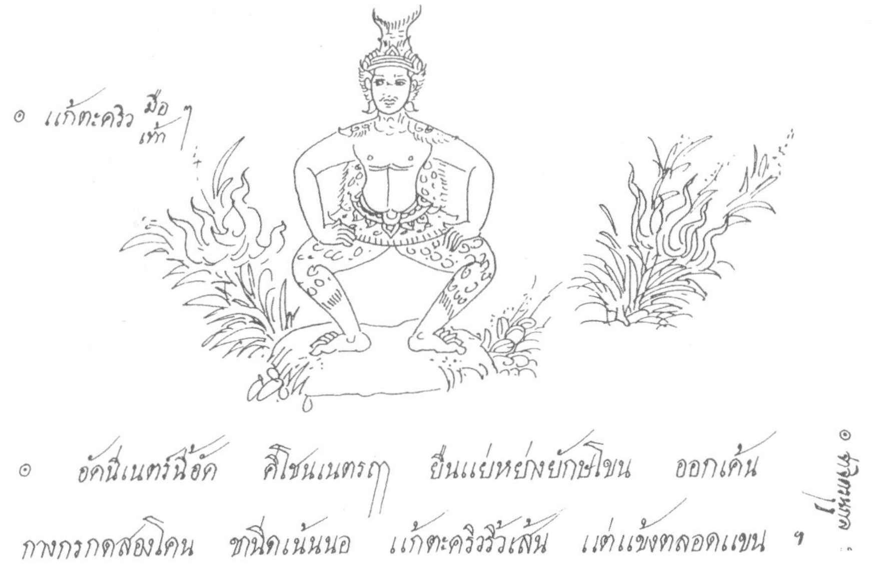

An archival drawing of Jivaka performing a remedy for cramps in the hands and feet, accompanied by a lyrical description of the posture in the ancient Thai language

RUESRI DAT TON: THE HERMIT'S ART OF HEALING

Thai yoga is based on the drawings and statues of Jikava practicing the exercises. These representations are based on iconographies and ancient texts that have since been lost. They are very important to the correct understanding of the exercises and are contemplated at length by those who wish to improve in the practice of this discipline. Each drawing holds a wealth of detail and useful information for comprehension of the techniques.

Descriptions of the exercises were composed in verse. This lyrical text makes great use of metaphor, which gives indirect information about the dynamics of the movements. For example, the description of the exercise shown above reads as follows:

From burning eyes
Of live flames,
Of the giant mask,
Assume the dance pose.
With outstretched arms,
Push hands on hips.
This is the remedy for cramping
In the hands and feet.

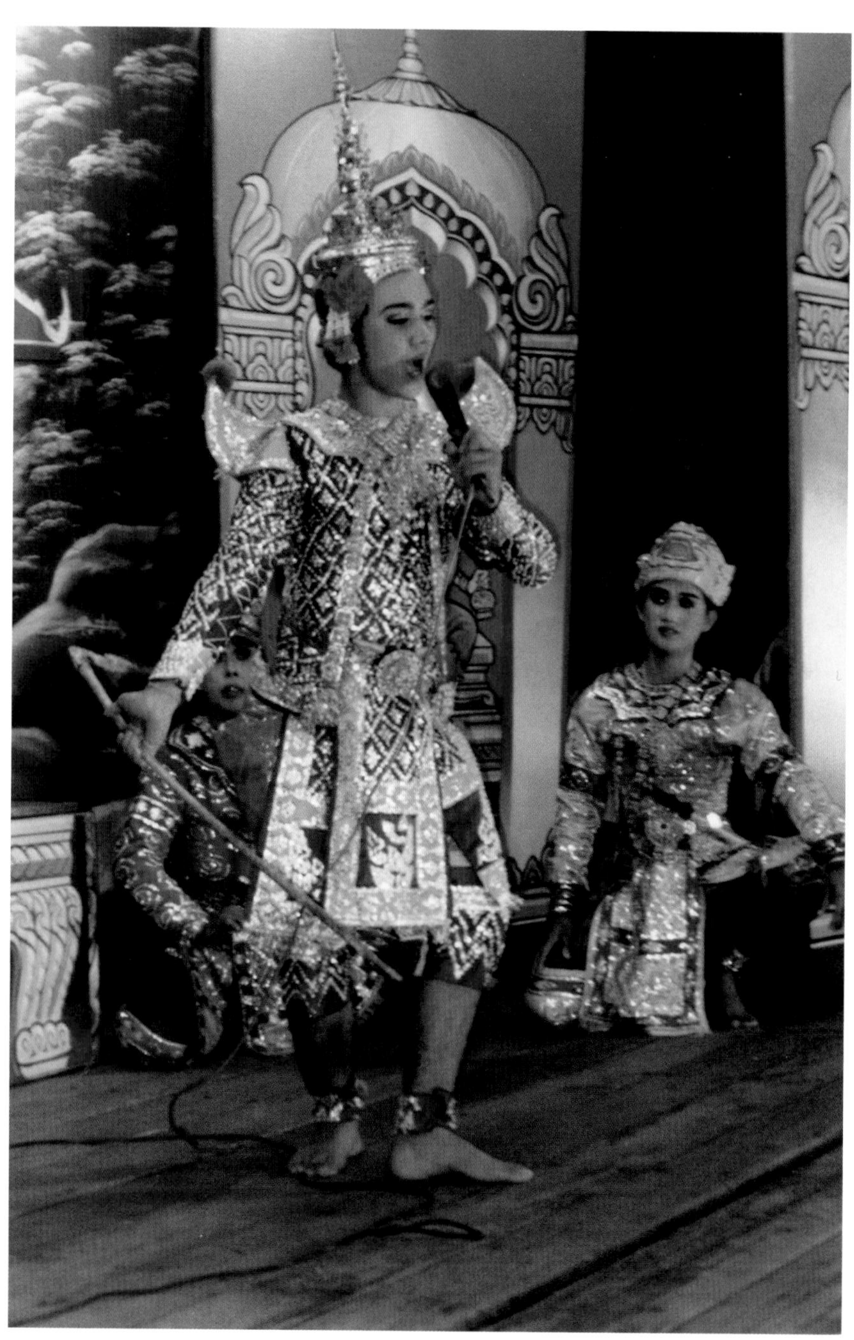

Thai dance is a derivative of traditional Thai yoga exercises.

Thai yoga, the hermit's art of healing, was once practiced mainly inside the temples of Buddhist monks. In recent times, though, it has spread throughout Thailand. One of the disciplines derived from the hermit's exercises, Thai dance, has become very popular. According to some, even Muay Thai (Thai boxing) is derived from Thai yoga exercises.

TWO

Principles and Benefits of the Practice

THE SEN ENERGY SYSTEM

The theoretical foundation of Thai medicine is based on the sen energy system. The sen are ten energy channels found throughout the body. The objective of Thai medicine, whether it is active or passive, is to reestablish the function of the body's systems by rebalancing the flow of energy in the sen. This practice is capable of curing and preventing numerous ailments by emphasizing the body's self-healing process.

Thai yoga and traditional Thai massage work in different ways, though along the same lines, to bring about the same final result. Both disciplines are based on the sensitivity of the person who uses them. Emphasis is always put on the sensation that the techniques give. In other words, it is the "feeling" produced by the massage or the exercise that determines the therapeutic results.

Because Thai yoga postures are practiced with a particular breathing technique, each posture evokes and channels energy, which is momentarily stored throughout the sen system. The practitioner must inhale deeply while moving into the posture. In this fashion, he or she introduces oxygen, which may be considered an energy container. Then the practitioner holds his or her breath for three seconds while maintaining the posture. Finally, the practitioner exhales and returns to the starting position. At completion, the exercise produces a benevolent

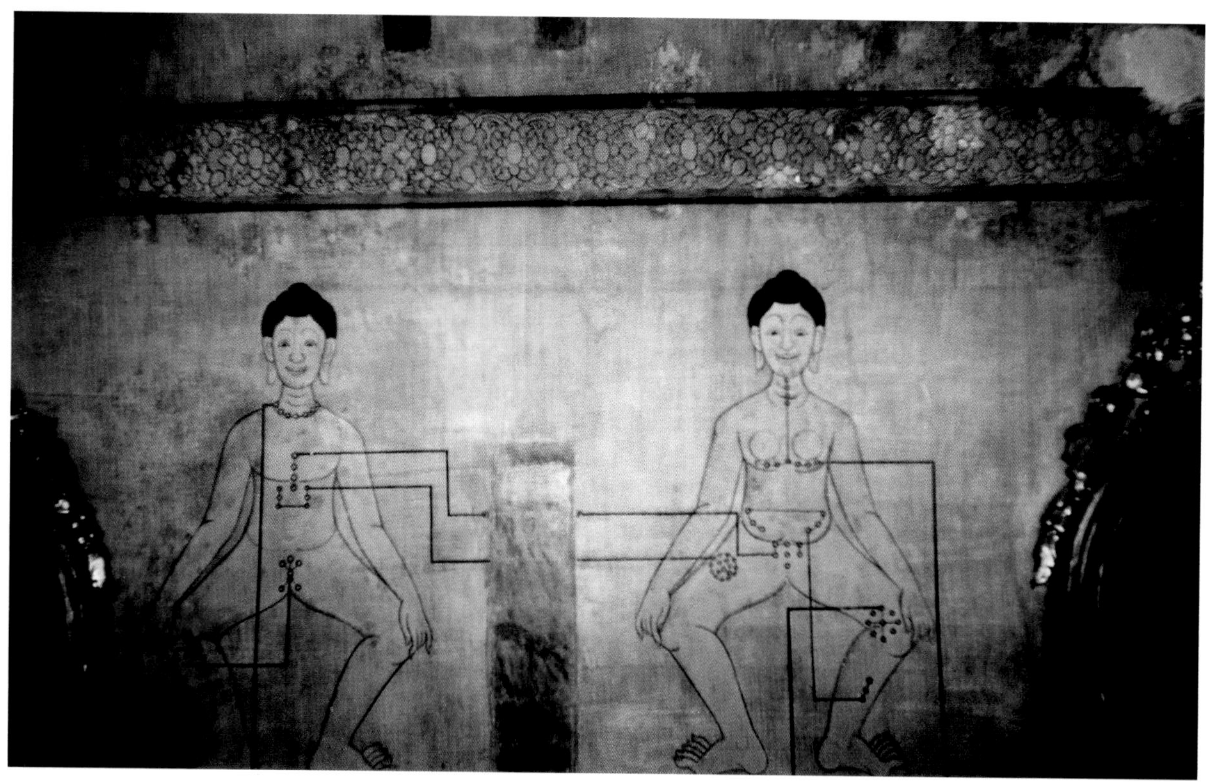

A representation of the sen energy system on a wall of the temple of Wat Pho in Bangkok, showing pressure points along the sen lines

and pleasantly warm sensation throughout the channels that have been used.

As you may gather, this particular type of breathing exercise is the most important part of the yoga discipline. The basic idea of the technique is to hold this energy for a few moments and guide it to where it is needed. An outside observer might think that these exercises are incapable of stimulating important areas of the body. However, when you put them into practice, you realize that while using the aforementioned breath-holding technique, every single movement puts muscles, glands, and internal organs into intense and profound traction, which is a surprisingly pleasant sensation. Furthermore, the dynamics of these exercises enable the body to carry out two distinct actions at the same time whereby one part of the body is flexed or stretched while the rest of the body remains completely relaxed. This peculiarity facilitates the energetic changes that the exercise works to produce, eventually balancing the entire system.

As you can see, practicing traditional Thai yoga allows the practitioner to easily trigger the sen system by himself without having to understand all the ways in which it functions. This is the main distinction between Thai yoga and Thai massage. To gain the benefits of Thai massage you need the help of a skilled Thai massage therapist who knows how to balance the sen channels by means of acupressure, compression, and passive stretching.

Thai yoga is an easy discipline and is suitable for anybody. Whoever has the chance to practice it can discover its enormous benefits. In order to improve and become a master of the techniques (especially if you want to teach them to others) we recommend that you learn how to work on the sen system with Thai massage. The knowledge of this discipline, especially in its more advanced therapeutic forms, enables you to understand the all of the dynamic functions of the sen system, including the exact therapeutic points along its channels and the curative function associated with each channel.

A thorough knowledge of the sen system it is not necessary, however, in order to simply practice traditional Thai yoga for your own health. As long as you follow the directions for each exercise carefully and pay attention to the sensations in your own body, you will reap all the benefits of this ancient healing system.

BENEFITS OF THE POSTURES

Each Thai yoga exercise is accompanied by a description of the benefits it offers in terms of curing or preventing various ailments, as indicated by the statues and drawings handed down from Jivaka. The ailments and their symptoms are described according to the medical concepts of the period in which the discipline was developed—concepts that are still used today by traditional Thai physicians. However, Thai yoga exercises represent a self-healing mechanism capable of curing and preventing much more than is indicated in the individual exercises. The rebalancing of the sen system is capable of treating a vast range of ailments.

One of the most difficult tasks for any physician or therapist, no matter which school he or she belongs to, is to diagnose an exact pathology and its causes. In Thai medicine diagnosis of illness is extremely simplified and is based on the evident symptoms. Musculoskeletal pain (as associated with articulation, lumbago, and so on), an excess of air in parts of the abdomen, or an oppressive sensation in the chest are only some examples of the symptoms that the "hermit's technique" proposes to treat. In Thai medicine, these simple symptomatic indications are able to show which parts of the sen system are not working correctly; they do not require further diagnostic research. The therapy concentrates on rebalancing the sen system that is connected to the ailment in question, without necessarily looking for the intrinsic cause of the pathology.

In this practice, intervening with the energy channels relevant to the ailment includes work on organs and systems that may appear to be irrelevant to the ailment. In fact, these organs and systems are connected to the zone of the ailment by the energy channels; they too may suffer from energy imbalance in the sen or could even be the cause of the imbalance. This type of therapeutic approach allows the practitioner to address not just symptoms but pathologies, even those whose existence may be unknown. If, for example, a person suffers from pain in the knee, perhaps he or she also suffers from an ailment of the liver, which is connected to the knee by an energy channel. It is probable that a liver malfunction has had a disharmonic effect on the sen channel that, in turn, has produced pain in the knee.

As a final analysis, the hermit's art of healing, like the other Thai medicine disciplines, addresses the more evident and obvious symptoms to treat pathologies that can be difficult to diagnose, whether because they relate to internal organs or because they are complex.

As mentioned above, by rebalancing the sen system, Thai yoga has an almost limitless potential for curing and preventing illness. It is worth listing the most common benefits:

- Alignment of the skeletal system
- Relief of pain and tension in the muscles and tendons
- Relief of range-of-motion disorders (lumbago, joint pain, cervical spine problems, and so on)
- Greater flexibility
- Muscular toning
- Improvement of venous and lymphatic circulation
- Expulsion of toxins
- Increased lung capacity
- Regulation of diaphragm functioning
- Promotion of weight loss, reducing levels of both adipose tissue and retained water

PRECAUTIONS

Thai yoga is not intended to be a painful discipline. Some exercises can cause intense sensations, such as stimulus in the organs and muscles, but they should not cause acute pain or discomfort. If you experience pain or discomfort, stop the exercise and do not continue until the discomfort passes.

After each exercise, always wait for your breathing and heartbeat to return to normal before starting another exercise. If you become dizzy, lie down for a few moments and wait until the feeling passes before standing again. Trust your instincts. If you feel unwell or have a headache or other disturbing symptom that could impede the exercises, do not do them. Do not transform a light discipline into a heavy discipline. The final result should be a feeling of complete well-being.

CONTRAINDICATIONS

The exercises should never be undertaken by someone who has any of the following conditions:

- Cardiac problems (including anyone who has a pacemaker or has had coronary bypass surgery)
- Hypertension
- A currently high level of psychological or emotional stress

If you have any doubt about the danger the exercises may pose for you, consult your physician for advice, particularly if you suffer from any of the following:

- Slipped disc
- Osteoporosis
- A fracture that has not yet calcified

Other precautions are indicated in the directions for the individual exercises.

THREE

Basic Techniques of the Practice

The practice of the exercises requires that you know some essential techniques in order to gain the most benefit. Although some of the specific details may not appear to be so important, every one is fundamental for the correct execution of the techniques. Instructions for taking a particular position carry great importance in terms of activating the energy channels. Flexing the wrist, for example, is intended to stimulate the five sen present on each arm. For these reasons, although Thai yoga is generally quite simple to practice, you must take care during the practice of each exercise to follow the instructions exactly.

BREATHING

The breathing method is one of the characteristics that distinguishes this discipline from other types of yoga. The correct application of the breathing method is *fundamental* for the success of the exercises.

As you move from the starting position into the final position required for a particular exercise, you must inhale deeply. Hold your breath for three seconds, while holding the position. Finally you will exhale, while returning slowly to the starting position.

Some exercises are composed of two distinct movements. In this case, you will exhale during the first movement and inhale, hold, and exhale, as just described, for the second movement. To calculate the canonical breath-holding time of three seconds as well as possible, we advise practitioners to mentally count the seconds.

This breathing technique positively stresses the body's breathing apparatus. As mentioned earlier, you should take a break whenever you find your pulse or breathing rate has increased, resuming the exercises only when it has come back to normal. Many people, especially during the first sessions of practice, will find it necessary to take a breath between exercises. Over time, as you practice the exercises regularly, you will notice that your need for breaks between exercises will progressively lessen.

STARTING POSITIONS

Half Lotus

The half lotus is the most common starting position. It entails sitting with your legs crossed, with one foot on top of the opposite leg (A).

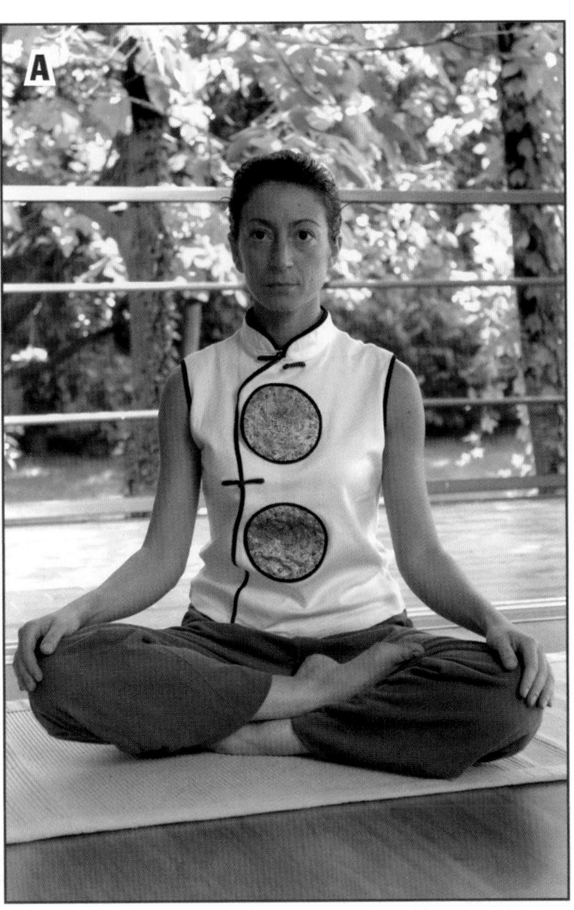

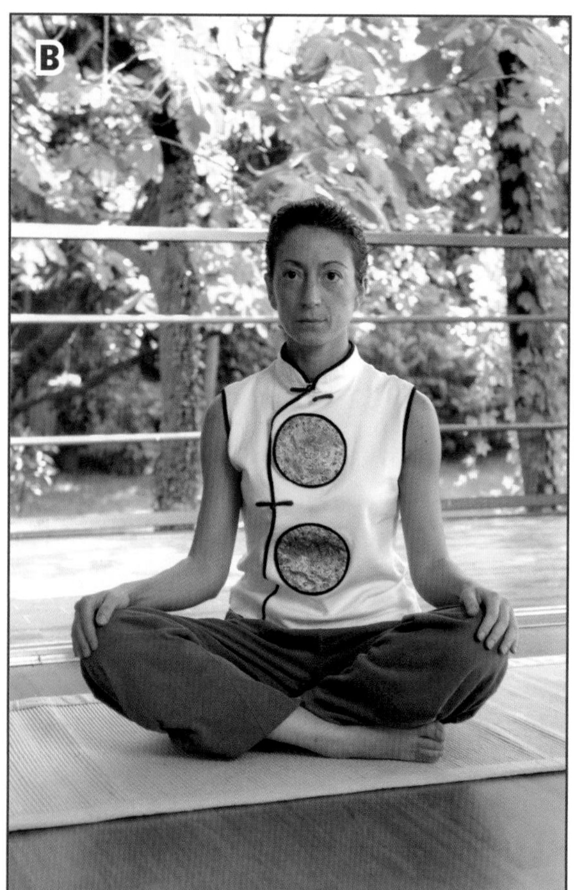

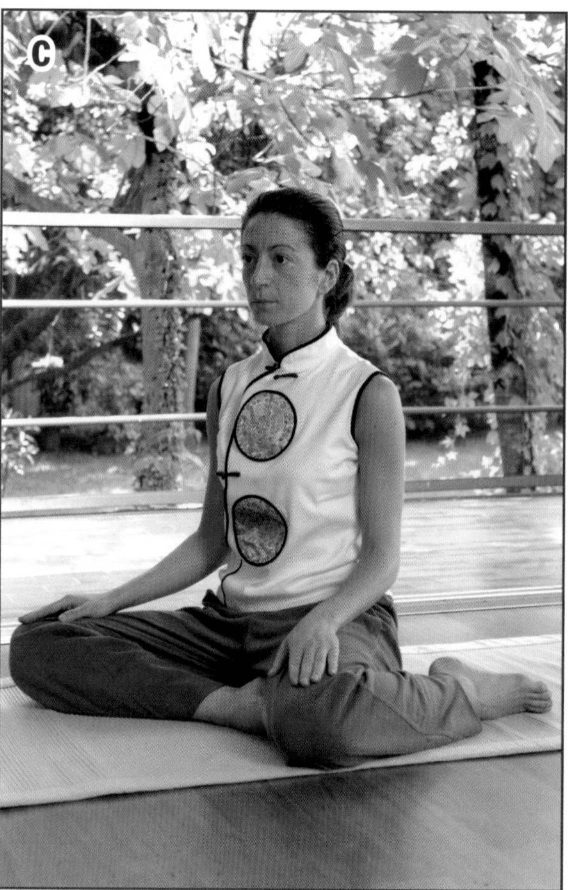

If you cannot assume the half-lotus position or if it is hard for you to hold it, you can assume the classic cross-legged position (B). Trying to assume the half-lotus position without having the necessary flexibility can damage the knees.

Thai Position

The Thai position calls for having one leg bent to the inside and the other bent outward (C).

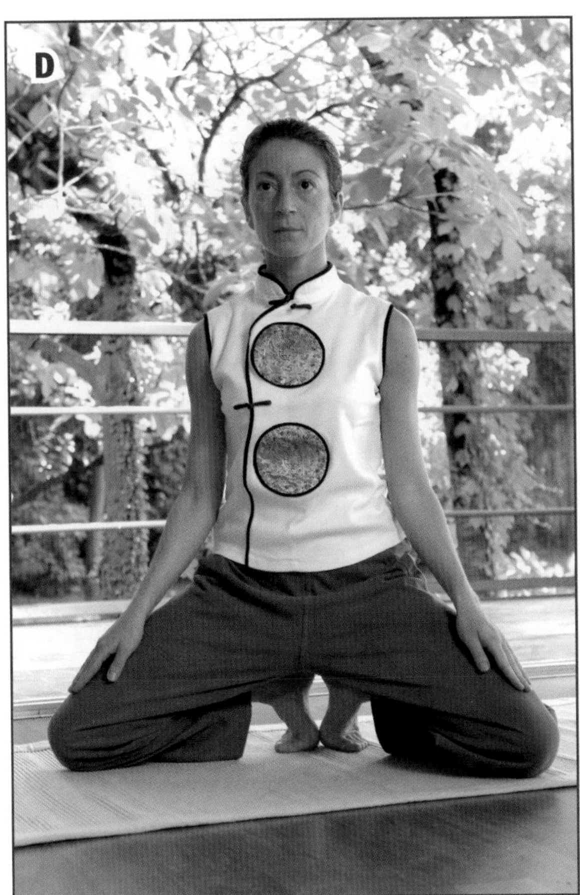

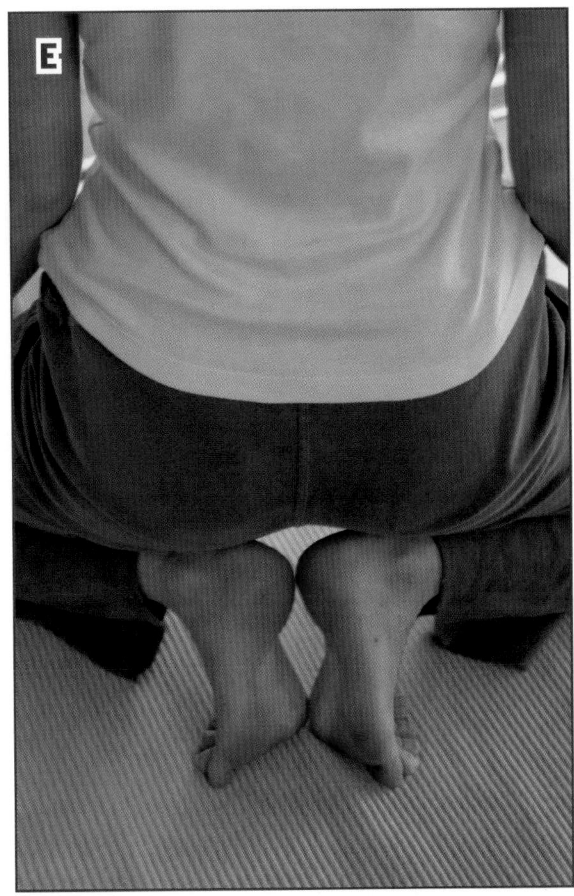

Sitting on Flexed Feet

In this position the feet are kept flexed and rotated to the outside as much as possible in order to let the heels and balls of the feet lean against each other. The legs stay open as much as possible (D) and the buttocks rest on the heels (E).

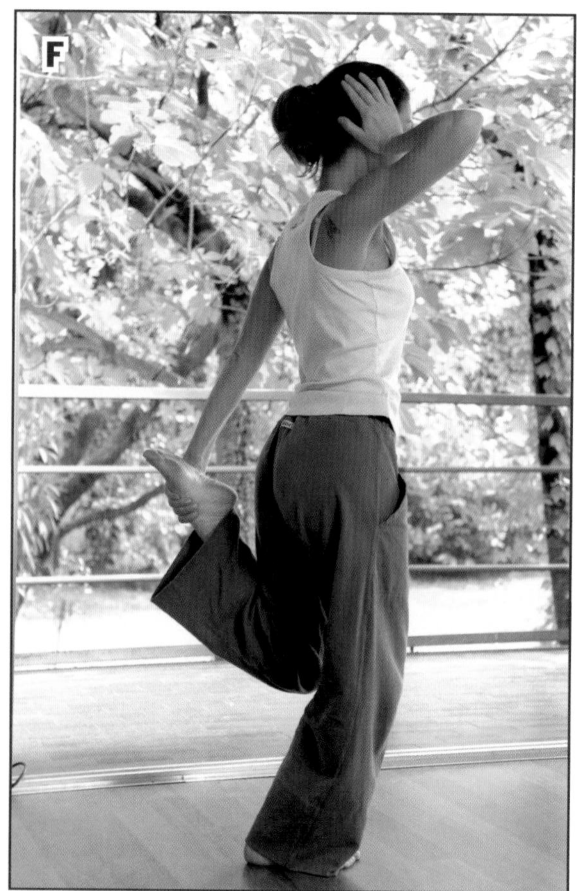

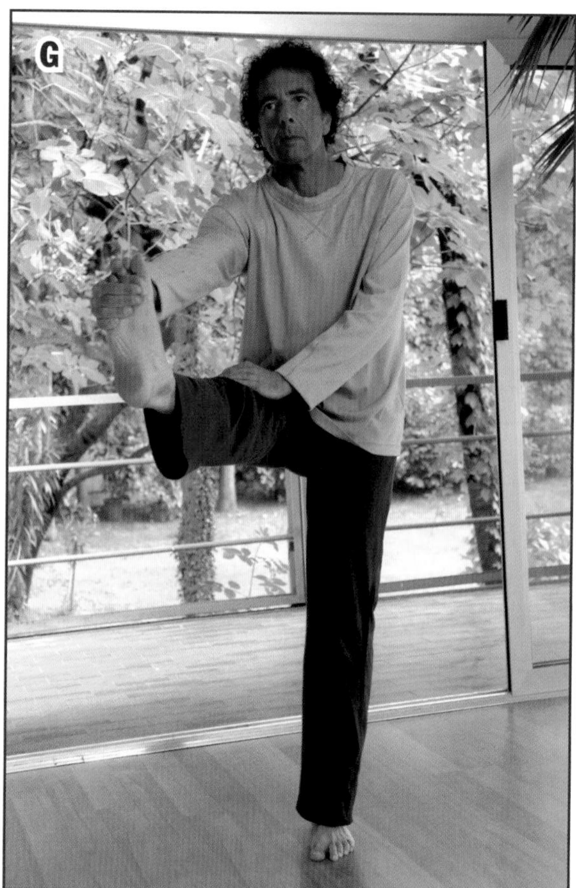

Balancing Positions

Some exercises call for balancing on one leg (F and G). At first you may have some difficulty holding your balance, and you might "hop about." A little patience and practice will quickly improve your ability to balance.

HAND POSITION

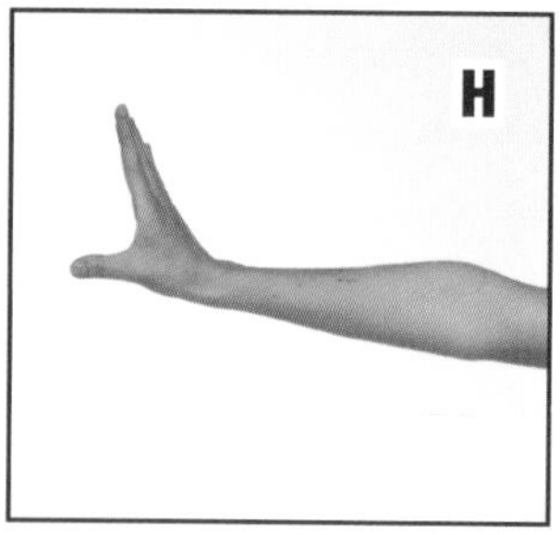

Although it may seem unimportant, hand position often determines the effectiveness of the techniques. Many exercises, as you will see, call for keeping the hands flexed backward. While the thumb stays outstretched forward, the other fingers are pushed backward as far as possible, thereby flexing the wrist (H). This traction, where called for, must be maintained for the duration of the exercise.

PRESSURE POINTS

Some techniques call for the practitioner to apply pressure on specific points. These points are located along the sen energy channels. The points are most often used in Thai therapeutic massage for the treatment of different pathologies.

Apply pressure with the fingertip of one or more fingers as instructed according to the exercise. The pressure applied must be quite deep, just below the person's pain threshold. To succeed in applying deep pressure without causing excessive pain, push with *rising strength*, that is, increasing the pressure as gradually as possible.

REPETITION, DURATION, AND ATTENDANCE

Each exercise should be repeated at least three times to achieve effective results from a therapeutic point of view, but it can be repeated up to five times. In cases where an exercise calls for bilateral application (on the right and the left), it should be repeated at least three times on each side.

Thai yoga can be practiced daily. One hour of practice is usually enough to obtain good results. You can, of course, practice for less time or do just those exercises that you feel are necessary or that you most enjoy practicing. Note, however, that the standing exercises generally require that you be warmed up, which you can achieve by practicing seated exercises or other exercises you know.

As described in chapter 2, a single exercise can benefit many organs and systems. Nevertheless, if you are going to practice one or more exercises to obtain the therapeutic results they are said to offer (for example, exercise 9, Remedy for Shoulder and Shoulder Blade Pain), it would be wise to practice the exercise regularly until the symptoms have disappeared or considerably weakened.

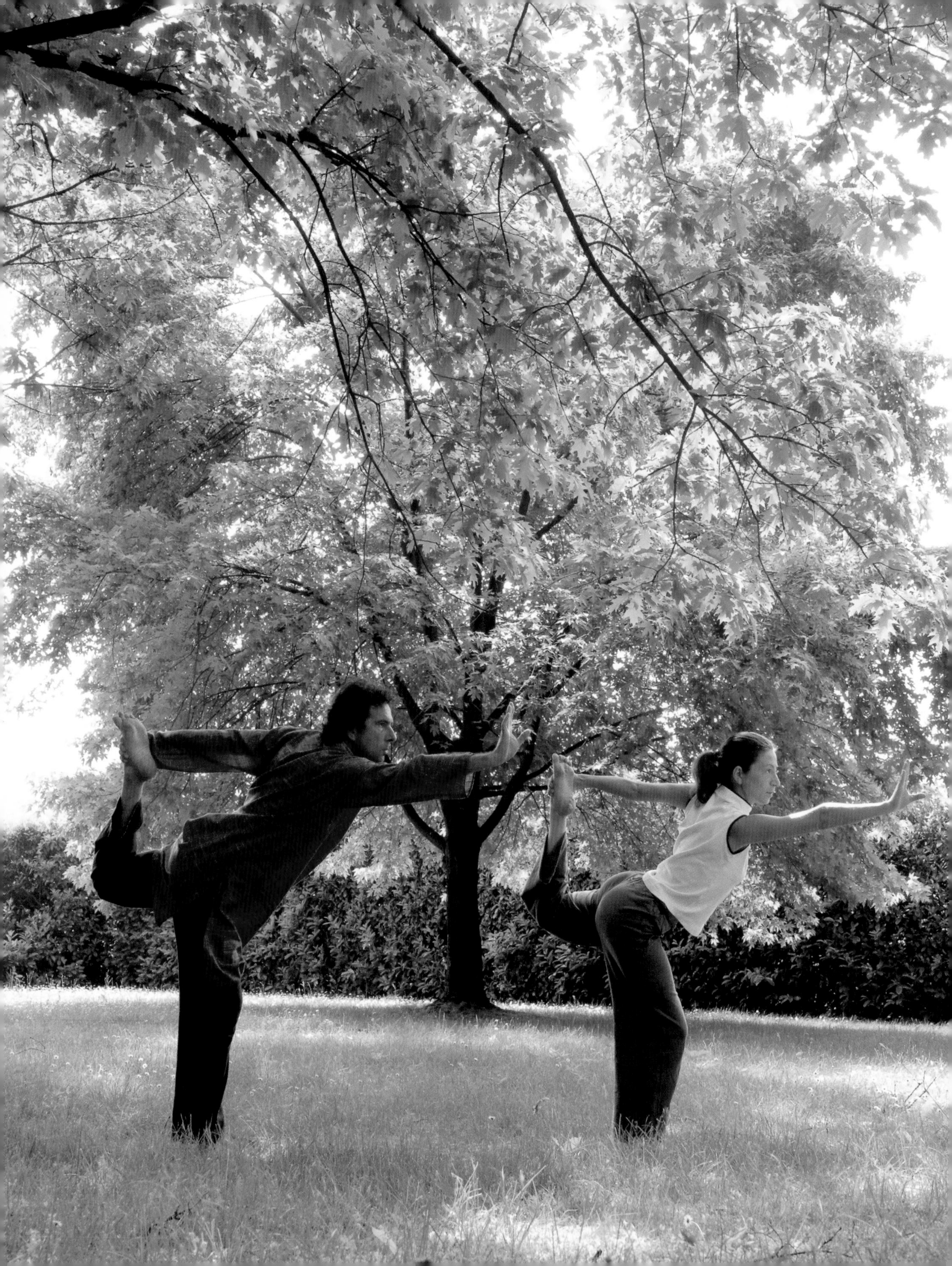

PART TWO

The Practice

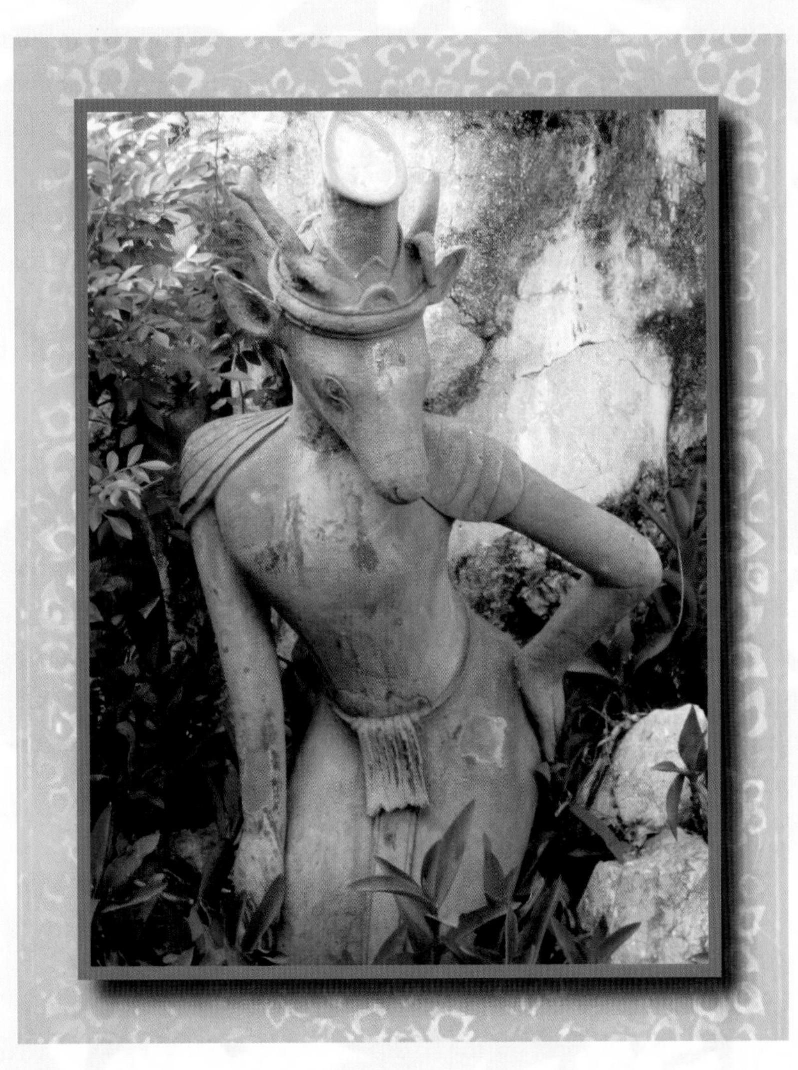

Welcome to the practice of Ruesri Dat Ton. In this part of the book you will find fully illustrated, step-by-step instructions for sixty traditional Thai yoga postures. You may be approaching this yoga practice with specific health problems that you would like to address in mind. If so, the titles of the exercises will tell you the primary health benefits of each, and the appendix will give you more information on the specific healing properties of all the exercises. You should also remember that each exercise has multiple benefits. In fact, most of the exercises actually provide at least some benefit to all ten of the sen channels. So you may approach the practice as a general health maintenance program as well. When selecting a number of exercises, it is recommended that you choose those with different starting positions in order to achieve a good balance among the techniques.

EXERCISE SEQUENCE

We have chosen to list the exercises in a head-to-toe order in this book, following Jivaka's original titles for the primary body parts affected by each posture. You will find postures that benefit the head, neck, and shoulders in chapter 4; postures that benefit the torso in chapter 5; postures that benefit the extremities—arms, legs, hands, and feet—in chapter 6; and postures that address more generalized problems of physical and mental health in chapter 7.

Occasionally Jivaka named widely divergent parts of the body in the same title, for example, exercise 12, Remedy for Shoulder and Leg Stiffness. These exercises have been listed in the chapter in which the first-named body part is covered. By that guideline, exercise 12 will appear in chapter 4, which focuses on the head, neck, and shoulders. Because legs are named in the title as well, you will also find a cross-reference to the exercise at the beginning of chapter 6, the extremities chapter.

Though Jivaka's titles point out the *primary* benefit of each exercise, each of these postures actually offers multiple health benefits. For this reason, we have provided a cross-referenced list of all the exercises in the appendix. There the exercise titles are grouped according to the ailments they are able to treat or prevent such as neck pain, middle and lower back pain, or hip pain. Under each heading we have listed all of the exercises that provide significant benefit to the area in question, whether or not that part of the body is mentioned in the exercise title. Always refer to chapter 3, "Basic Techniques of the Practice," for a better understanding of the positions and of the general features of the exercises.

PREPARATION FOR PRACTICE

The exercises that take place on the floor require a soft, but not too soft, support. A gym mat is a simple and effective option. The standing positions are best undertaken on a wooden floor or a very thin mat, such as a yoga mat. These standing exercises should be performed with bare feet.

Try to keep your focus throughout the exercises. Before beginning, close your eyes and try to relax, clearing your mind, letting go of worries, and releasing tension in your muscles. In Thailand, practice of the disciplines created by Jivaka is preceded by a request for help from Jivaka himself, sometimes accompanied by a prayer addressed to the "Father of Medicine." These traditional rituals express the gratitude that Thai people feel toward Jivaka, but they also undertake a technical function in that they allow practitioners to gather the concentration needed for the practice.

Remember, also, to be kind to yourself as you begin your practice. Ruesri Dat Ton should always be practiced in the spirit of loving-kindness, so have patience with yourself if some of the postures seem challenging at first. With repetition, they will soon become easier.

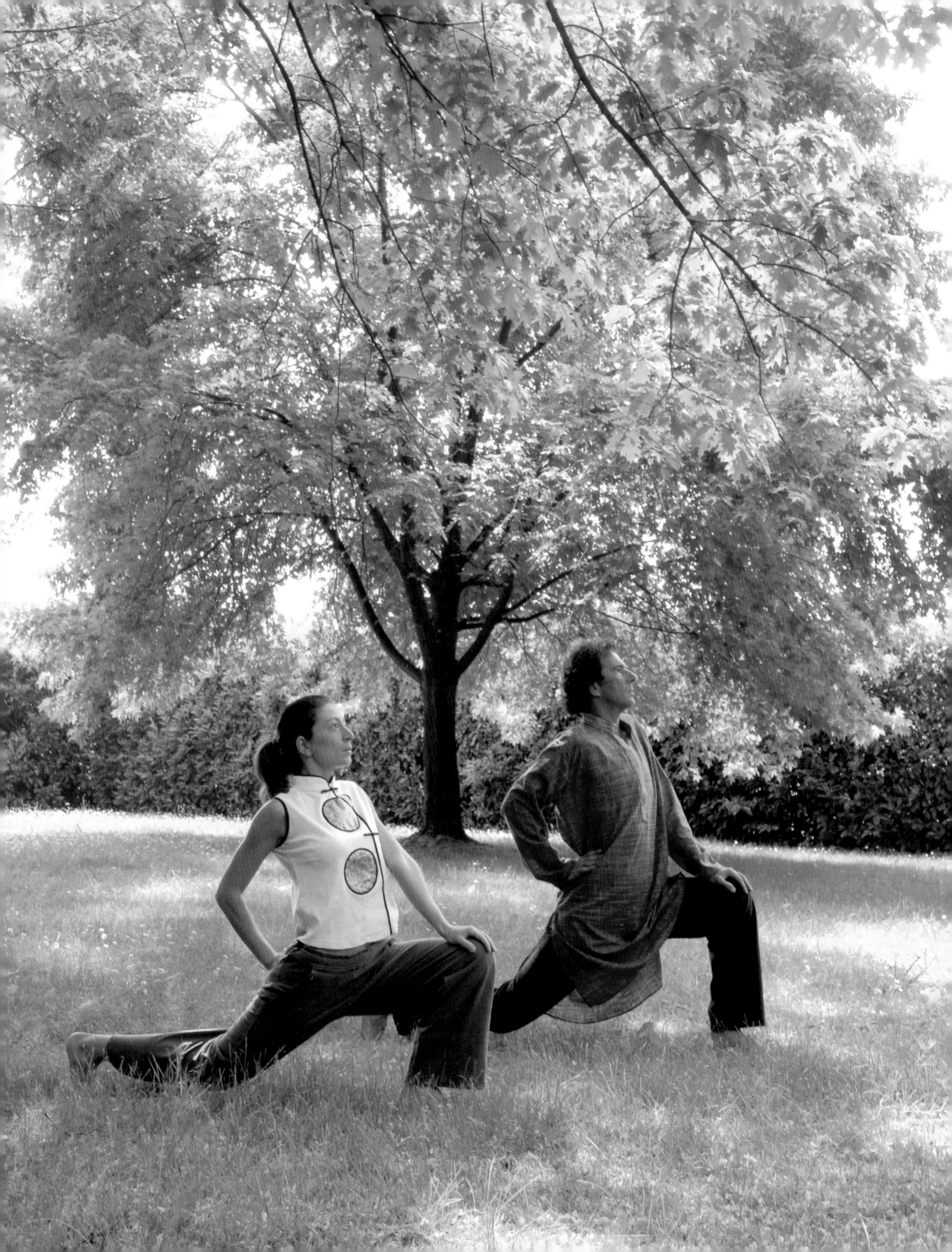

FOUR

Postures That Benefit the Head, Neck, and Shoulders

1. Remedy for Tension Headache
2. Remedy for Migraine Headache
3. Remedy for Sinus Congestion
4. Remedy for Neck Pain
5. Remedy for Neck and Shoulder Pain
6. Remedy for Neck and Shoulder Stiffness
7. Remedy for Shoulder Pain
8. Remedy for Shoulder Stiffness and Pain
9. Remedy for Shoulder and Shoulder Blade Pain
10. Remedy for Shoulder and Hip Pain 1
11. Remedy for Shoulder and Hip Pain 2
12. Remedy for Shoulder and Leg Stiffness

See also:

- Exercise 13, Remedy for Chest, Shoulder, and Abdominal Pain
- Exercise 19, Remedy for Abdominal Pain and Shoulder Blade Pain
- Exercise 43, Remedy for Leg and Neck Pain

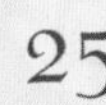

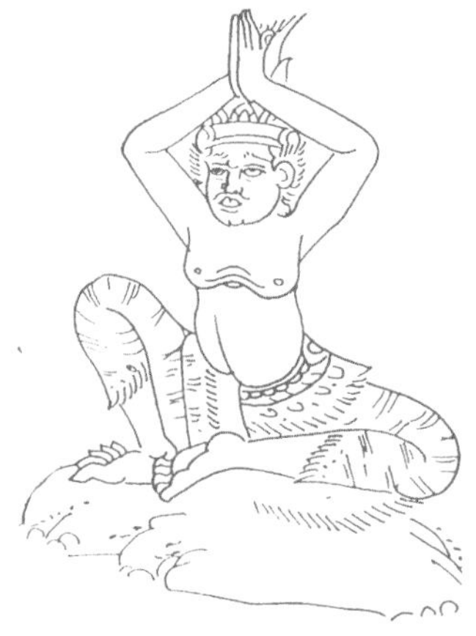

1 Remedy for Tension Headache

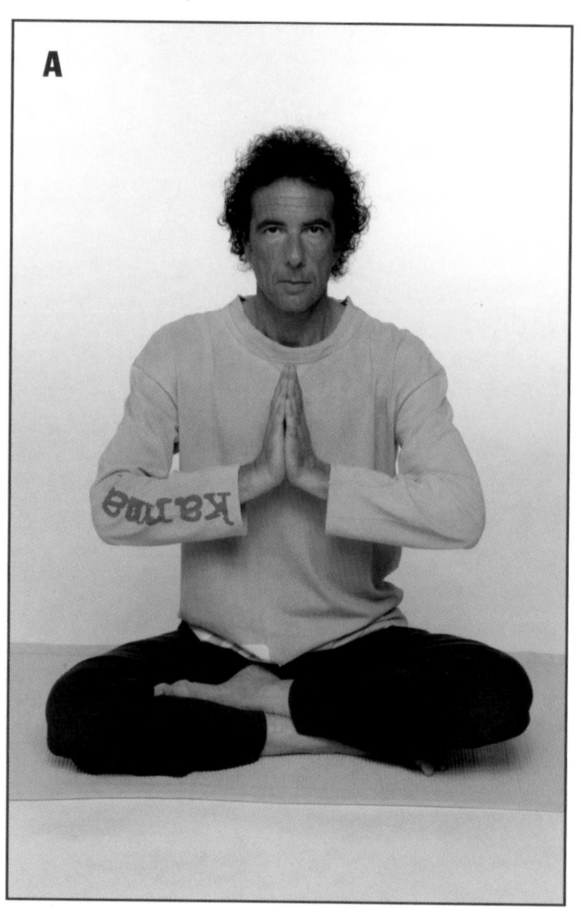
A

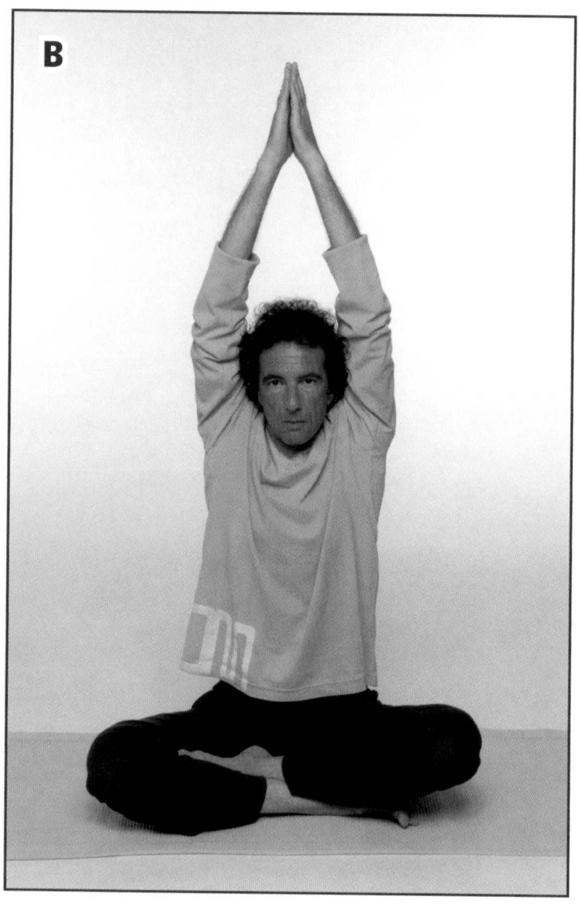
B

Sit in the half-lotus position or with your legs crossed. Join the palms of your hands in front of you, while keeping your shoulders relaxed (A).

As you breathe in, stretch your arms up as straight as you can, keeping the palms of your hands together (B).

Holding your breath, maintain this position for 3 seconds.

As you breathe out, return slowly to the starting position.

While breathing in, twist your body to the left as far as you can, while

๏ พระมโนชสำนักด้าว ดงยูงยางเฮย จิตรพรั่นหวั่นหวาดฝูง มฤคร้าย
กำเริบโรคขบสูง สังเวช องค์เอย นั่งดัดหัตถ์ขวาซ้าย นบเกล้าบริกรรม

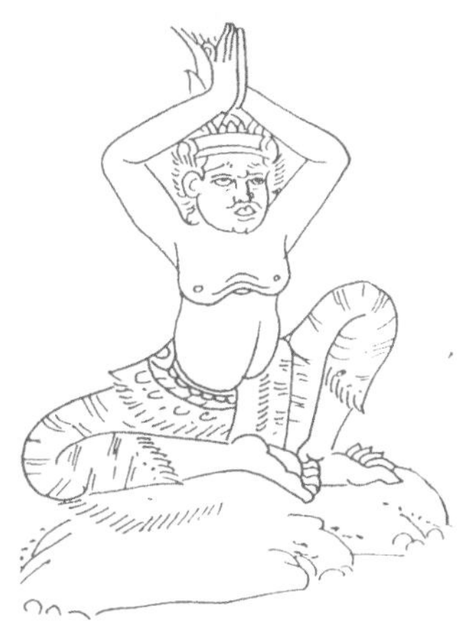

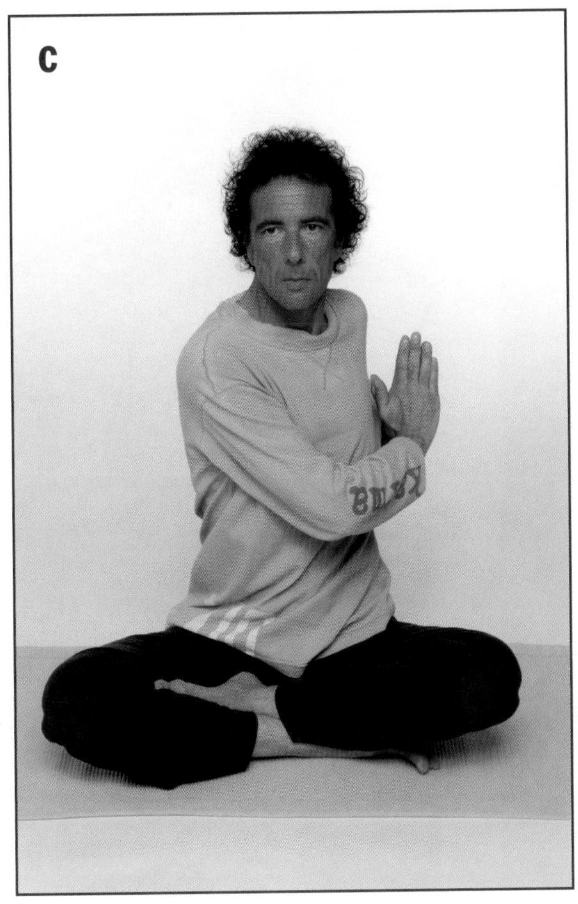

keeping your head facing forward. Help yourself twist by pushing your right hand against your left hand (C).

Holding your breath, maintain this position for 3 seconds.

As you breathe out, return slowly to the starting position.

Perform the exercise 3 to 5 times on the first side. Then practice the exercise on the other side.

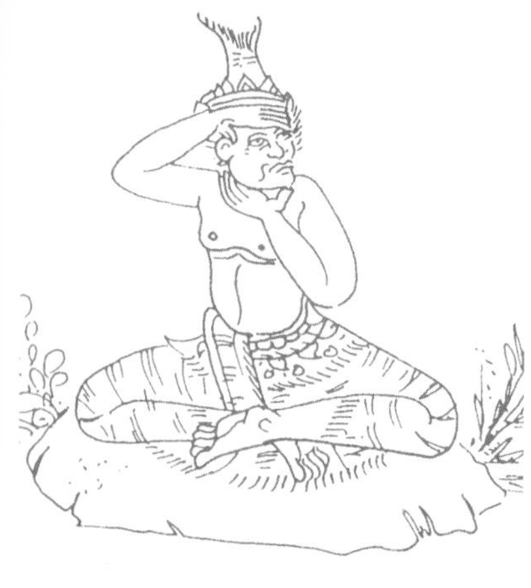

2 Remedy for Migraine Headache

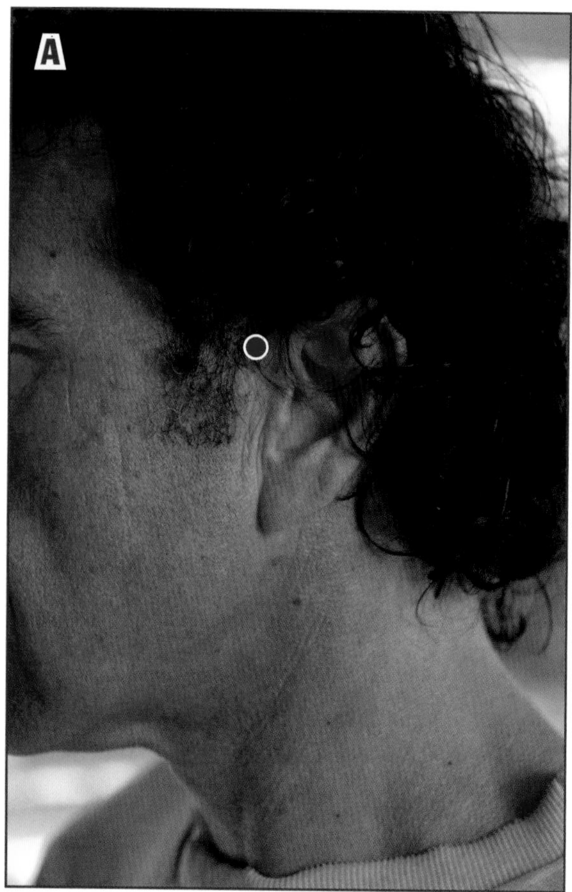

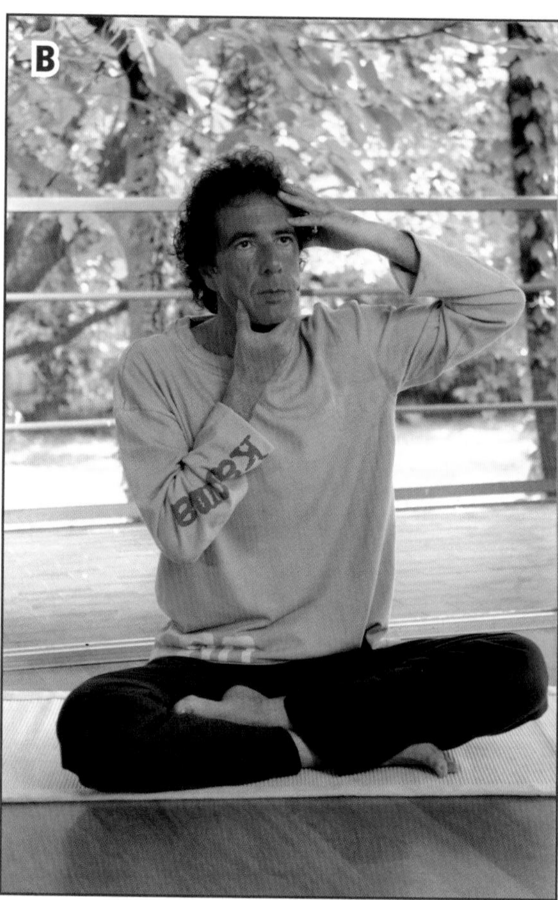

This technique requires finger pressure on a point located next to the upper side of the ear (A). You should apply gradually increasing pressure until you are pressing almost as hard as you can stand.

Sit in the half-lotus position and hold your chin with your right hand. Place your left hand on your forehead with your thumb on point 1 (B).

๏ กาลชฎิลดัดมล้าง ลมดุะ ไคลขมับจับหะนุ นวดเน่น

มึนเศียรมืดจักษุ เสื่อมส่างไข้แฮ ไว้ฉะบับบอกเส้น ประสิทธิ์แก้ลมปะกัง ฯ

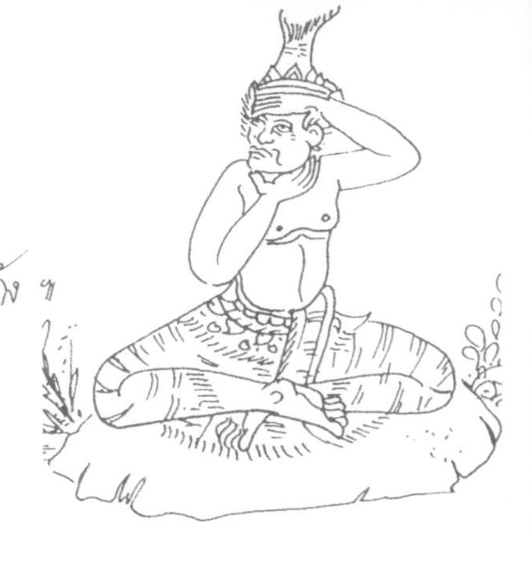

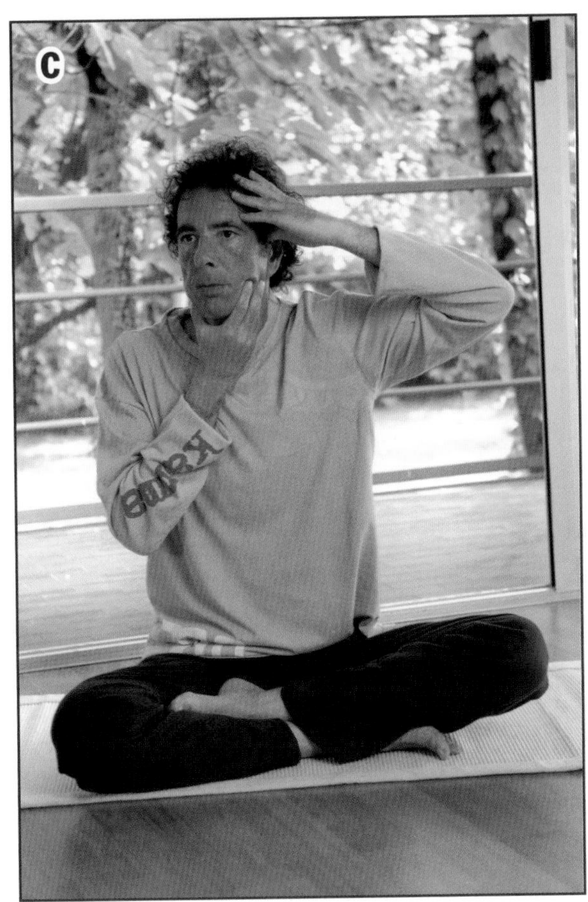

Turn your head slightly to the right. Keeping your neck relaxed, and holding your head completely still with your right hand, breathe in and push point 1 with your thumb (C).

Holding your breath, maintain this position for 3 seconds.

As you breathe out, return slowly to the starting position.

Perform the exercise 3 to 5 times. Then practice the exercise on the other side. If the symptoms persist, repeat the exercise 10 times on each side.

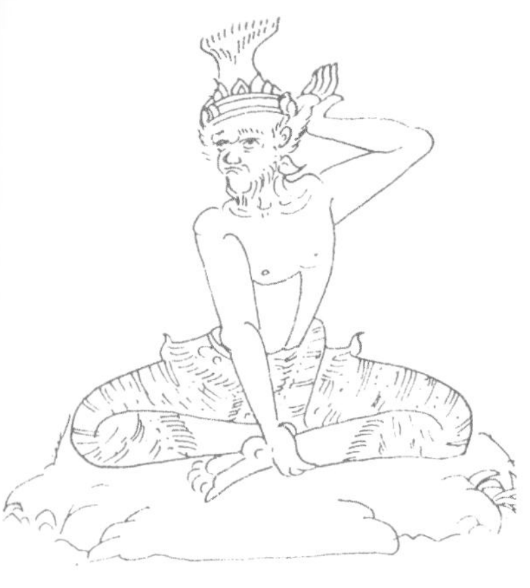

3
Remedy for Sinus Congestion

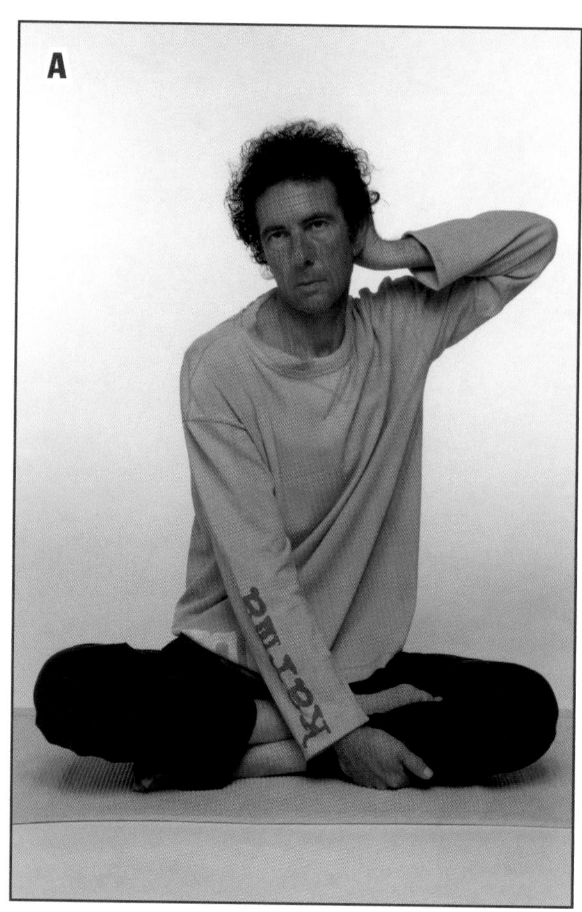

Sit in the half-lotus position. Hold your left leg near the knee with your right hand. Place your left hand just behind your left ear, with the heel of the palm under the occipital bone and your fingers pointing upward. Keep your left arm raised so that the elbow points outward (A).

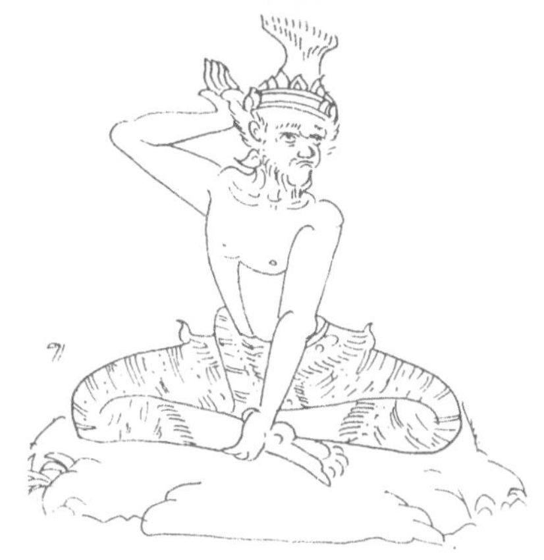

๏ พระบทธอักขระไว้ นามยุทธ สืบอักษรตราบสุด สิ้น
นั่งสมาธิหัดกำสัปรยุทธ เศียรเอิก แข้งนา เสมหะปทะต้นลิ้น ล่งล้างลำคอ ฯ

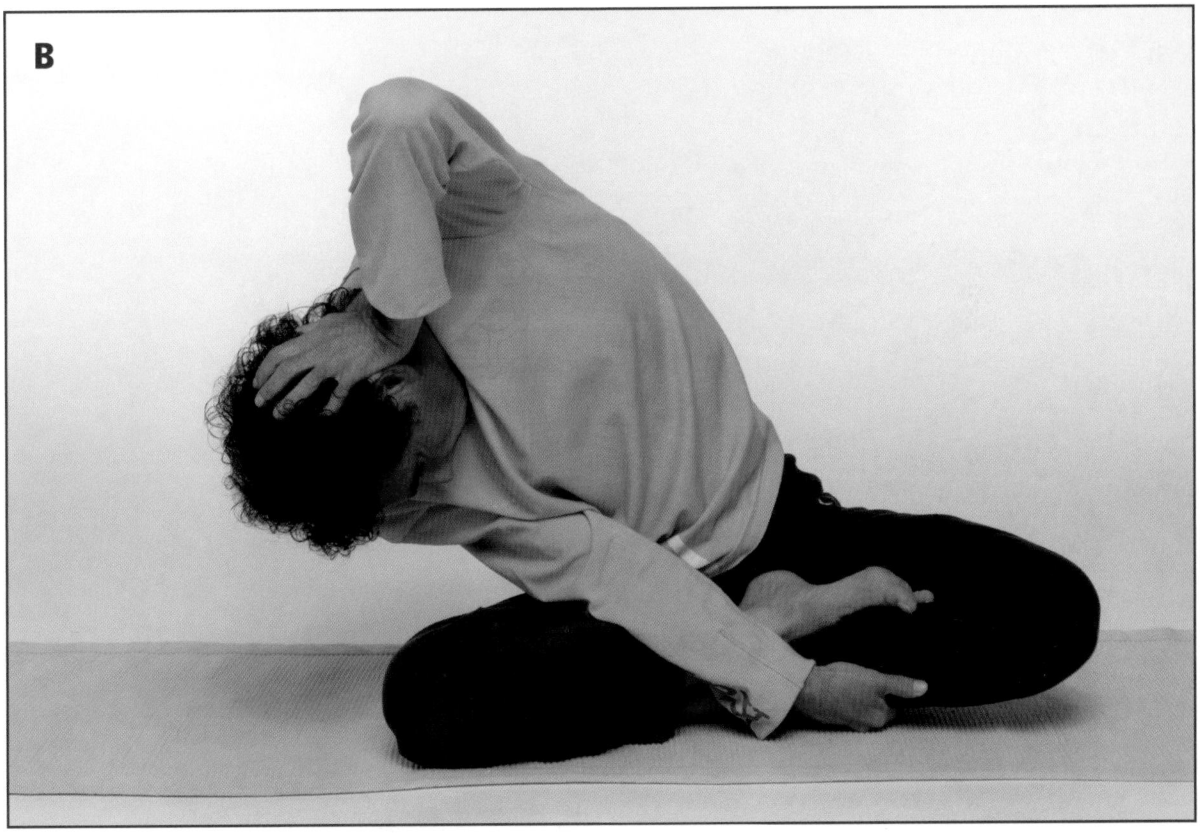

B

As you breathe in, push your head down with your left hand, bending your body to the side. Anchor your legs to avoid losing your balance (B).

Holding your breath, maintain this position for 3 seconds.

As you breathe out, return slowly to the starting position.

Repeat the movement on the other side, holding your right leg with your left hand and pushing against your head with your right hand.

Perform the exercise 3 to 5 times.

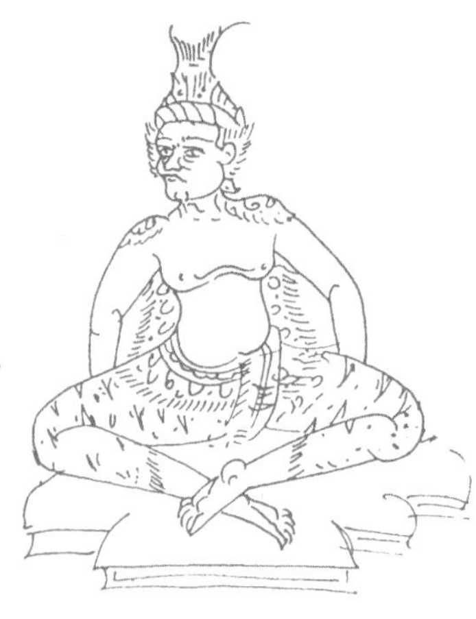

4 Remedy for Neck Pain

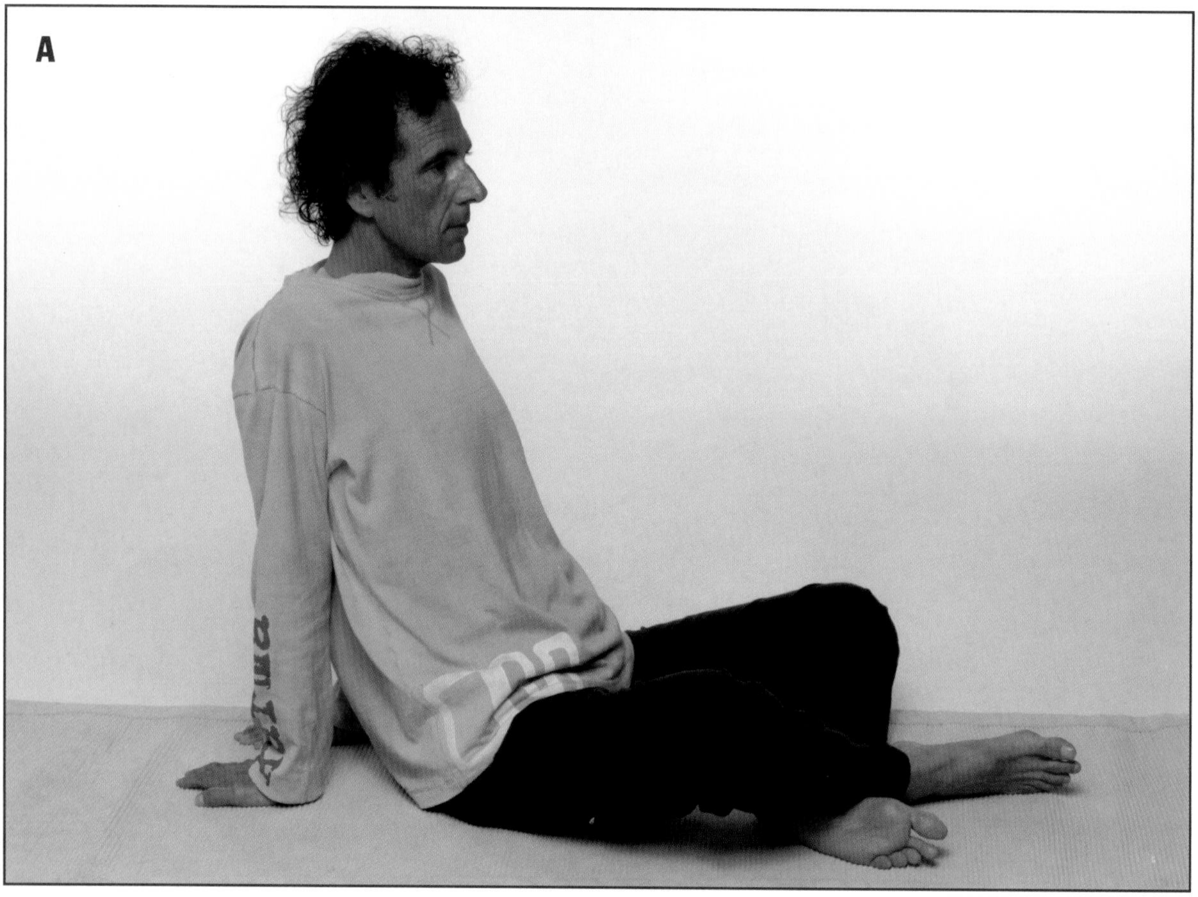

A

Sit with your legs crossed slightly away from you. Place your hands on the floor behind your back, with your fingers pointing away from your body (A).

๑ พระกาญจนลมเสียดเส้น สอเสียว เพื่อนตื่นบเดินเทียว เทียวง้อ
แก้ตอบิดตอเหลียว ลมเหือดหายแฮ คู่เข่าขก่อมก้อ หัดถ์เคล้นไคลขา ฯ

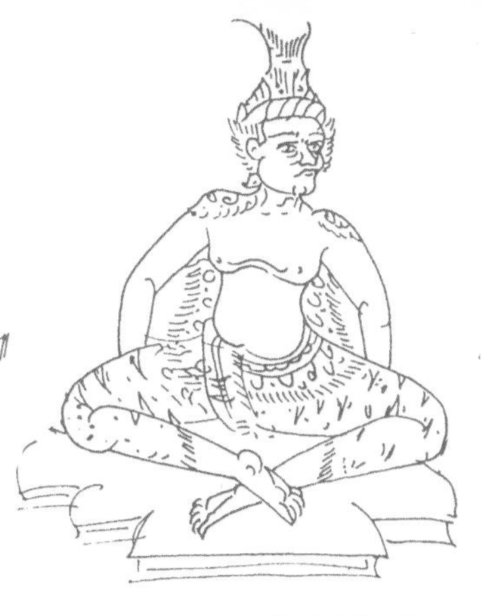

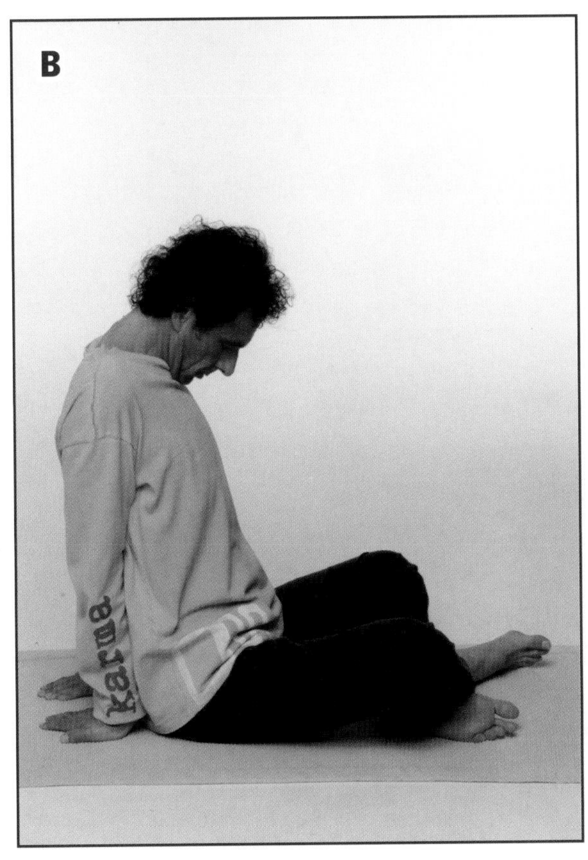

B

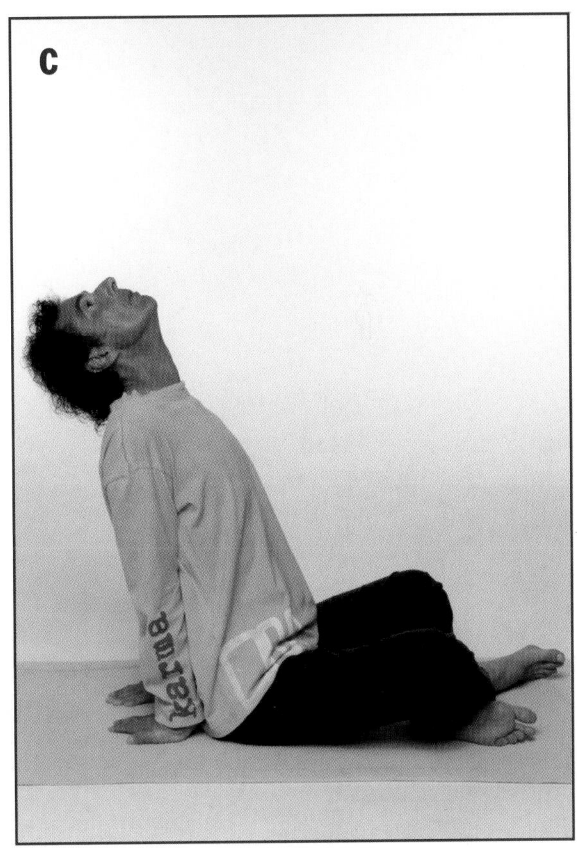

C

Breath in and bend your head toward your chest as far as possible (B).

Holding your breath, maintain this position for 3 seconds.

As you breathe out, return slowly to the starting position.

Breathing in, bend your head backward as far as possible (C).

Holding your breath, maintain this position for 3 seconds.

As you breathe out, return slowly to the starting position.

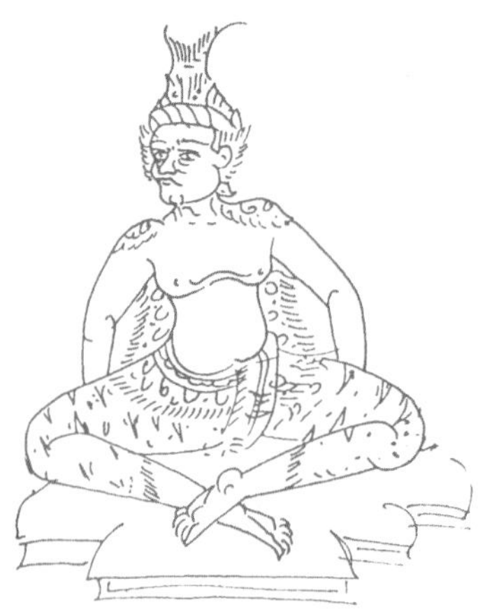

๑ พระกาญจนลมเสียดเส้น สอเสียว เพื่อนตื่นบเดินเทียว เทียวง้อ
แก้ตอปิดตอเหลียว ลมเหือดหายแฮ คู่เข่าขก่อมก้อ หัดถ์เคล้นไคลขา ฯ

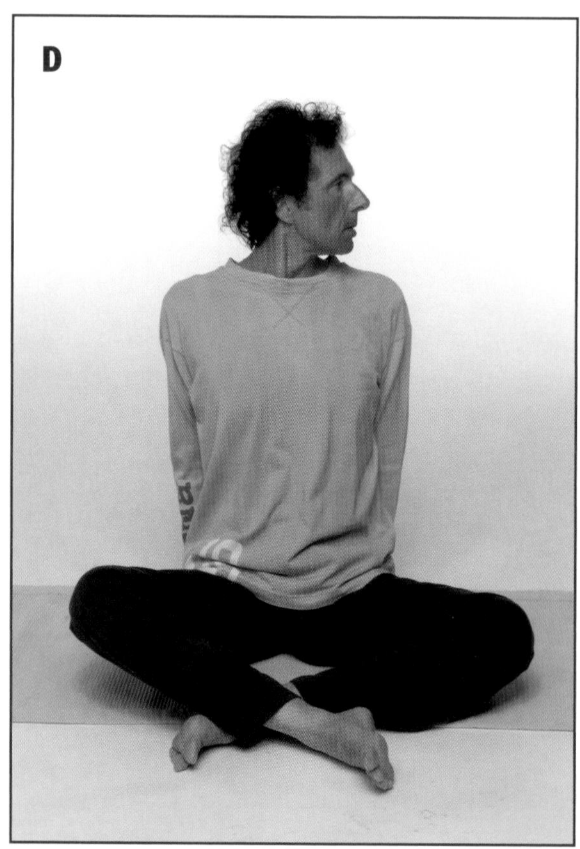

While breathing in, turn your head to the left as far as possible (D).

Holding your breath, maintain this position for 3 seconds.

As you breathe out, return slowly to the starting position.

Repeat the exercise, this time turning your head as far as possible to the right.

Perform the entire exercise sequence 3 to 5 times.

5

Remedy for Neck and Shoulder Pain

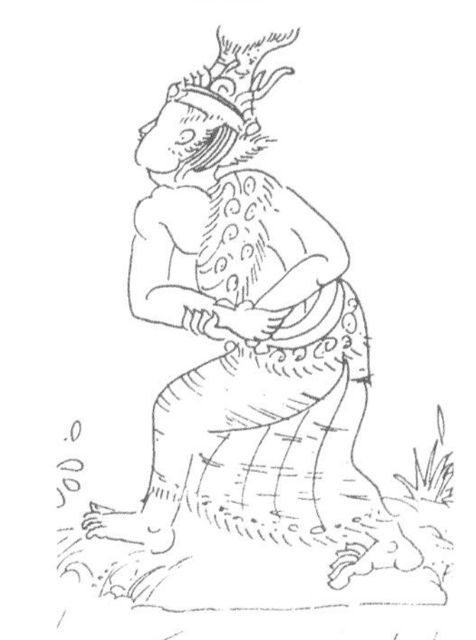

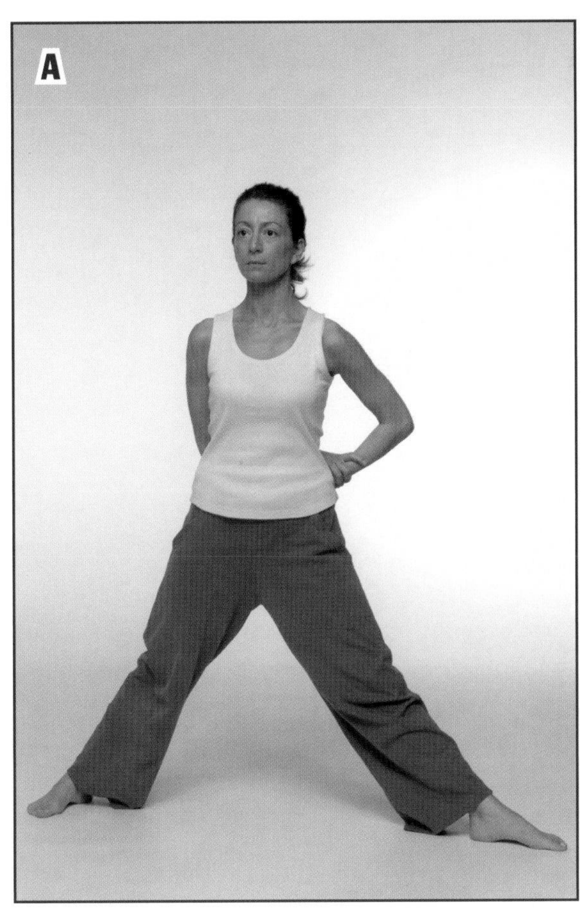

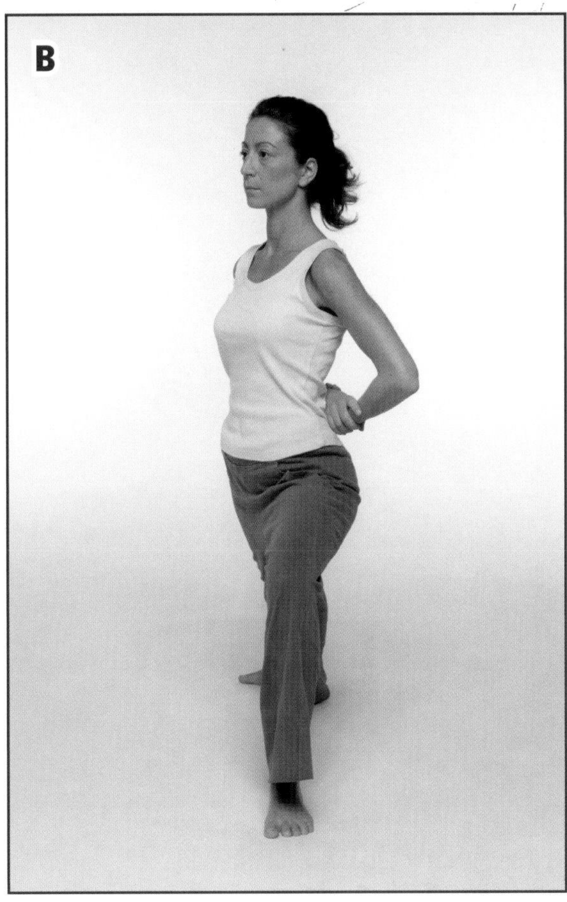

Stand with your legs apart. Pull your right leg back and point your left foot forward, so that your heels are aligned but your feet are perpendicular to each other. Cross your arms behind you and push them to the left as far as possible, keeping your chest to the front (A).

Breathing out, bend your left leg to a 90-degree angle, stretching your right leg behind you (B). Take care not to bend your knee beyond 90 degrees.

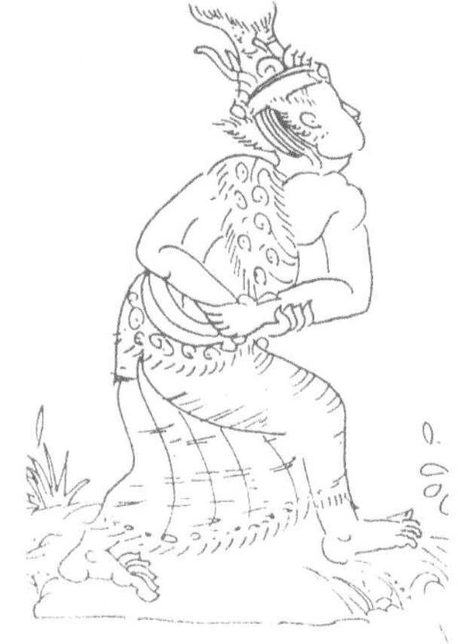

อิสิงค์ดาบศหน้ำ เปนมนุษย์ เชงอกเล่เศียรคาง ดั่งเนื้อ
คัดหัตถ์สองยุด กันกดเอวนา คอไหล่ไขว้รั้งเรื้อ โรคร้ายริ้งถอย

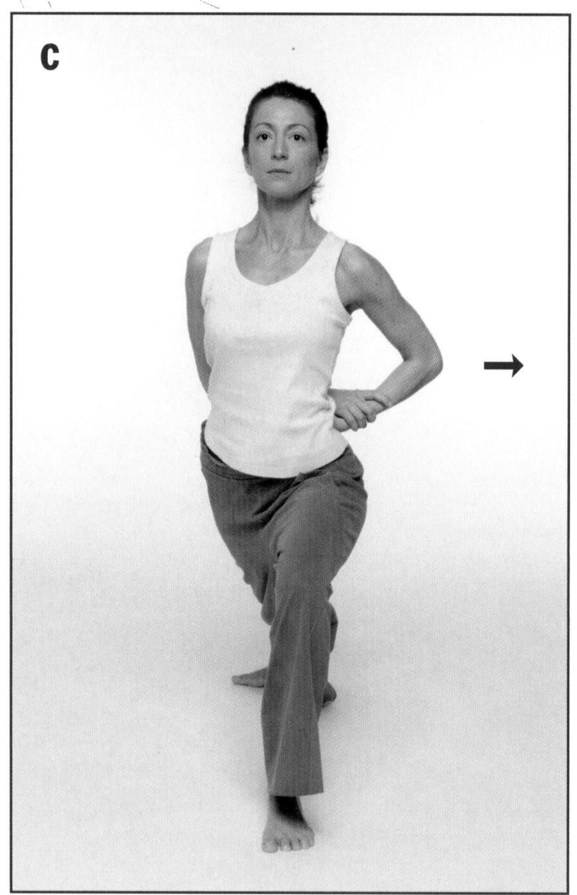

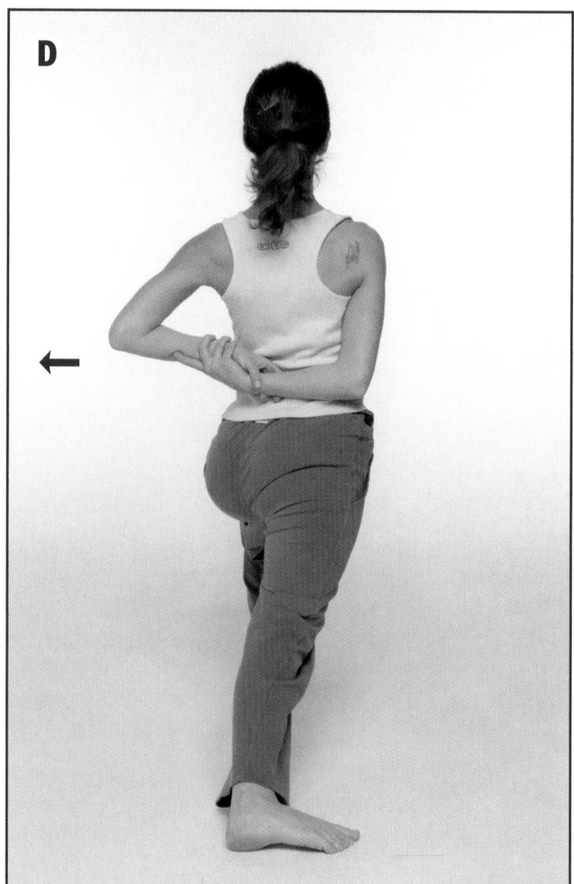

As you breathe in, keep your head slightly lifted and use your left arm to pull your right arm to the left as far as you can. The traction of the arm and shoulder will make your chest turn to the right (C).

Holding your breath, maintain this position for 3 seconds (D).

อิสิงค์ดาบศหน้า เป่นมนุษย์ เชงอกเล่เศียรคจ ดั่งเนื้อ
ดัดหัตถ์สองยุด กันกดเอวเถ ตอไหล่ไข้รั้งเรื้อ โรคร้ายริ์งถอย

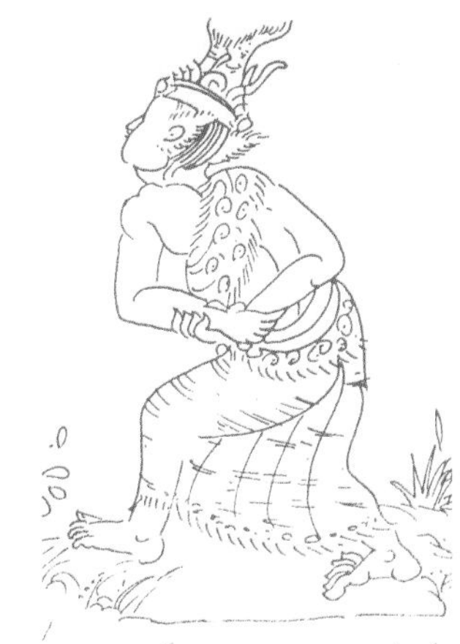

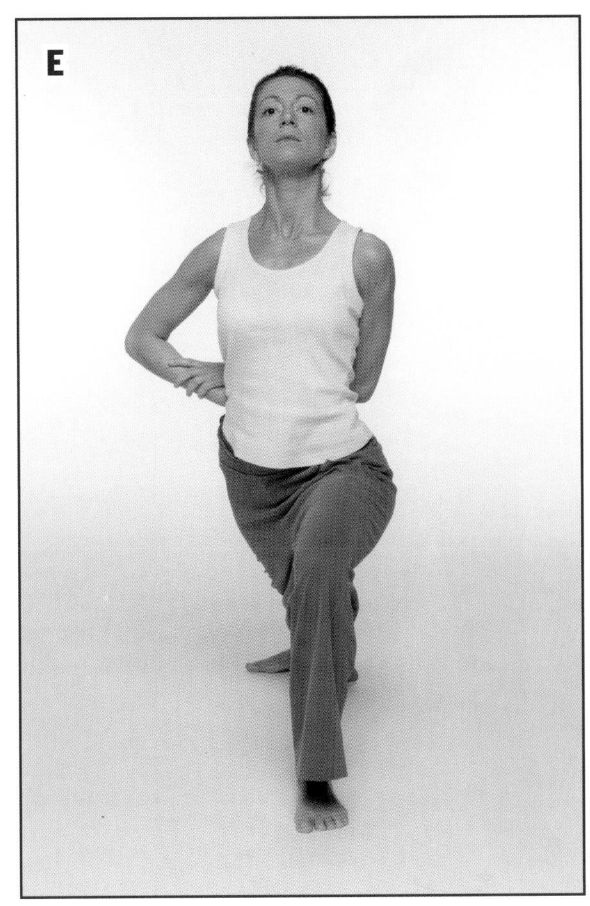

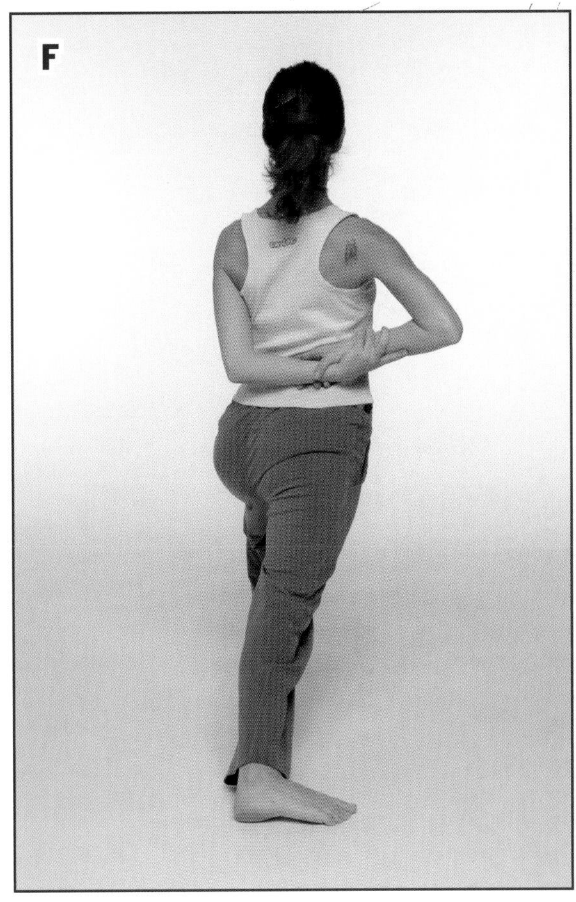

As you breathe out, release the pull on your arm, and slowly return to the starting position.

Repeat the sequence, now pulling your arms to the right (E and F).

Perform the exercise 3 to 5 times. Then practice the exercise on the other side, with the right foot now pointing away from your body; start by pulling your arms to right and then alternate, as before.

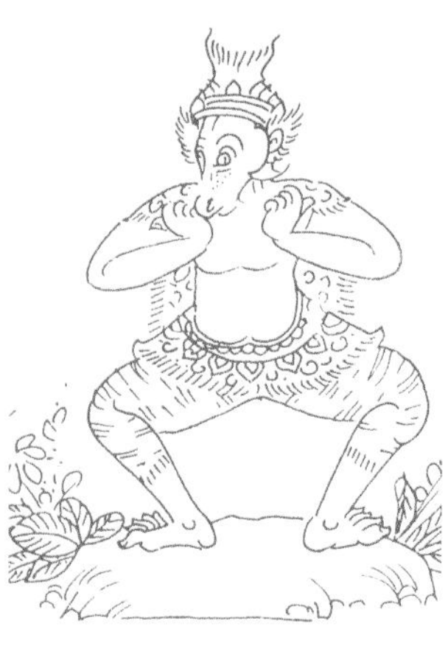

6

Remedy for Neck and Shoulder Stiffness

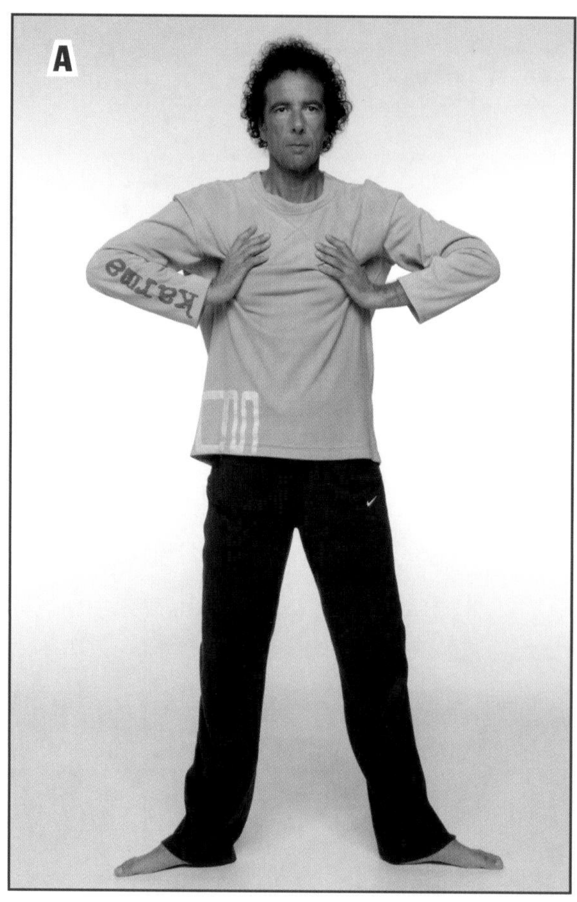

Stand with your feet 1 foot (30 cm) apart, pointing your toes outward as much as possible without losing balance. Place your hands on your sides, just under your armpits (A).

๏ นักพรตภักตร์เพศม้า มีแผนพม่านา ชื่ออัศวมุขิแขน ค่ค้
ขุ ปุ
ท่าอัดดัดเหลี่ยมแบน แบะเข่า ตอเคล็ดแคลงไหล่หล้ ในลกแก้ทลอดกัน ฯ
ปุ

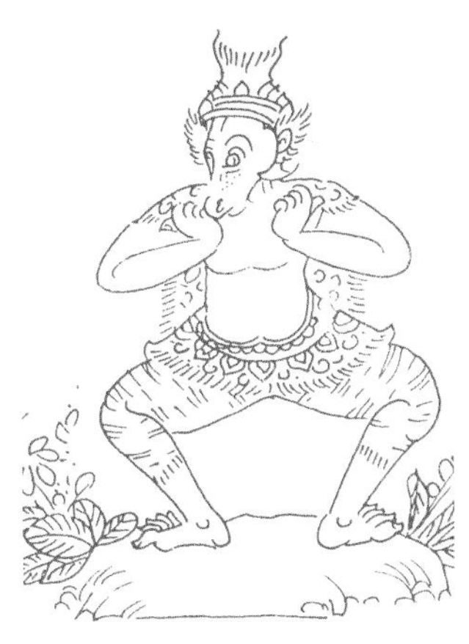

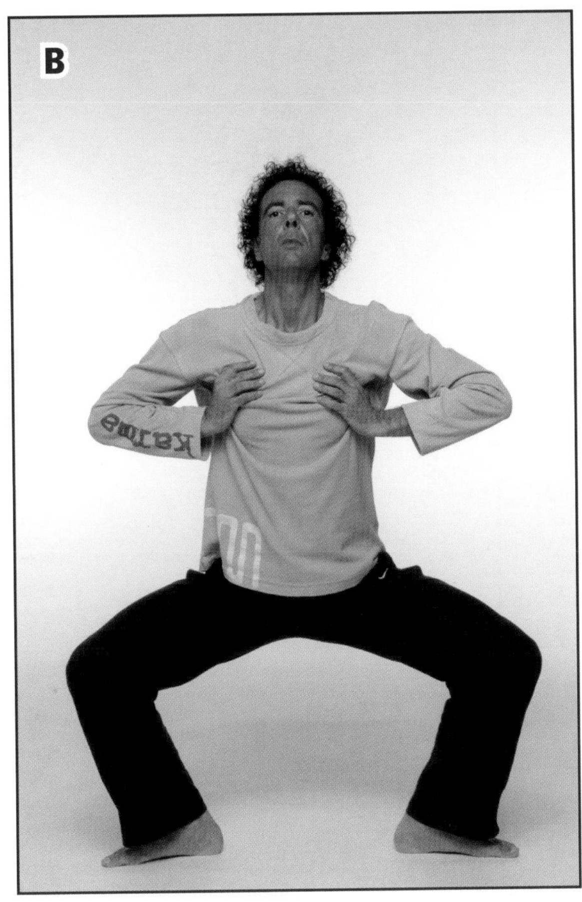

While breathing in, bend your legs outward, lowering yourself as far as possible. As your chest expands, compress it with your hands (B).

Holding your breath, maintain this position for 3 seconds.

As you breathe out, return slowly to the starting position.

Perform the exercise 3 to 5 times.

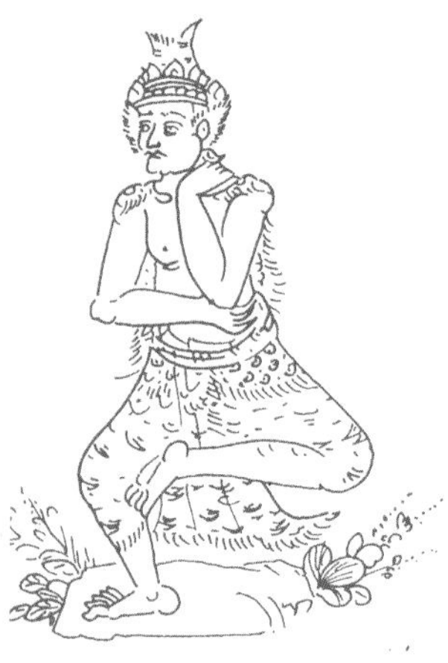

7
Remedy for Shoulder Pain

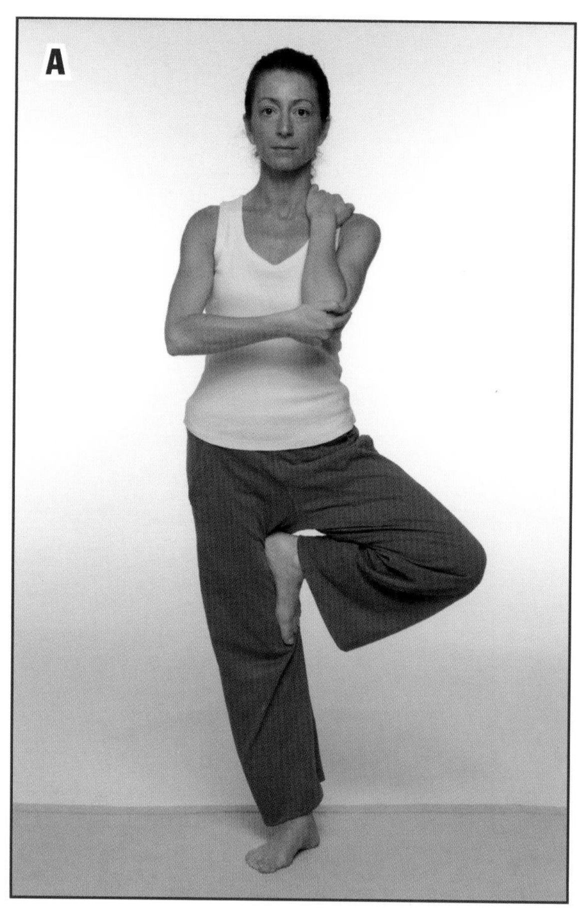

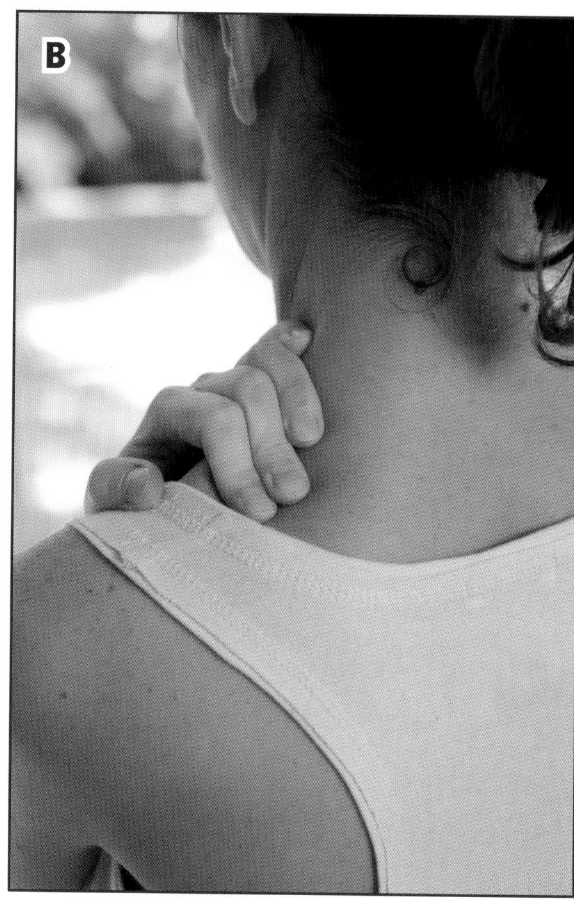

Stand on your right leg with your left leg bent inward, resting your foot against the inner part of the right thigh. Place your left hand on your left shoulder, supporting your elbow with your right hand (A).

Place the fingers of your left hand on the trapezius muscle next to the neck (B).

๑ เพชฎองการย่อเท้า เบื้องขวายืนเฮย เท้าหนึ่งยกยันขา กดเส้น
หัตถ์หนึ่งเหนี่ยวอังษา นิ้วรีดเส้นแฮ กรหนึ่งกุมศอกเคล้น ไหล่เท้าลมถอย ฯ

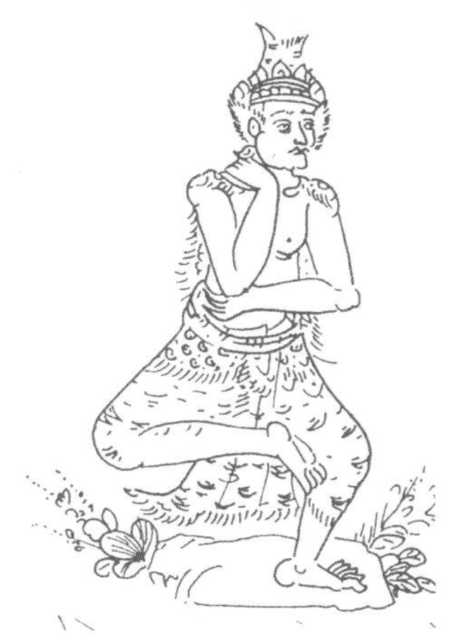

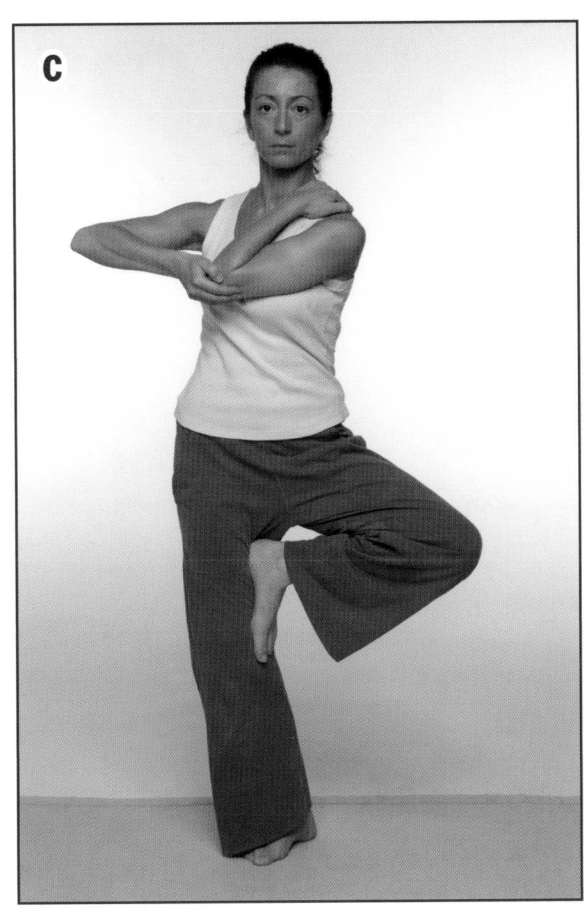

As you breathe in, bend your right leg slightly, pull your left elbow to the right with your right hand, and press the trapezius muscle with the fingers of your left hand (C).

Holding your breath, maintain this position for 3 seconds.

As you breathe out, return slowly to the starting position.

> Perform the exercise 3 to 5 times. Then practice the exercise on the other side.

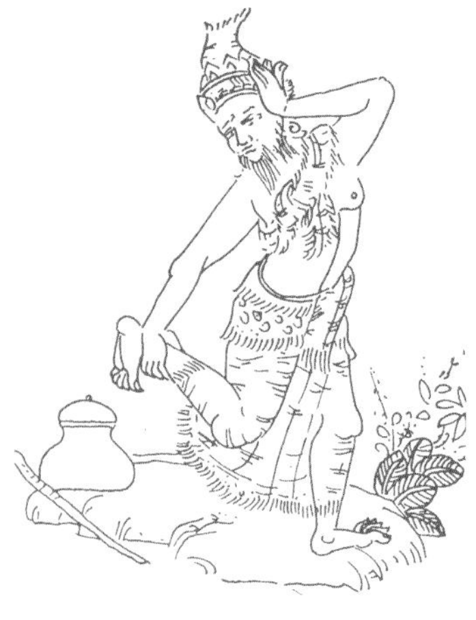

8
Remedy for Shoulder Stiffness and Pain

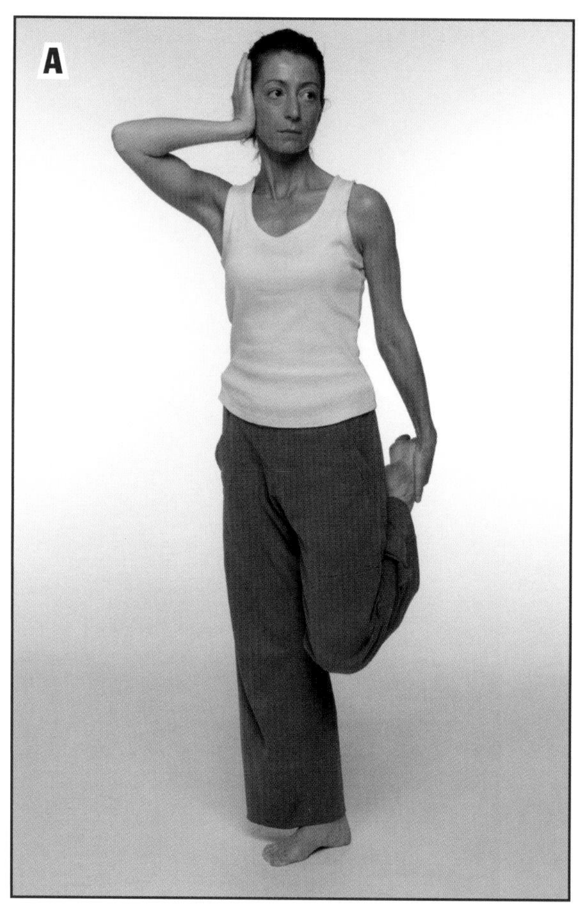

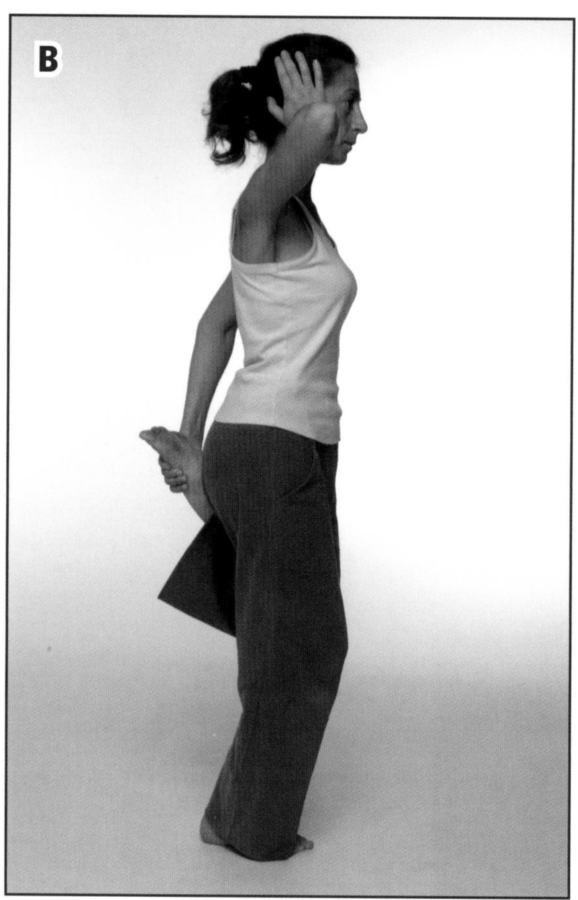

While standing, bend your left leg and seize the ankle with your left hand. Place your right hand against your right ear, with your fingers pointing upward (A).

While breathing out, bend your right knee (B).

๏ ดาบสเทวบิดนี้ นักงาน น้ำนา ตักส่งสมศิวญาณ อยู่เกล้า
กายป่มป่วยพิกาล ปัดฆาฏตคริวเฮย ยืนดัดเศียรเย่อเท้า ท่านแก้กลหมอ ๚

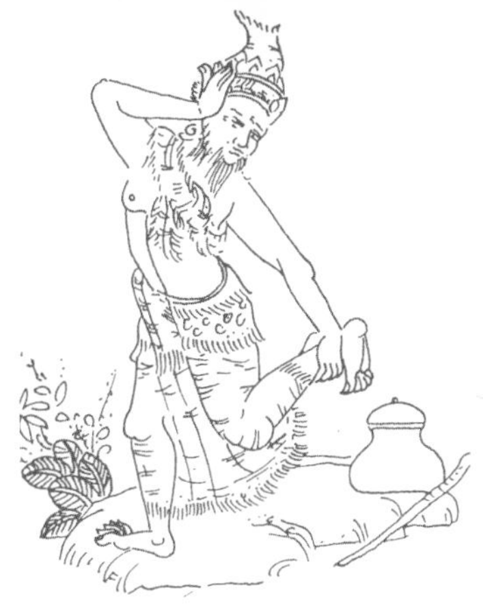

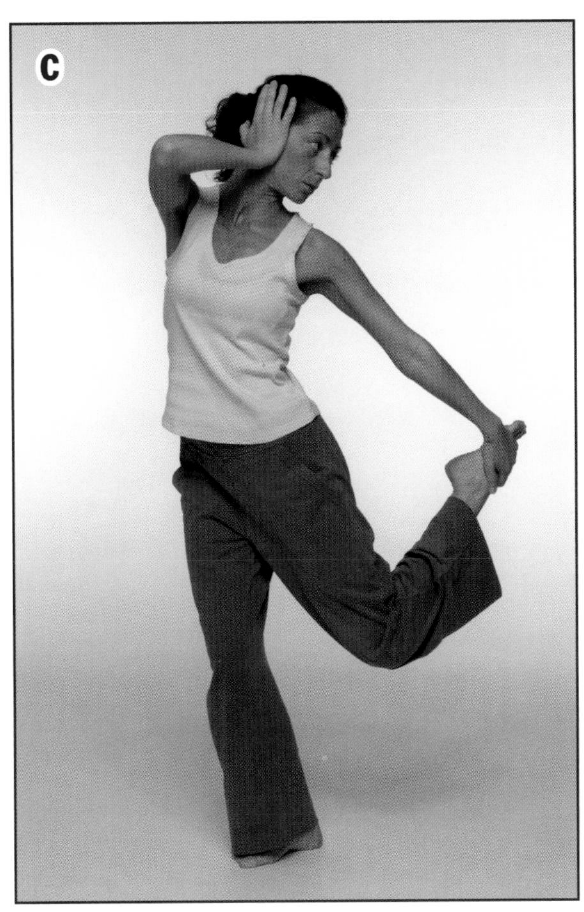

As you breathe in, stretch your left leg and bend and turn your head to the left, pushing it with your hand (C).

Holding your breath, maintain this position for 3 seconds.

As you breathe out, return slowly to the starting position.

Perform the exercise 3 to 5 times. Then practice the exercise on the other side.

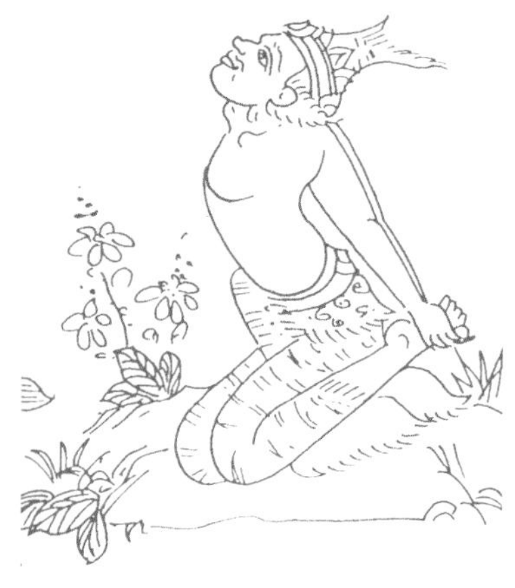

9
Remedy for Shoulder and Shoulder Blade Pain

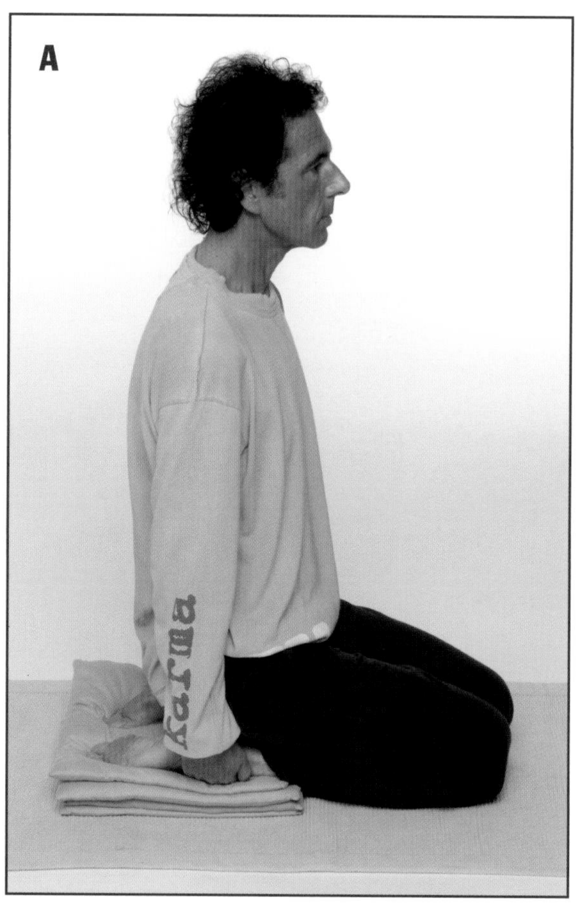

Kneel with your feet on a thin cushion or folded-up blanket, so that your legs slope down. Sit on your heels and hold your feet with your hands (A).

๏ หัดถ์หน่วงนิ้วเท้าพับ ชงฆชิดเพลาเฮย แก้สลักไหล่เพื่อพิศม์ ผ่อนน้อย
จะตันตะตระบะฤทธิ์ มฤครัก ท่านแอ มีแม่ไคหาร้อย หยอดนำมถวาย ฯ

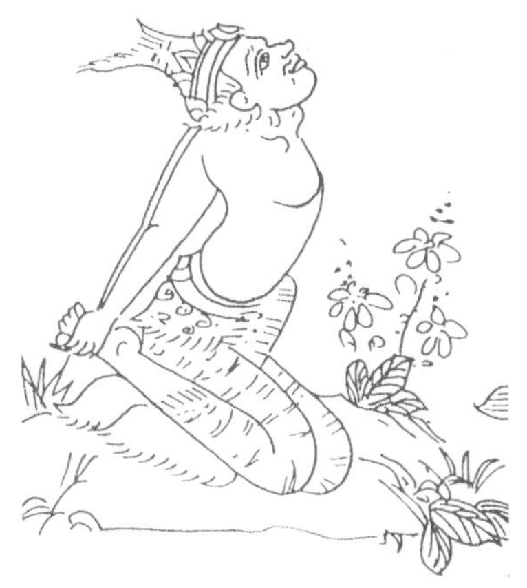

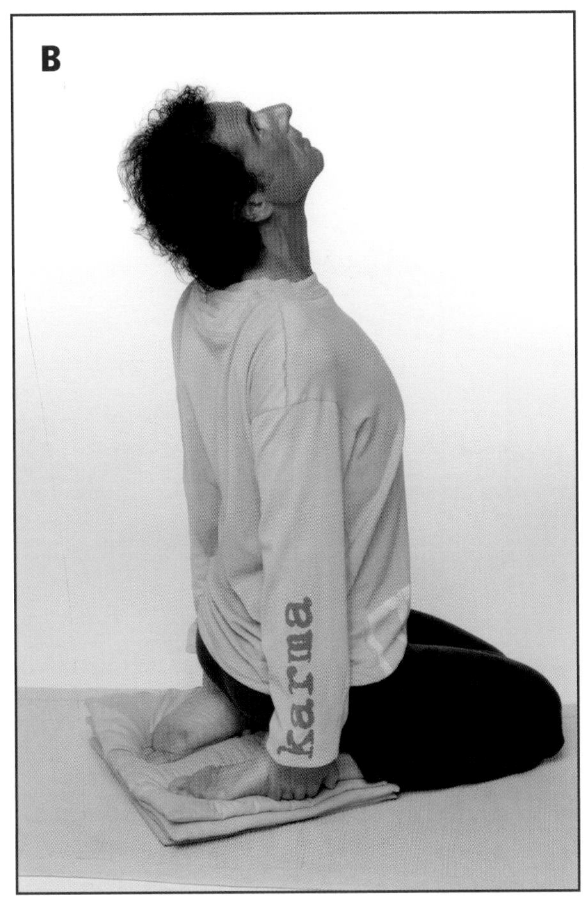

While breathing in and while keeping yourself anchored to your feet, bend your head and shoulders backward, stretching your chest (B).

Holding your breath, maintain this position for 3 seconds.

As you breathe out, return slowly to the starting position.

Perform the exercise 3 to 5 times.

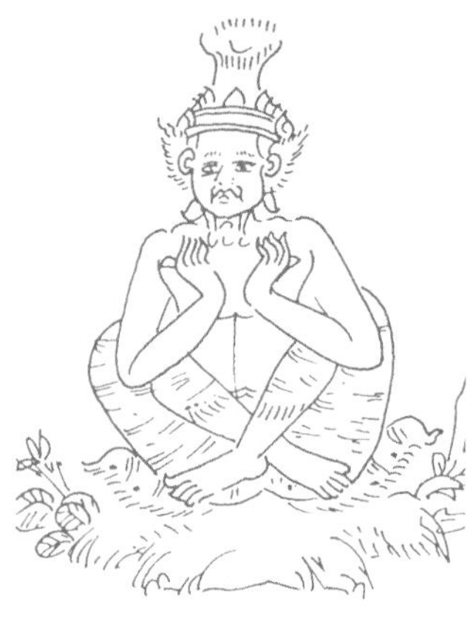

10
Remedy for Shoulder and Hip Pain 1

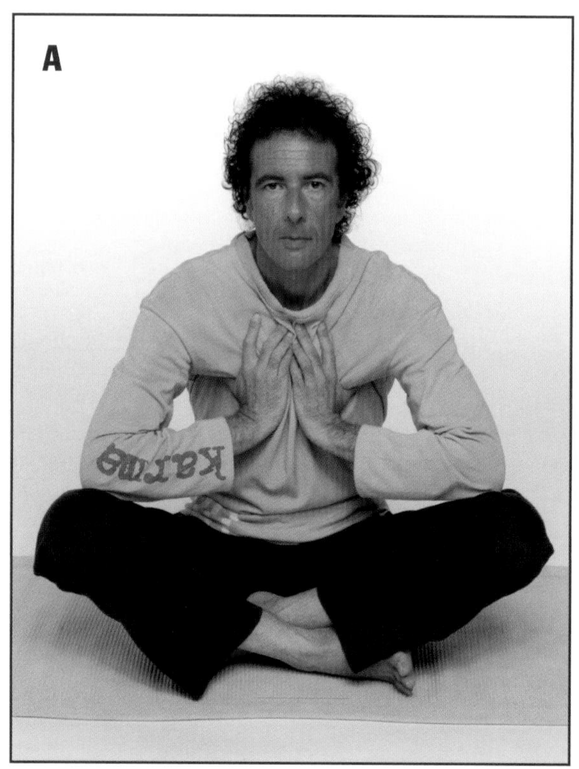

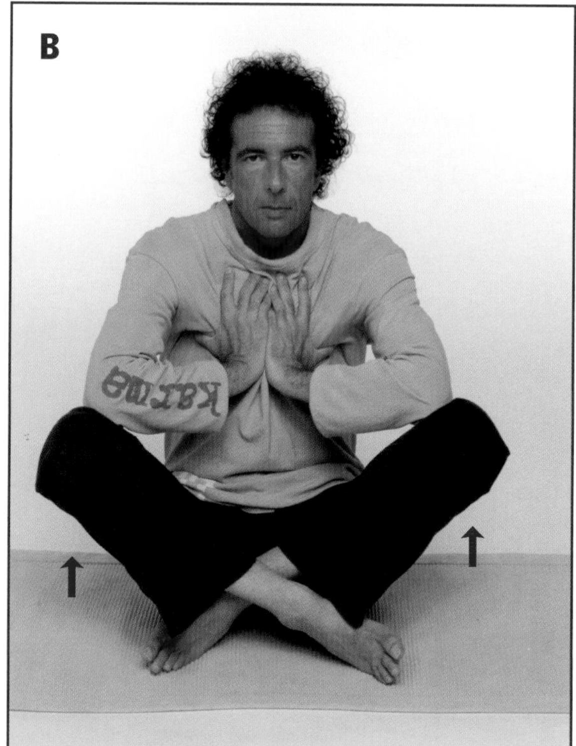

PART ONE

Sit with your legs crossed and knees slightly lifted. Place your elbows on your inner thighs, approximately 1½ inches (4 cm) up from your knees, and hold your chest with your hands (A).

As you breathe in, lift your legs, pushing your hands against your chest (B).

Holding your breath, maintain this position for 3 seconds.

As you breathe out, return slowly to the starting position.

Perform the exercise 3 to 5 times.

๑ พระชนกนักสิทธินี้ ชนะมาร ไตรเพทไตรพิธญาณ ย่อมแจ้ง
เอกไหล่ยอกโตรภกษ์าน ปี้นป่ากอยู่นอ คู้เข่าศอกกดแข้ง หัดถ์เคล้นโคลท

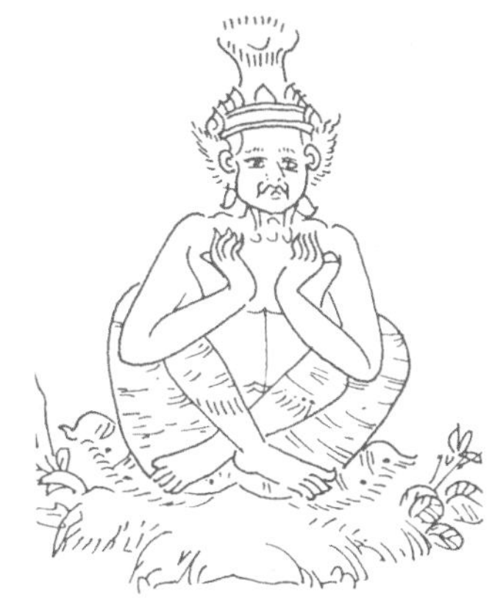

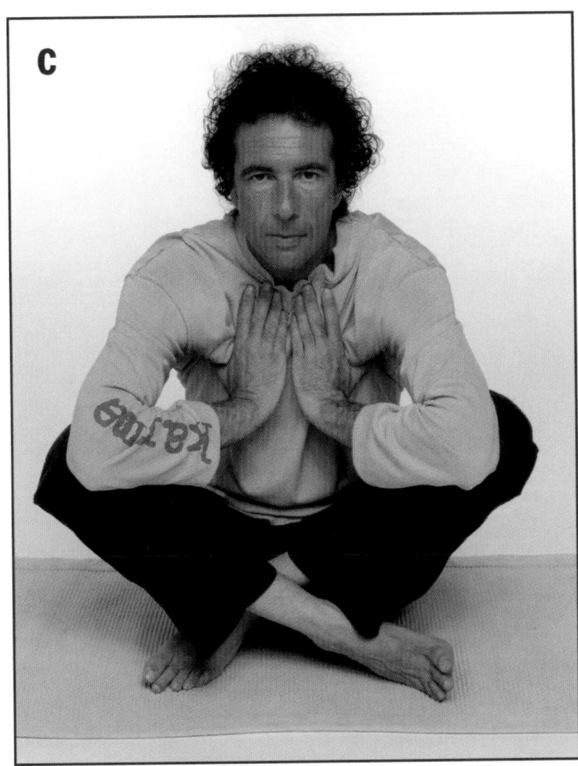

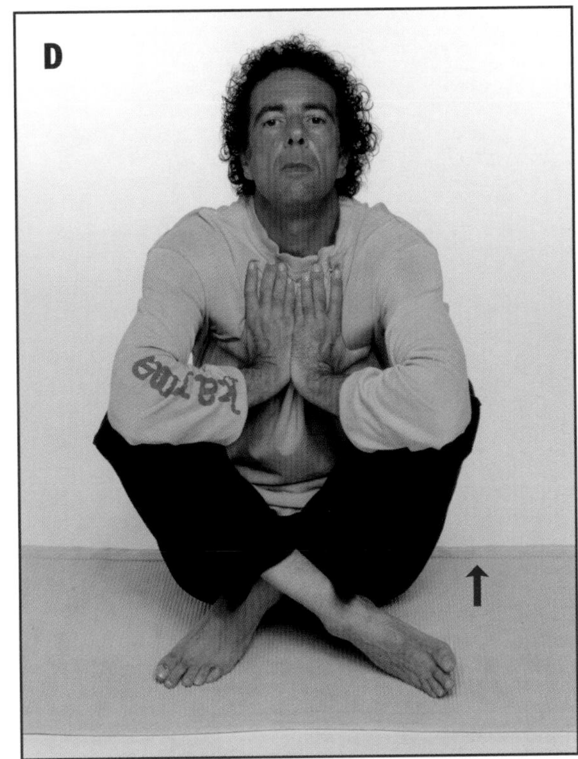

PART TWO

Hook your elbows over your knees, with your forearms on your upper shins, while keeping your hands on your chest (C).

While breathing in, lift your legs as high as possible, using your arms to help lift your legs (D and E).

Holding your breath, maintain this position for 3 seconds.

As you breathe out, return slowly to the starting position.

Perform the exercise 3 to 5 times.

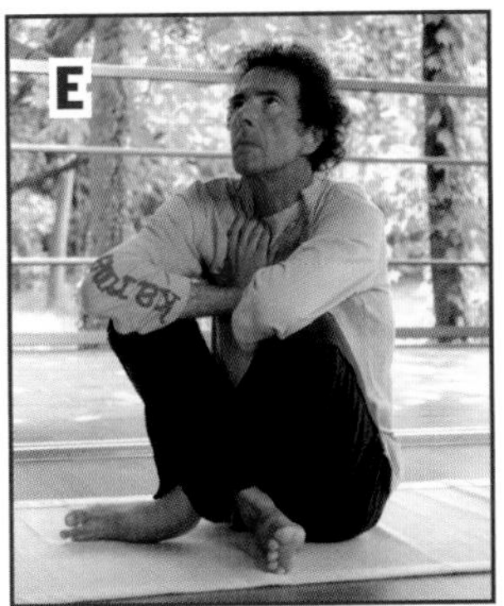

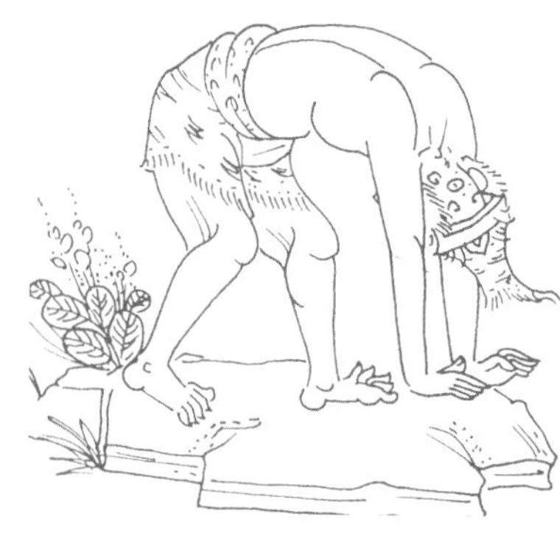

11 Remedy for Shoulder and Hip Pain 2

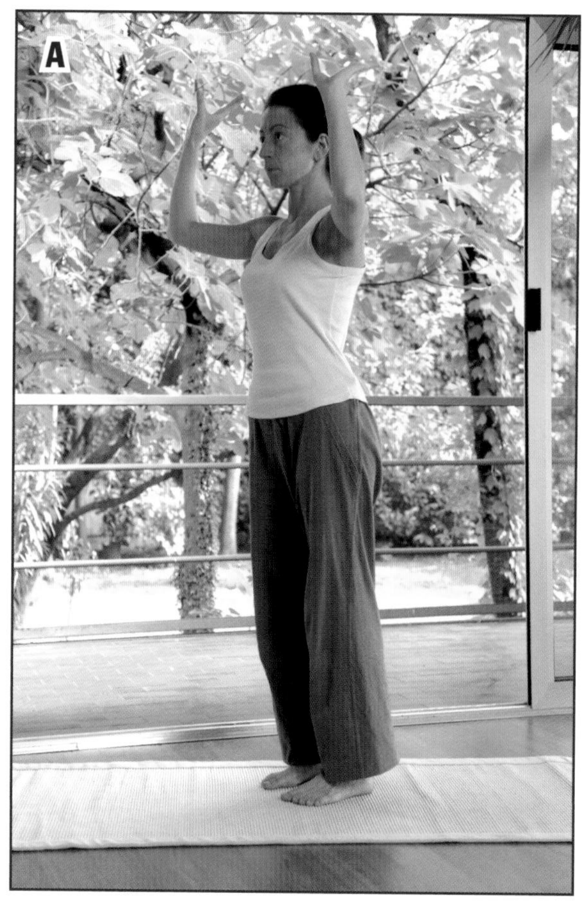

While standing, lift your arms and flex your wrists backward (A).

พระอัลกัปะกะเปื้อง บรรพ์รบินนั้นฤา รู้ฤกษบนมนตร์พิณ ผะเหลาะข้าง

กหัดกิจรดดิน ยื่นหย่งเย่นฯ แก้ไหล่ตะโภกเกลี่ยวข้าง เข่าแข้งขาหาย ฯ

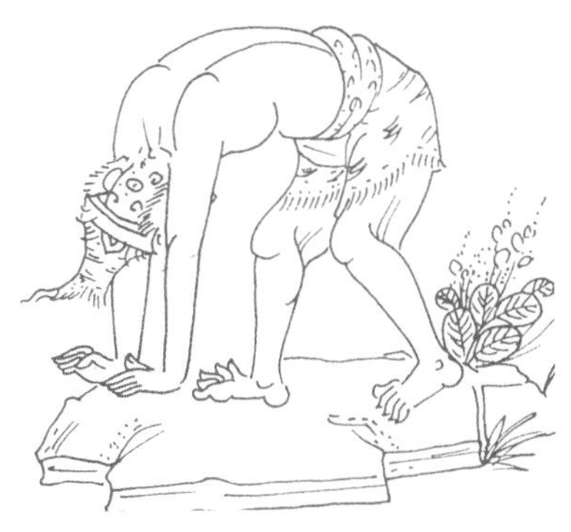

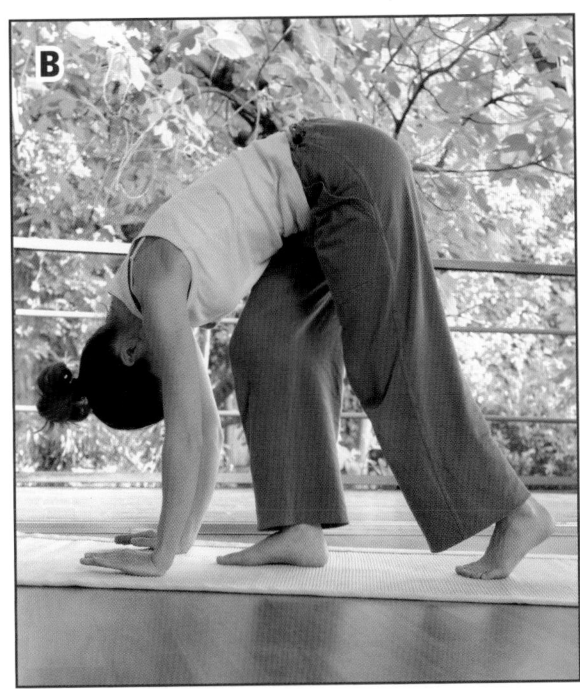

While breathing out, step forward with your right leg, and bend forward to place your hands on the floor, keeping your wrists well flexed so that your fingers don't touch the floor. Keep your right knee bent and your left leg and foot flexed (B).

Breathe in deeply and, holding that breath, maintain this position for 3 seconds.

As you breathe out, return slowly to the starting position. (It's important to return to the starting position very slowly in order to avoid becoming dizzy.)

Perform the exercise 3 to 5 times. Then practice the exercise on the other side.

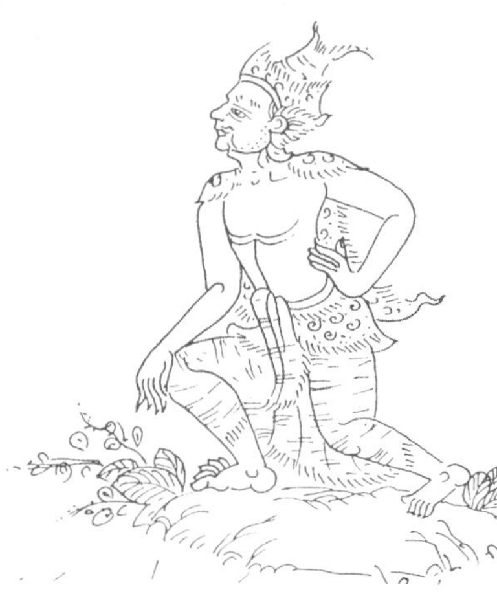

12

Remedy for Shoulder and Leg Stiffness

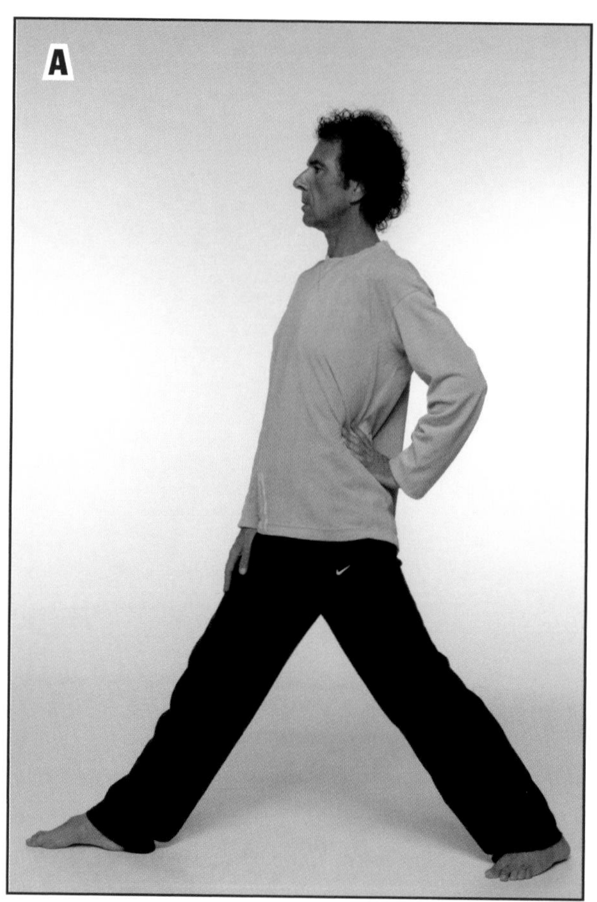

Pull your left leg back to stand with your legs apart and your heels aligned. Point your right foot forward and turn your left foot out at a 45-degree angle. Put your right hand on your right leg and your left hand on the small of your back, with your fingers pointing upward (A).

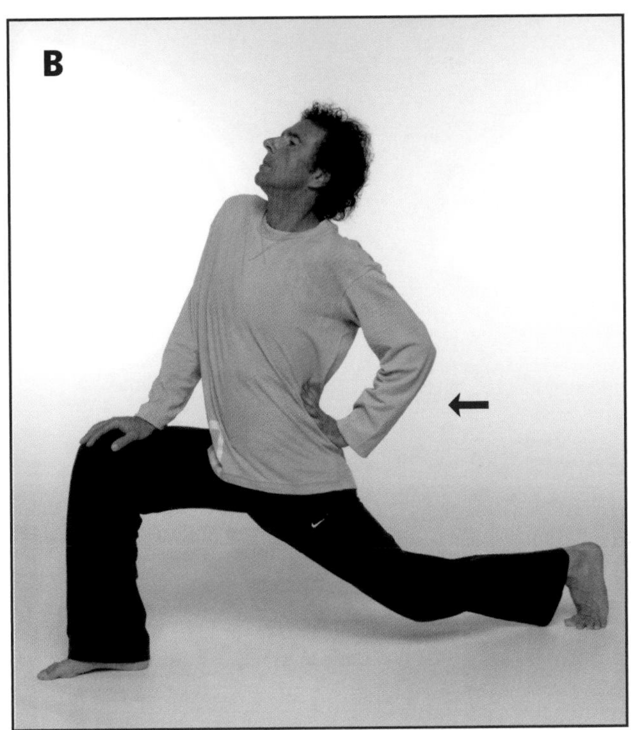

While breathing in, turn your left foot to align it with the right one, bending your right leg and flexing the left one. Keep your right arm on your right leg, sliding it down to your knee. Push against your back with your left hand in order to increase the stretch (B).

Holding your breath, maintain this position for 3 seconds.

As you breathe out, return slowly to the starting position.

Perform the exercise 3 to 5 times. Then practice the exercise on the other side.

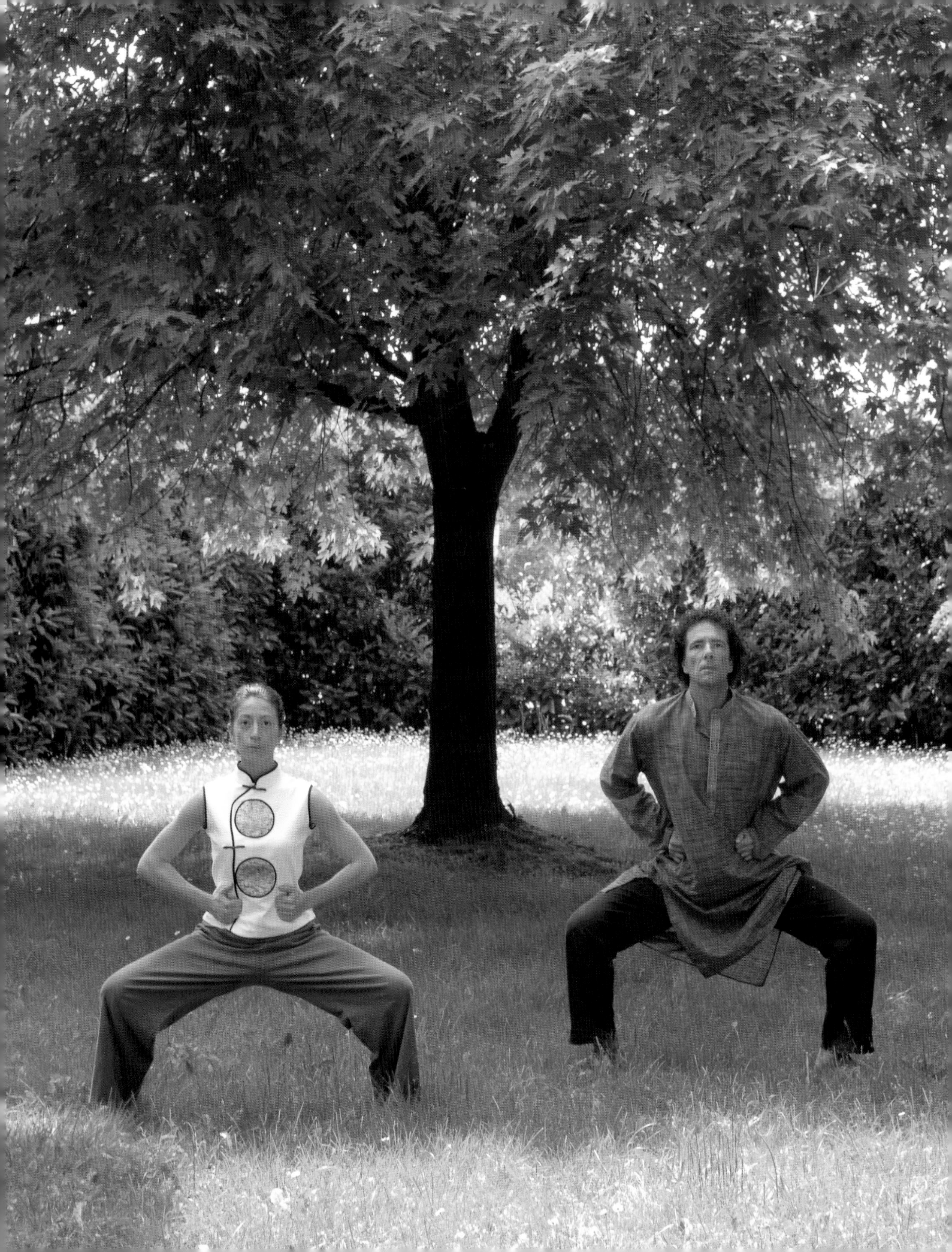

FIVE

Postures That Benefit the Torso

13. Remedy for Chest, Shoulder, and Abdominal Pain
14. Remedy for Painful Pressure in the Chest
15. Remedy for Pressure in the Chest 1
16. Remedy for Pressure in the Chest 2
17. Remedy for Heartburn
18. Remedy for Intercostal Pain
19. Remedy for Abdominal Pain and Shoulder Blade Pain
20. Remedy for Abdominal Pain
21. Remedy for Sharp Pain at the Waist
22. Remedy for Abdominal Pain Caused by Gaseous Indigestion
23. Remedy for Stomach Troubles
24. Remedy for Abdominal Pain and Ankle Pain
25. Remedy for Lower Back Pain
26. Remedy for Lower Back and Hip Pain
27. Remedy for Lower Back and Leg Pain
28. Remedy for Hemorrhoids
29. Remedy for Abdominal Distension and Pain in the Genital Area
30. Remedy for Lower Abdominal Pain and Scrotal Discomfort
31. Remedy for Pain in the Testicles and Difficult Urination

See also:

- Exercise 42, Remedy for Knee, Leg, and Chest Problems

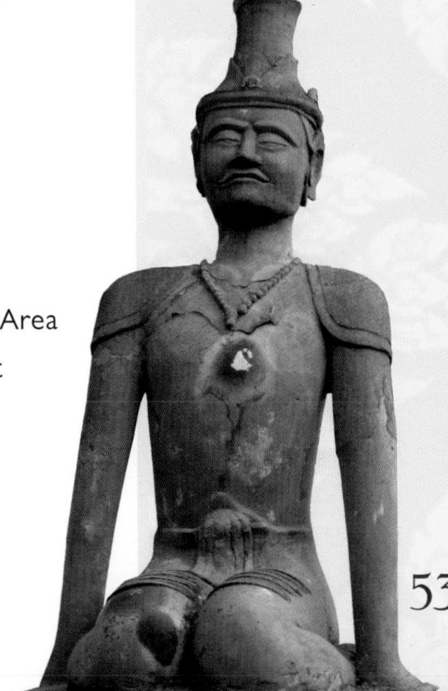

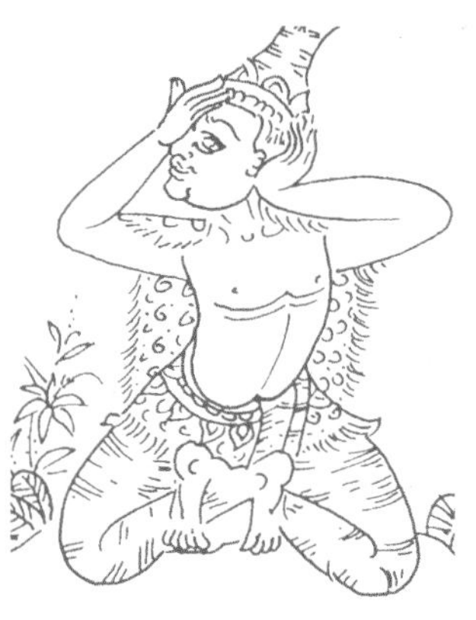

13
Remedy for Chest, Shoulder, and Abdominal Pain

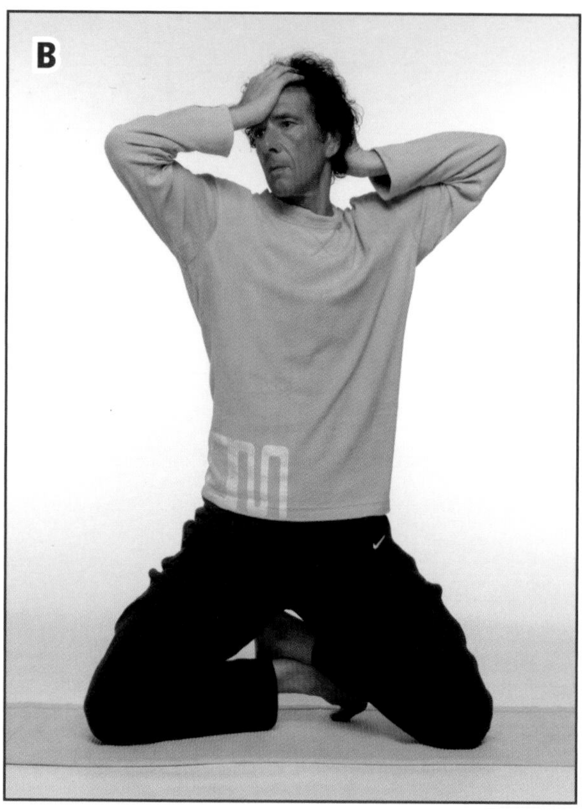

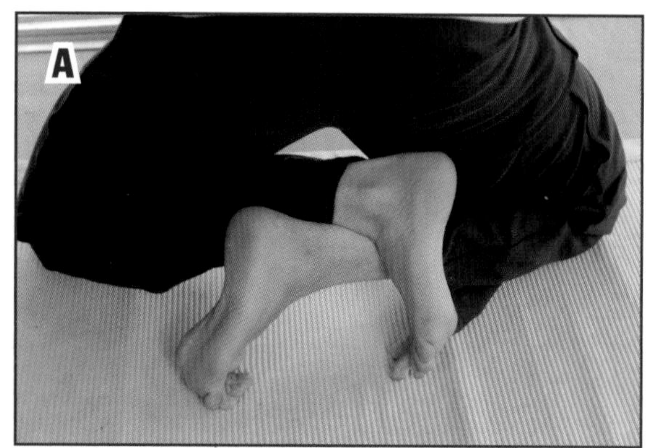

Kneel with your feet flexed and crossed beneath you (A).

Place the ball of your left hand immediately under the occipital bones next to the ear and the palm of your right hand on your forehead, between the eyebrows. Keep the fingers of both hands pointing up (B).

As you breathe out, slightly twist your chest to the left.

๑ นักสิทธิ์สมาบัติสร้าง สร่างเกลศ กาละกุรักขรปื่อเกช เพรียกพร้อง
กดผากกดท้ายเกษ บาทขัดคุกแอ่ มับโรคลมไหล่ท้อง อุระด้วยดั่งแผน

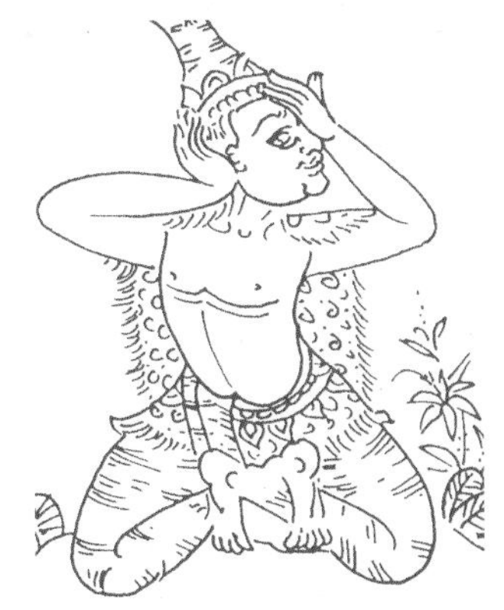

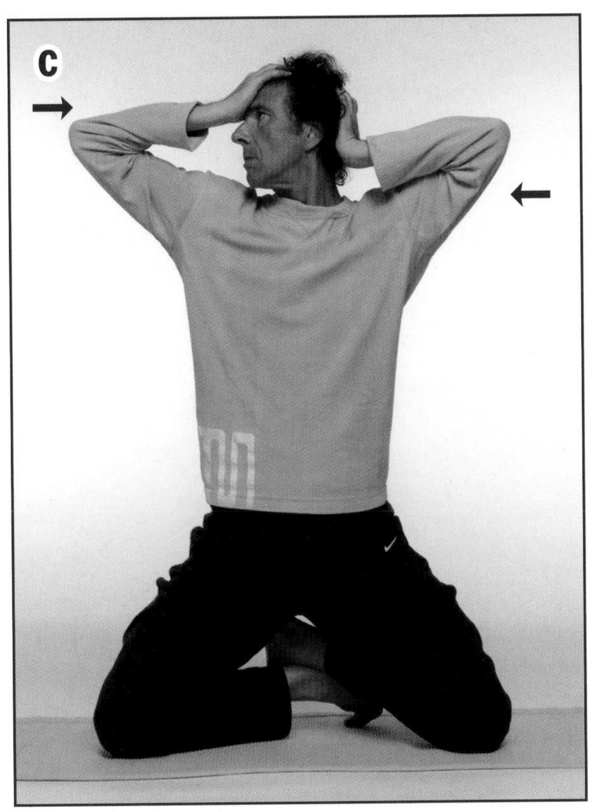

Breathing in, turn your head to the right as much as possible and at the same time, press into your head with both hands (C).

Holding your breath, maintain this position for 3 seconds.

As you breathe out, return slowly to the starting position.

Repeat this sequence in the opposite direction, now turning your head to the left and pressing with your left hand on your forehead and your right hand on the back of your head.

Perform the exercise 3 to 5 times.

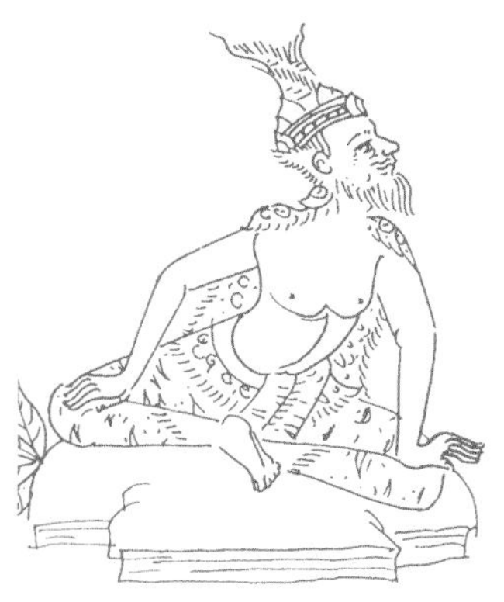

14
Remedy for Painful Pressure in the Chest

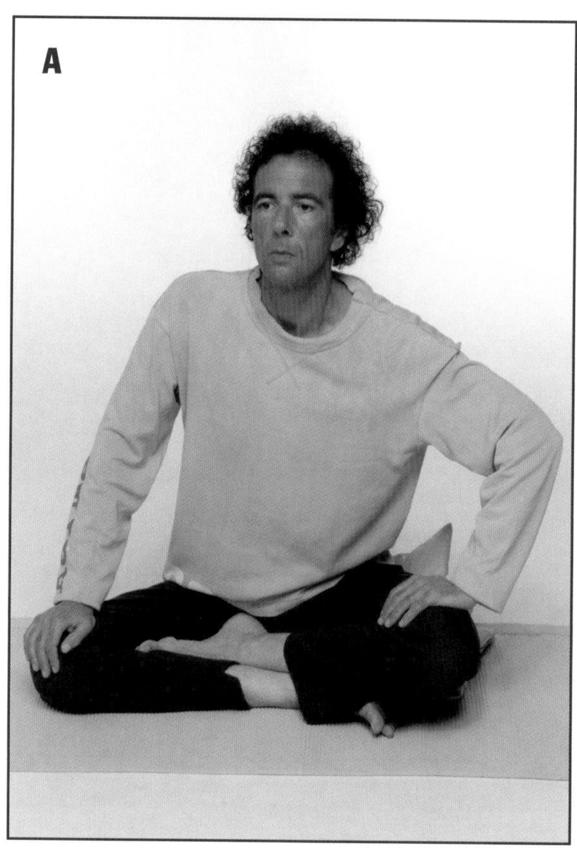
A

This exercise is more effective if performed on a slightly sloping base. Use a few cushions or blankets in order to obtain it.

Sit in the half-lotus position with just your buttocks on the cushions, with your right leg under the left and sloping downward. Place the palm of your right hand above your right knee, with your fingers pointing down over the outside of the knee. Place the palm of your left hand above your left knee, your fingers pointing down toward your body. Having your hands in the correct position is important in order to keep your shoulders in the proper position (A).

๏ สัจพัณฑ์นักสิทธิ์ผู้ สถิตย์สัจพัณฑ์เอย ลมเสียดทรวงอกอัด โรคเรื้อ
ประจงสองพระหัตถ์กดคัด ดันเข่าสองนา นรชาติใครได้เชื้อ นวดเท้าอธิษฐาน ฯ

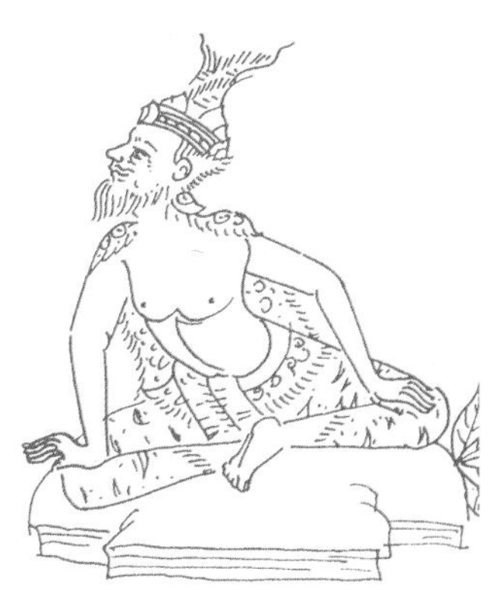

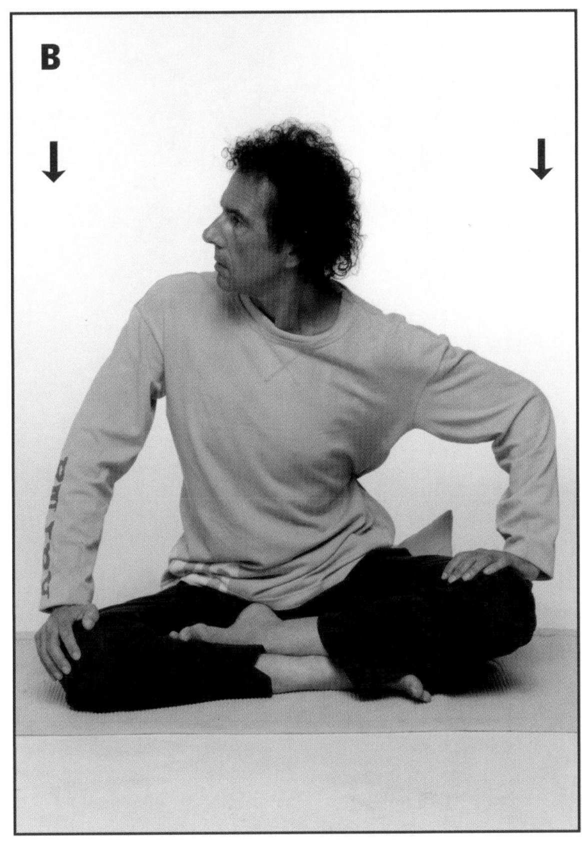

As you breathe in, push down on both legs with your hands. At the same time slightly turn your head and chest to the right (B).

Holding your breath, maintain this position for 3 seconds.

As you breathe out, return slowly to the starting position.

Perform the exercise 3 to 5 times on the first side. Then practice the exercise on the other side.

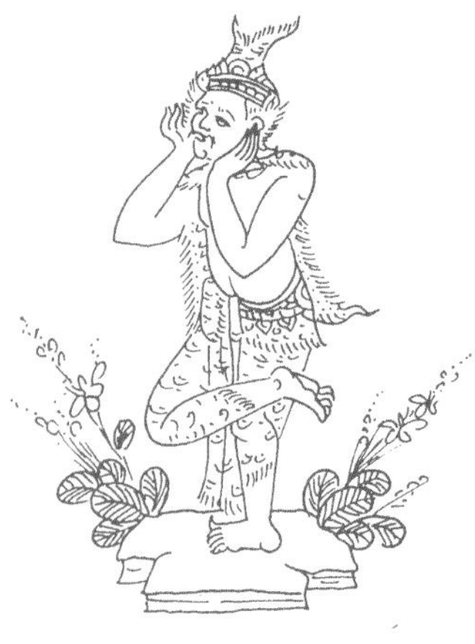

15
Remedy for Pressure in the Chest 1

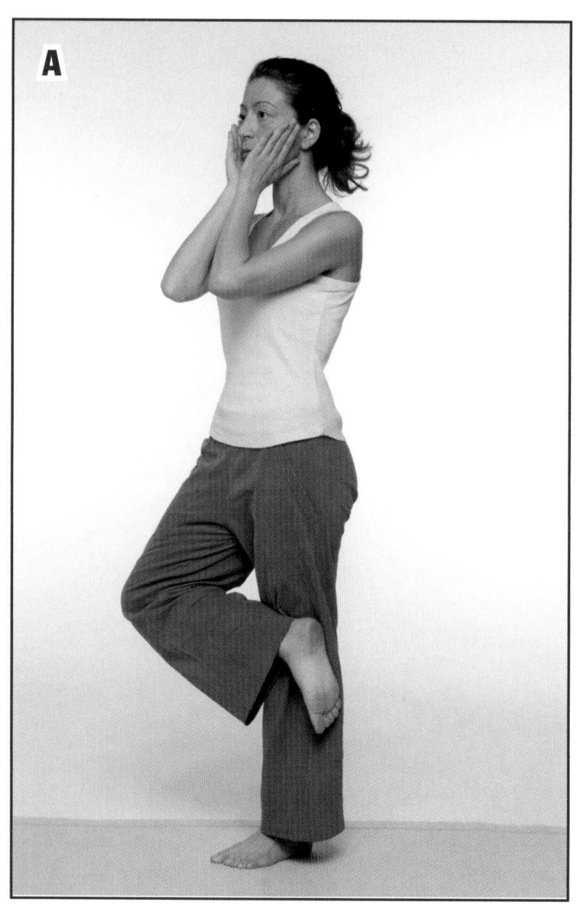

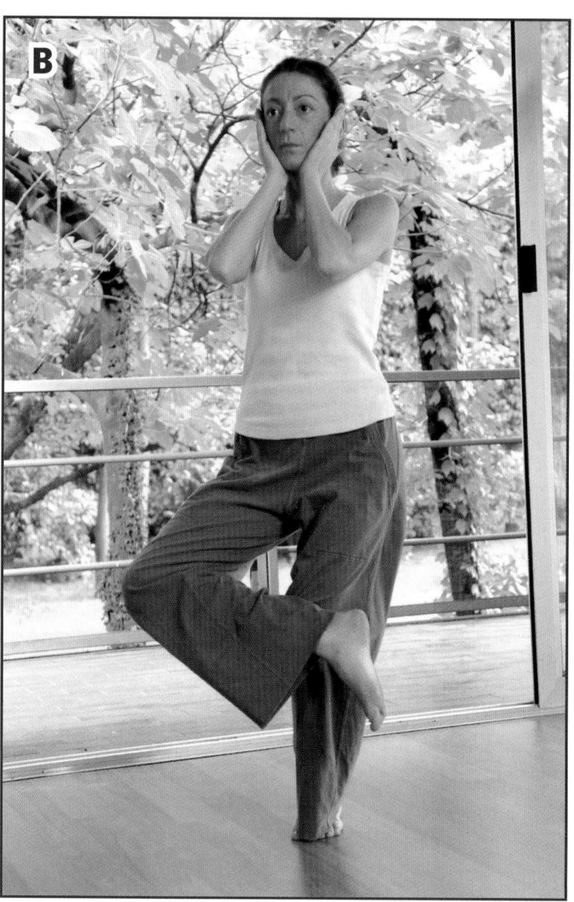

While standing, bend your right leg and place it over the left knee. Place the palms of both hands against the jaw (A).

Breathe out and bend your left knee (B).

๑ ฤๅษีสำมิทธิ์แม้น ครูหมอนวดฯ ยืนหยัดยกเท้างอ ไขว่ไว้
สองมือดัดคางคอ เข่งยืดตัวแฮ แก้แน่นหน้าอกได้ เสียดเส้นลมหาย ฯ

พญาไชยวิชิต ๖

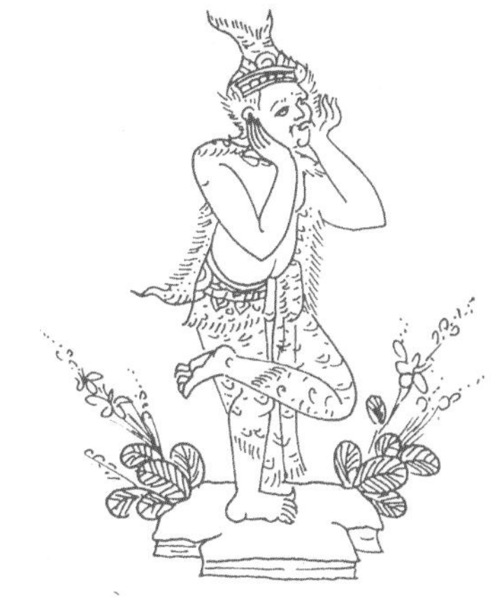

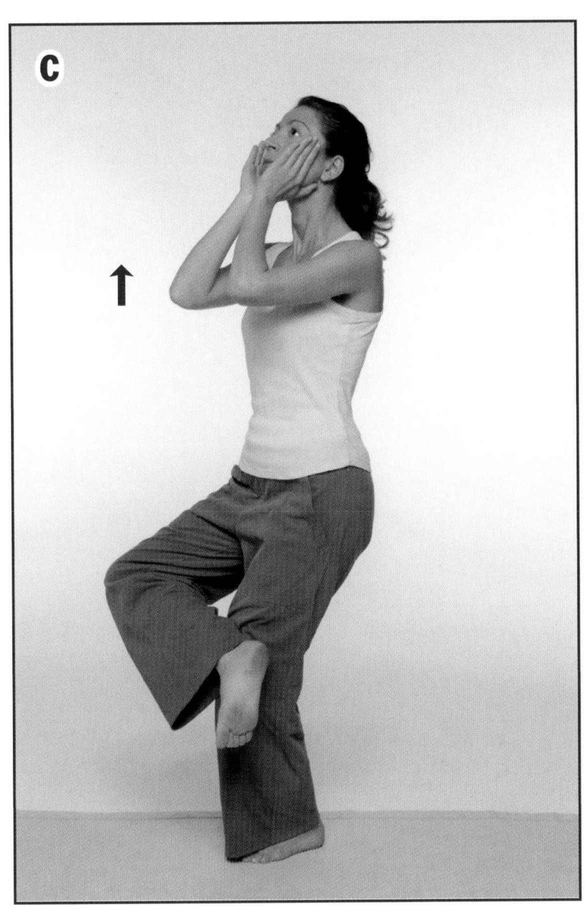

As you breathe in, push your head backward with your hands (C).

Holding your breath, maintain this position for 3 seconds.

As you breathe out, return slowly to the starting position.

Perform the exercise 3 to 5 times. Then practice the exercise on the other side.

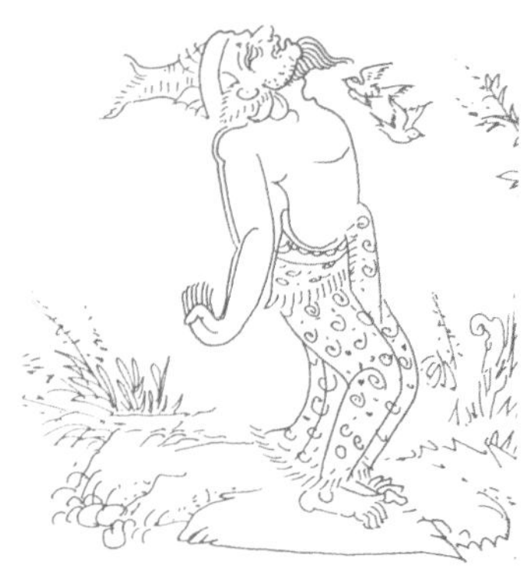

16

Remedy for Pressure in the Chest 2

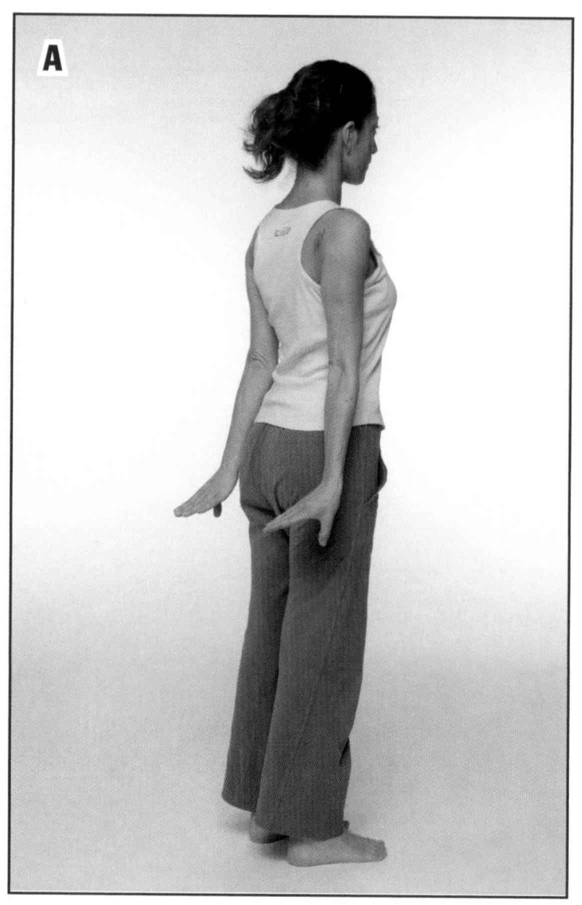

A

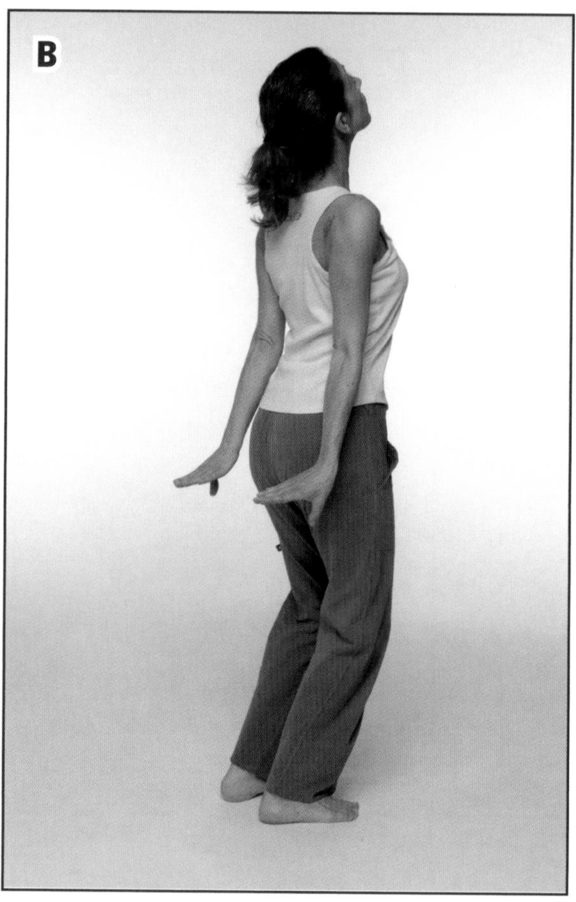

B

Stand with your feet close together and your arms stretched behind you, with your wrists well flexed (A).

Breathing in, bend your knees slightly, extend your chest upward, and flex your head backward, keeping your wrists flexed as much as possible (B).

Holding your breath, maintain this position for 3 seconds.

As you breathe out, return slowly to the starting position.

Perform the exercise 3 to 5 times.

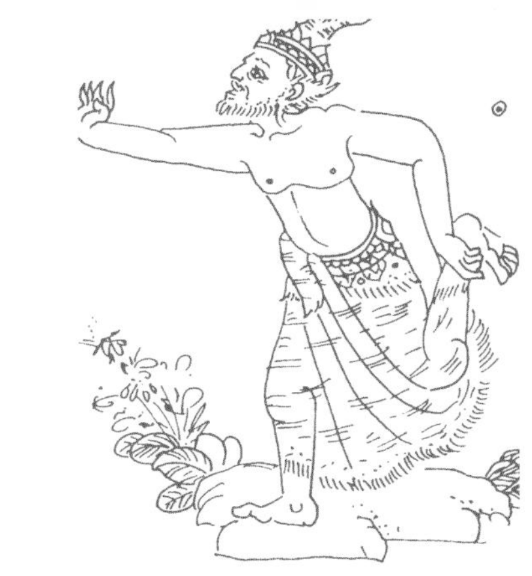

17 Remedy for Heartburn

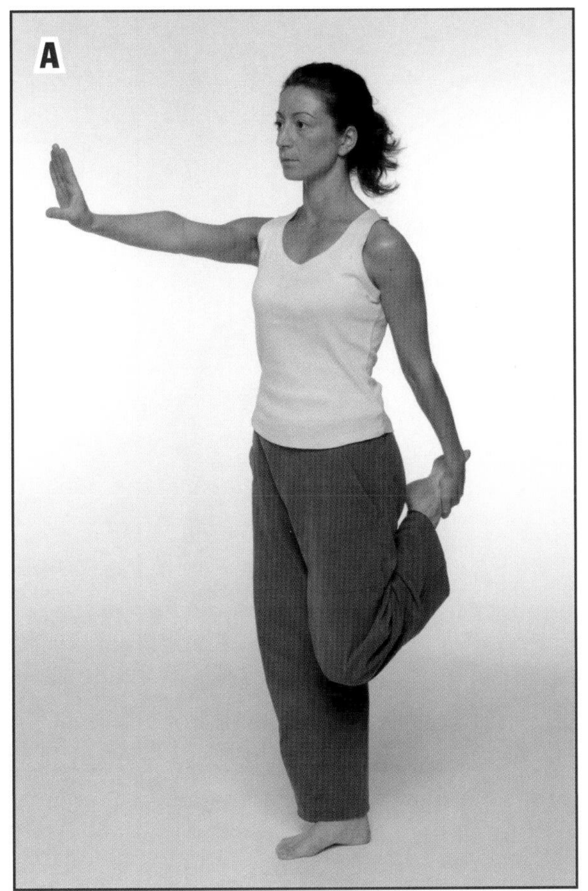

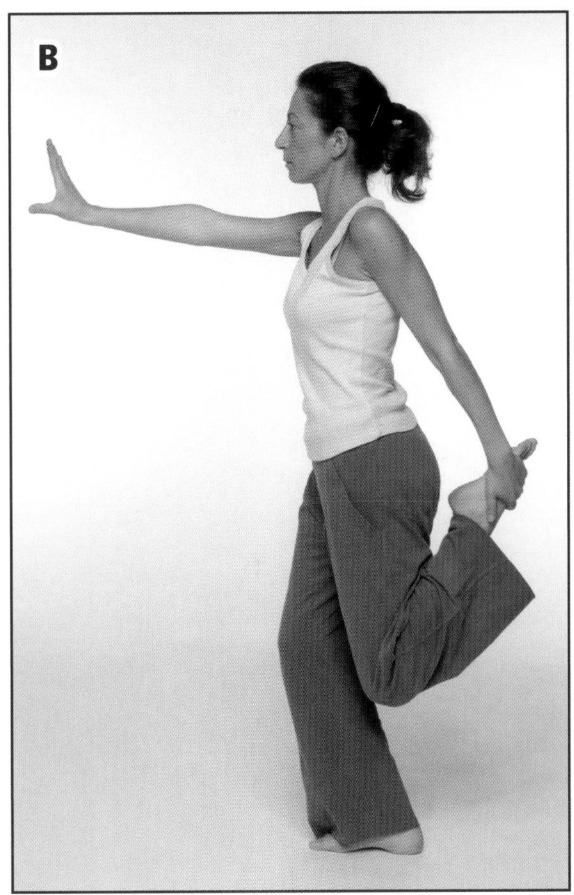

While standing, bend your left leg back and grasp the ankle with your left hand. Stretch your right arm out in front of you, keeping the wrist well flexed (A).

While breathing out, bend your right knee (B).

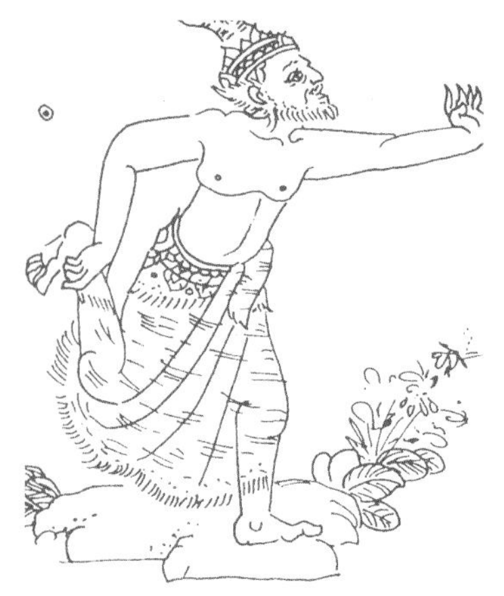

๏ ยืนเหนี่ยวค่อเท้าเชอด หัดถ์เห็นยกแย แก้เสียดทรวงเส้นเอ็น ขอดได้
นรทเสกไม้เป็น ปลิงเกาะกระบี่พ่อ ยิ้มเยาะวานรให้ เหือดร้ายรังแก ฯ

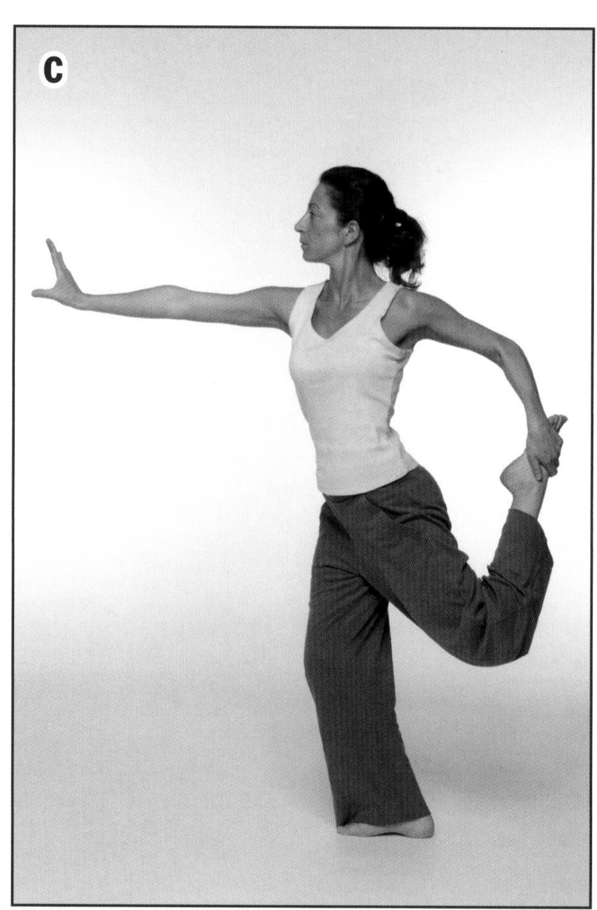

As you breathe in, push your left foot against your left hand. The traction between your hand and foot will pull your arm and shoulder back, causing your chest open to the left (C).

Holding your breath, maintain the position for 3 seconds.

Breathe out, and slowly return to the starting position.

๏ ยืนเหนี่ยวค่อเท้าเชอด หัดถ์เหิ้นยากแฮ แก้เสียดทรวงเส้นเอ็น ขอดได้
นารทเสกไม้เป็น ปลิงเกาะกระบี่พ่อ ยิ้มเยาะวานรให้ เหือดร้ายรังแก ฯ

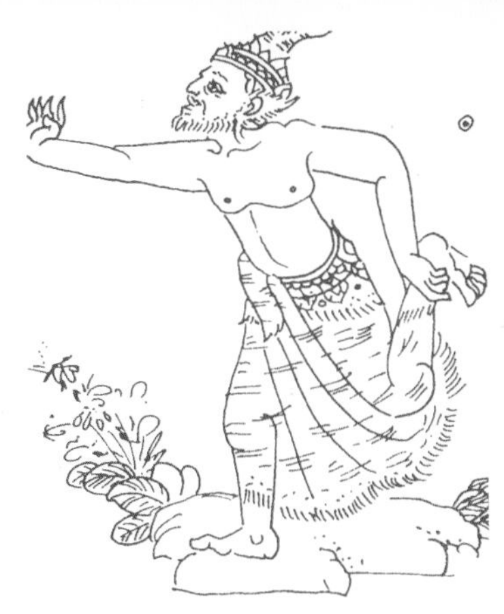

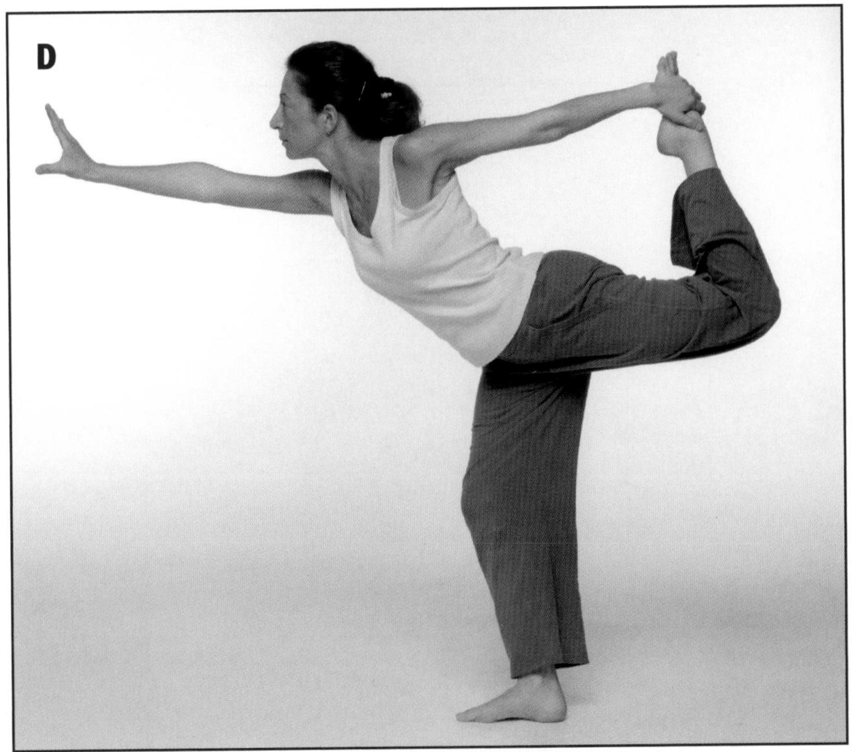

After taking a breath, bend your right knee again while breathing out (B).

This time as you breathe in, lift your left leg back as far as possible and stretch your arm and chest forward as a counterbalance (D).

Holding your breath, maintain this position for 3 seconds.

As you breathe out, return slowly to the starting position.

Perform the entire exercise 3 to 5 times. Then practice the exercise on the other side.

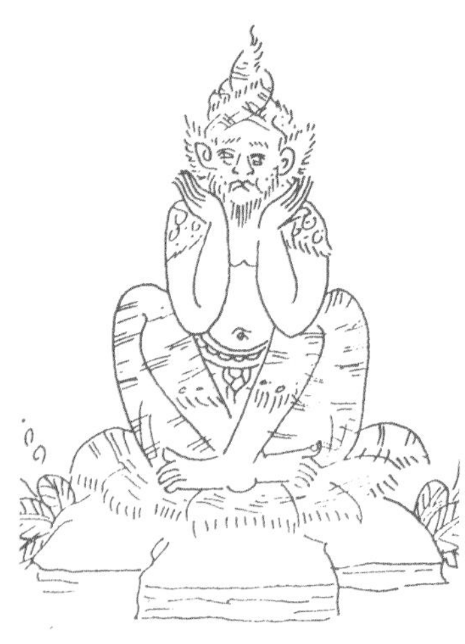

18

Remedy for Intercostal Pain

(Pain in the Muscles between the Ribs)

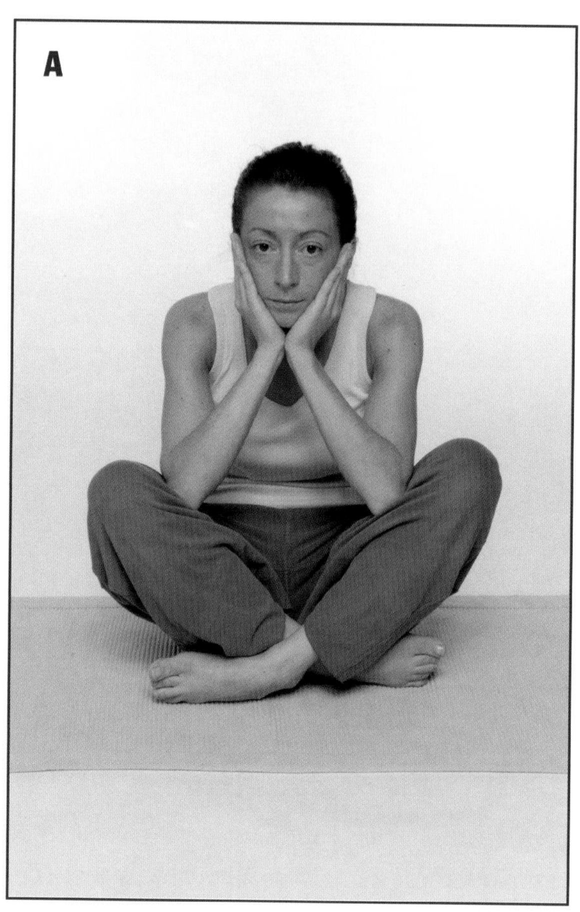

Sit cross-legged, with your knees lifted. Place the palms of both hands over your jaw, and rest your elbows on your inner thighs (A).

๏ โยคีอะแหม่เม้น แขกพราหมพรตแฮ มือสิบเบ็ดนิ้วสลาม ศีรษะไท้
แก้ลมอัณหวาตหาม ลำแล่นเสียวนา คู้เขาเท้าสองไขว้ หัดถ์เคล้นไคลหอ ฯ

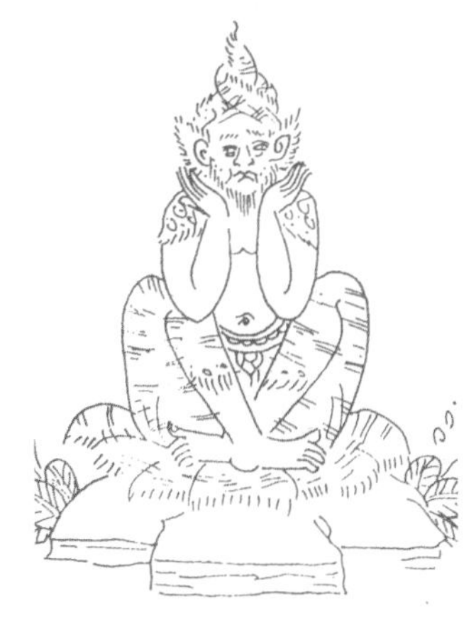

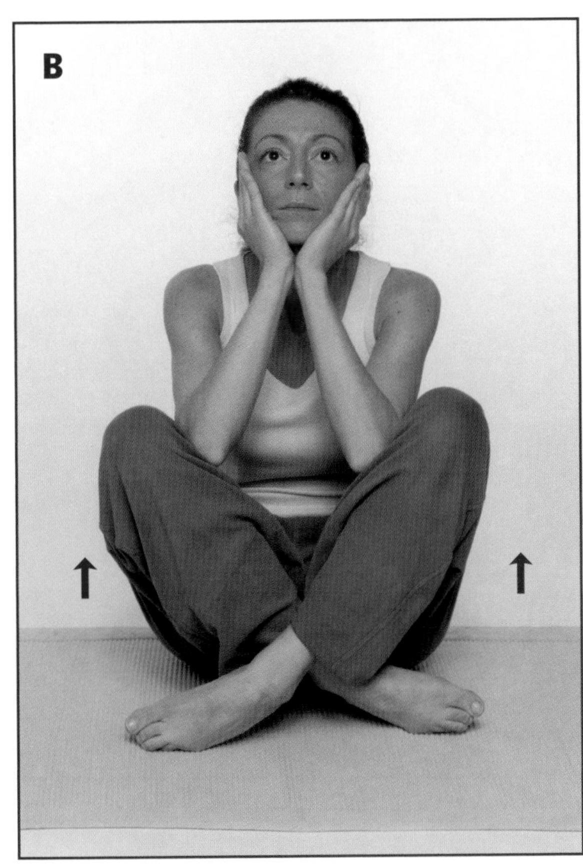

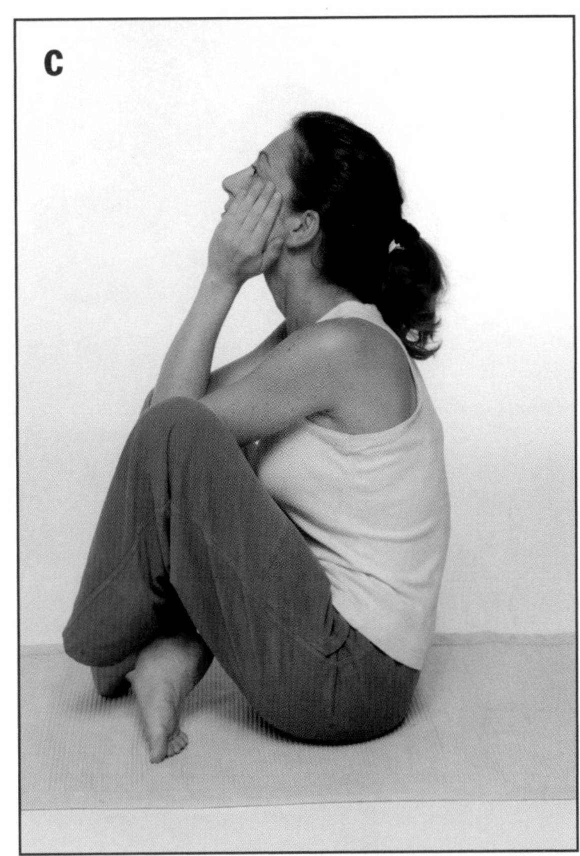

While breathing in, lift your knees. The knees will then lift your arms, which will slightly lift your head backward (B and C).

Holding your breath, maintain this position for 3 seconds.

As you breathe out, return slowly to the starting position.

Perform the exercise 3 to 5 times.

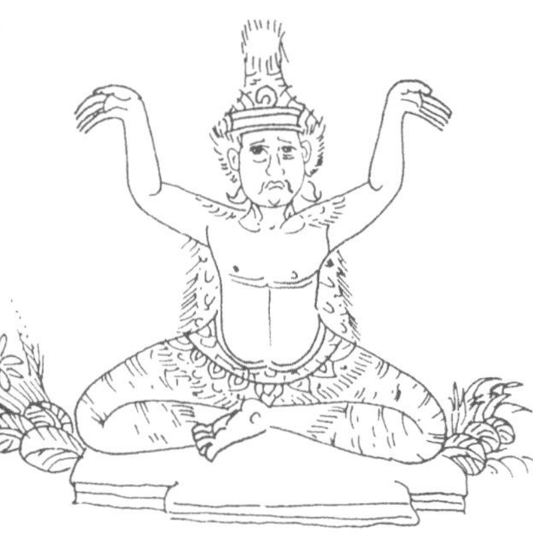

19 Remedy for Abdominal Pain and Shoulder Blade Pain

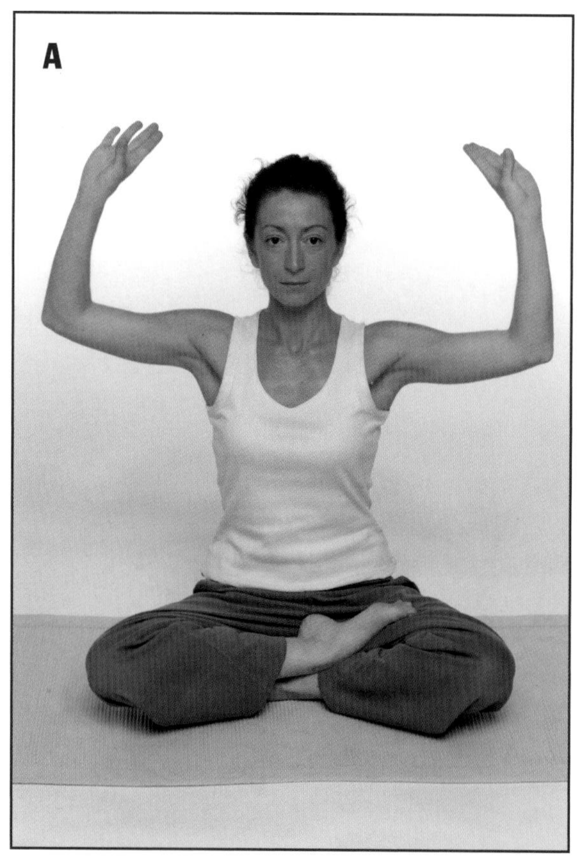

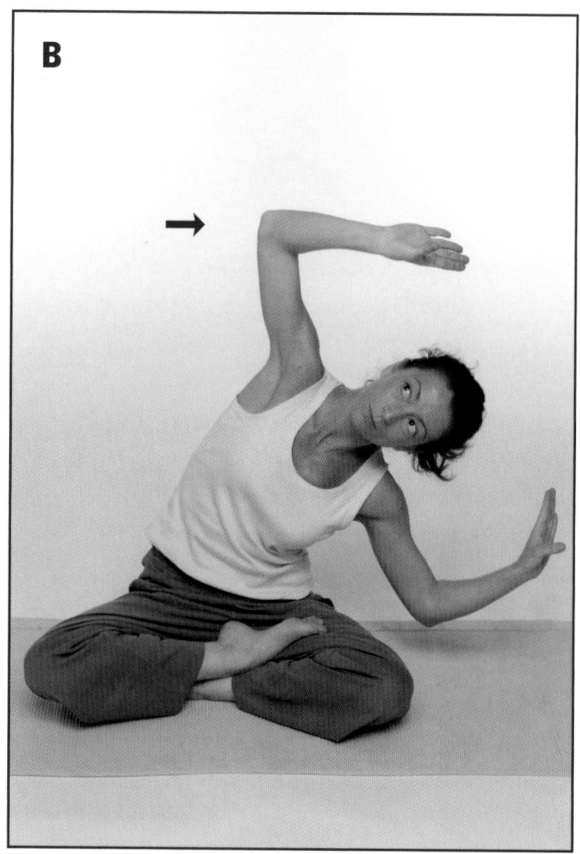

Sit in the half-lotus position. Hold your arms bent upward at your sides, as if you were holding a tray over your head, and keep your wrists well flexed (A).

As you breathe in, bend to the left as far as you can, keeping your arms in the starting position (B).

Holding your breath, maintain this position for 3 seconds.

As you breathe out, return slowly to the starting position.

Repeat the bending sequence, now bending to the right.

๏ ธรงนามยามหญุนี้ เนกพนาเวศนา ชูเชอดสองพาหา หัตถ์ช้อย
นั่งแบะฝ่าบาทา ซ้อนทับกันแฮ แก้ป่วนปวดท้องน้อย อีกเส้นสบักจม ฯ

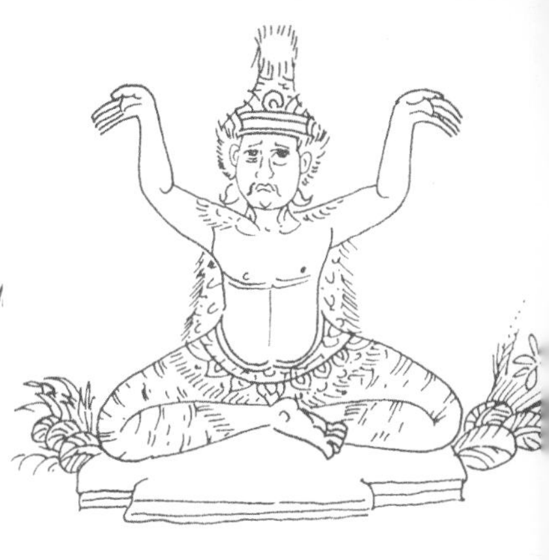

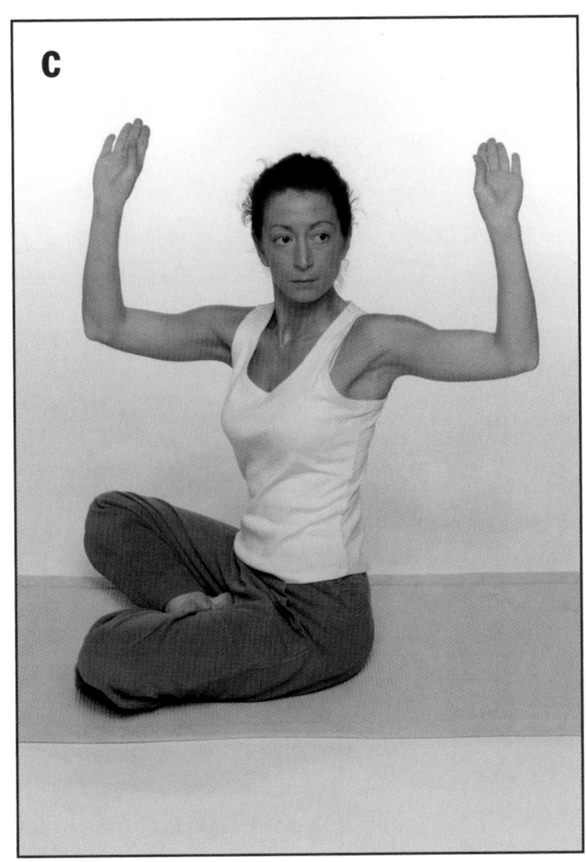

From the starting position, breathe in and turn your body to the left as far as possible, helping yourself to turn by pulling with your left arm (C).

Holding your breath, maintain this position for 3 seconds.

As you breathe out, return slowly to the starting position.

Repeat the turning sequence, now turning to the right.

Perform the entire exercise sequence 3 to 5 times.

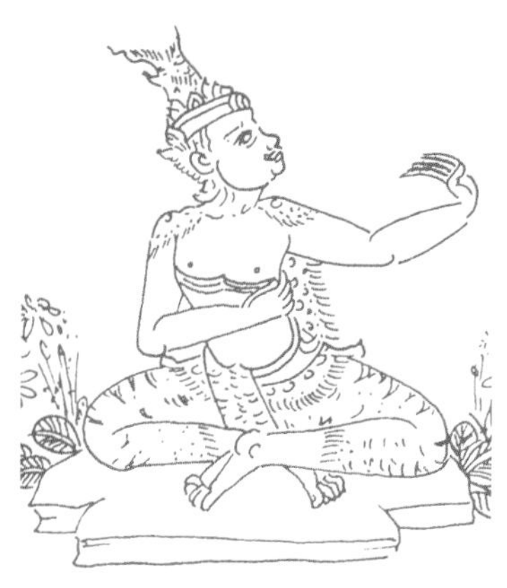

20
Remedy for Abdominal Pain

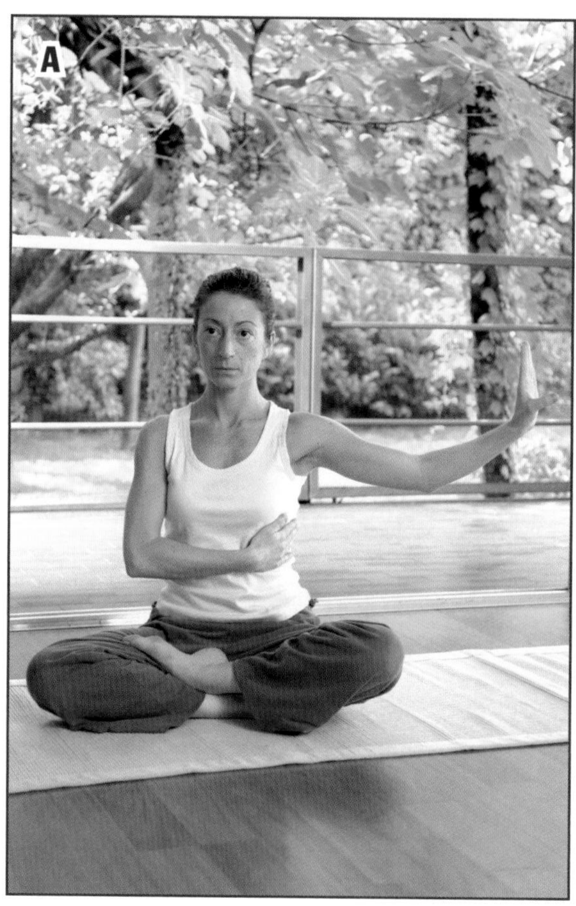

Sit in the half-lotus position. Raise your left arm at your side, keeping it slightly bent and the wrist well flexed. Place your right hand on the left side of your rib cage (A).

พระไชยทิศเชื้อ ชฎิลดง ลมเสียดเส้นสเอวองค์ ขดค้อม

นั่งสมาธิ์ถวัดคม กรเวียดเอวแฮ เหยียดหัตถ์ดัดตนน้อม เหนี่ยวแก้สกลกาย ฯ

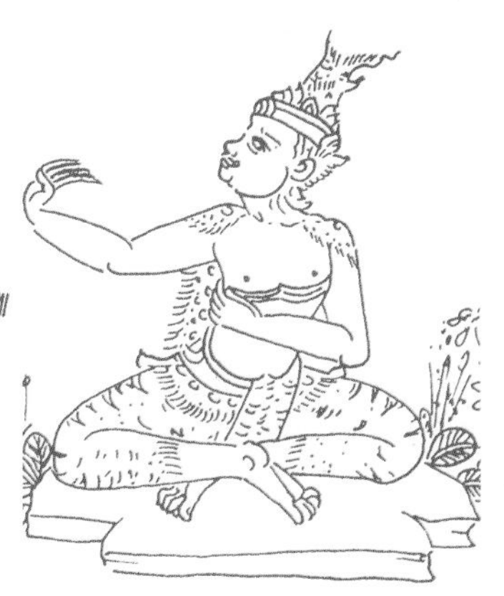

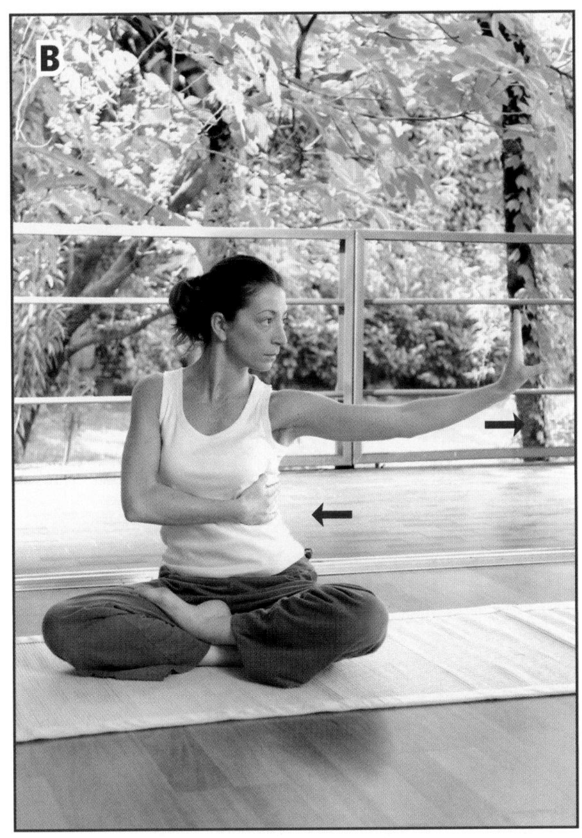

Breathing in, lift your right shoulder, and slightly bend your rib cage toward the right, helping yourself by pressing with your right hand. At the same time stretch out your left arm and increase the flexion of the wrist (B).

Holding your breath, maintain this position for 3 seconds.

As you breathe out, return slowly to the starting position.

Perform the exercise 3 to 5 times. Then practice the exercise on the other side.

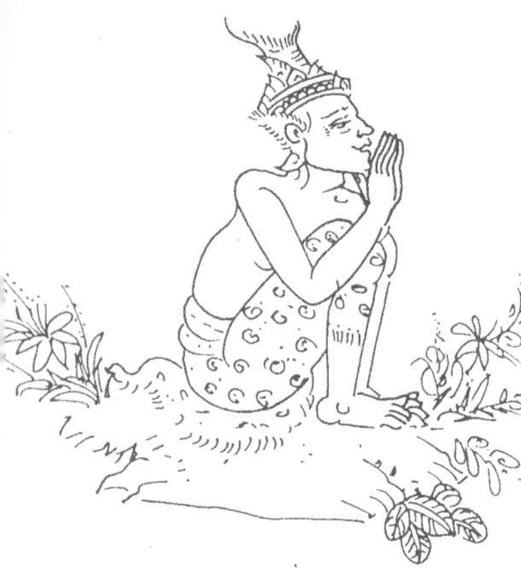

21

Remedy for Sharp Pain at the Waist

(Pain Brought on by Overexertion such as Running)

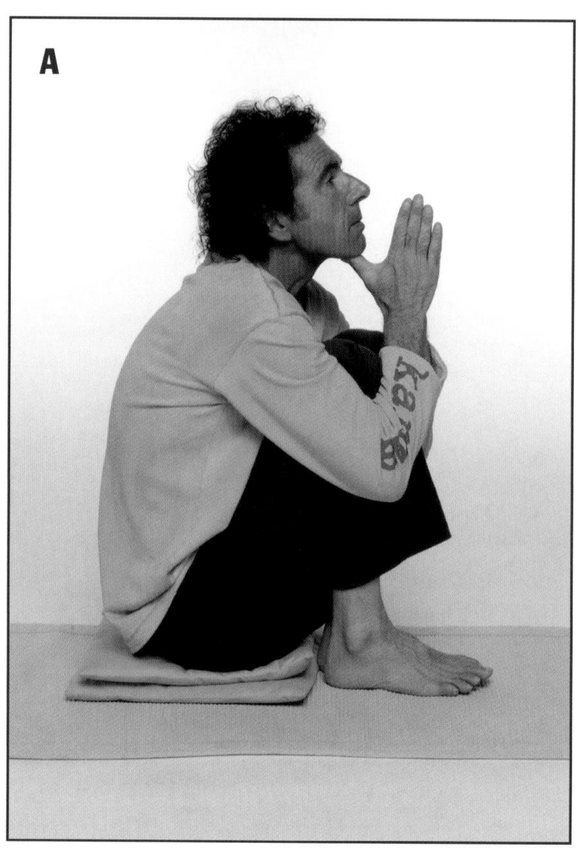

Sit on a cushion or folded-up blanket with your legs bent and your knees pulled as close to your chest as possible. Bending your arms, keeping them outside your legs, place your palms together and extend your thumbs so that they support your chin (A).

๑ พระวัชมฤคเลี้ยง บุตรลบ นั่งหยองสองมือจบ เจอดหน้า
แก้เส้นสะดุ้งขบ เอวยอกหาบนอ ใครอย่าหมิ่นประหมาทถ้า ท่านท้าให้ลอง

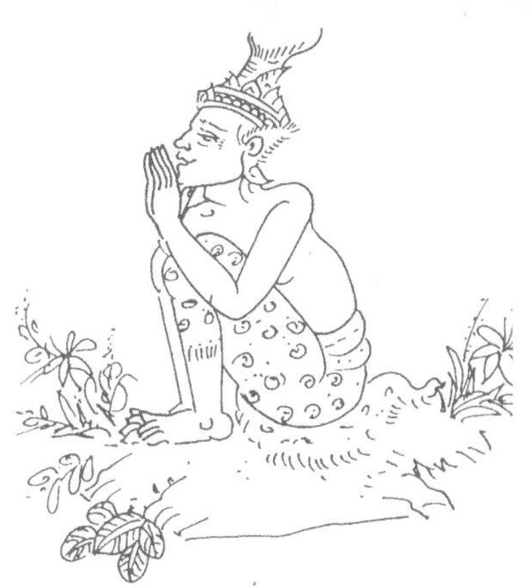

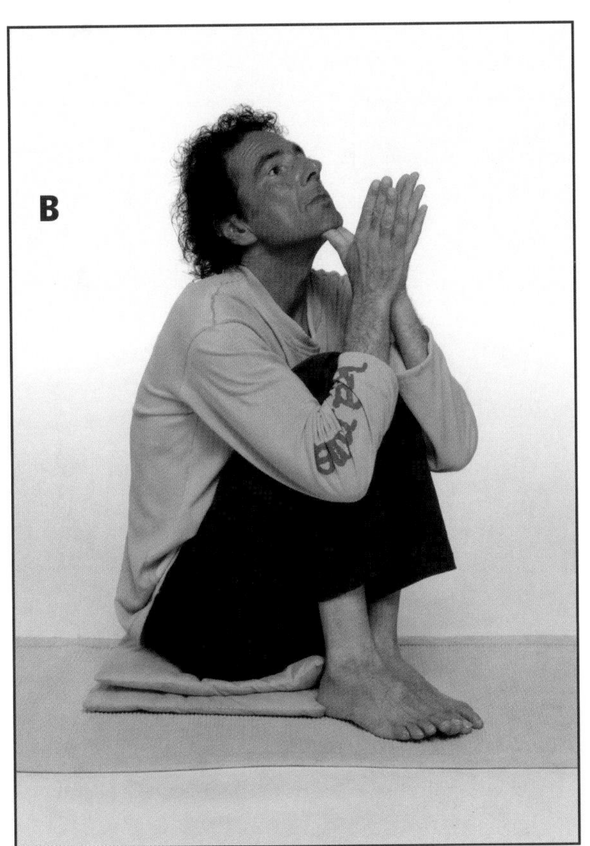

While breathing in, press in with your arms in order to squeeze your legs together, and press your thumbs against your chin, pushing your head backward (B).

Holding your breath, maintain this position for 3 seconds.

As you breathe out, return slowly to the starting position.

Perform the exercise 3 to 5 times.

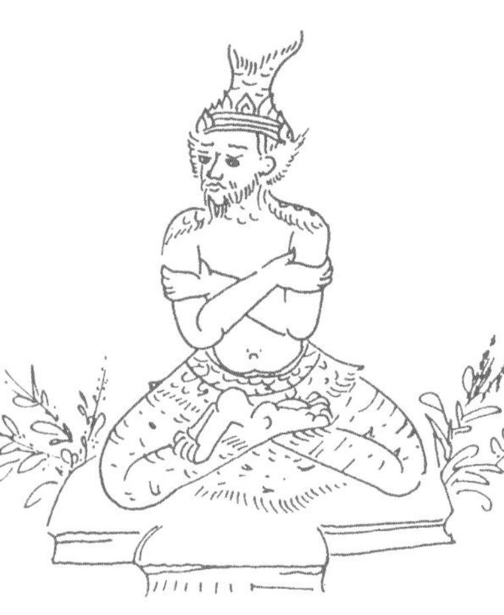

22 Remedy for Abdominal Pain Caused by Gaseous Indigestion

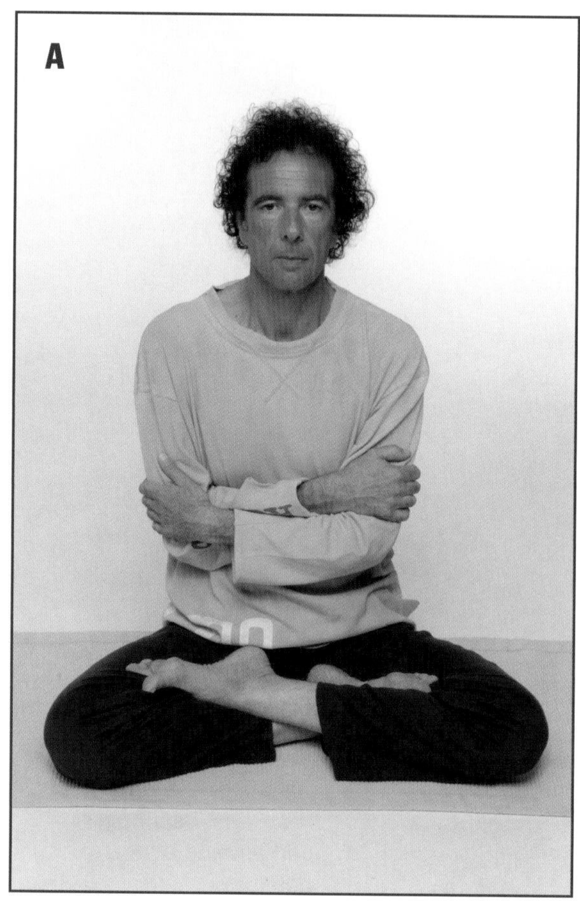
A

Sit on a cushion in the lotus position (if you cannot sit in a full lotus, then sit in the half lotus or cross-legged). Crossing your arms in front of you, seize each arm just above the elbow with the opposite hand (A).

๑ นักสิทธิ์สันโดษฐ์ค้น แดนดง นามพุทธชฎิลทรง ตำหรับแหร้
ไขว่หัตถ์รัดอกองค์ สมาธิเพ็ดนั่งนา จุกเสียดสรรพางค์แก้ กอปด้วยดัดหาย ฯ

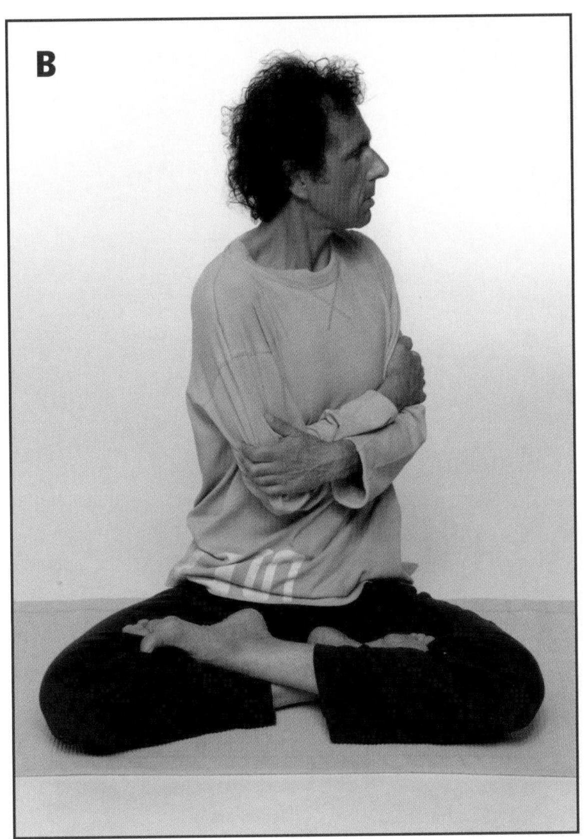

As you breathe in, hold your arms tightly against your chest, and at the same time turn your chest to the left, pushing with your hands to extend the turn (B).

Holding your breath, maintain this position for 3 seconds.

As you breathe out, return slowly to the starting position.

Repeat the exercise, now turning in the opposite direction.

Perform the exercise 3 to 5 times one each side, alternating from side to side as you practice.

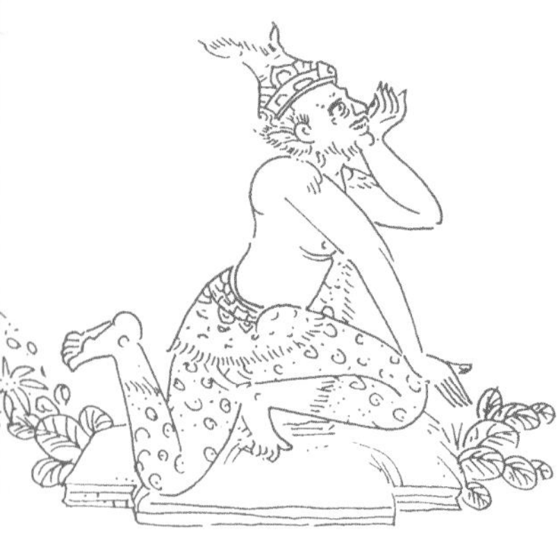

23
Remedy for Stomach Troubles

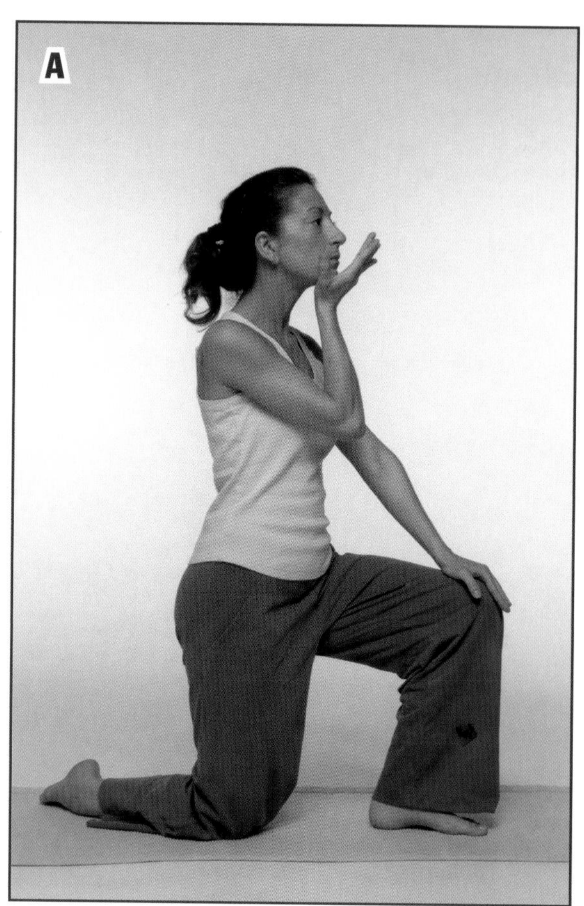

PART ONE

Kneel on your right knee, with your left leg bent in front of you. Place your left arm on your left knee and the palm of your right hand under your chin (A).

๏ พระภะรัตะดาบศไพ้น ภากเพียรนักนอ ตำหรับปะหรอดเรียน รอบรู้
โรคลมจุกเสียดเบียน บำบัดองค์เฮย นั่งคุกกดเข่าคู้ หัดถ์ค้ำคางหงาย ฯ

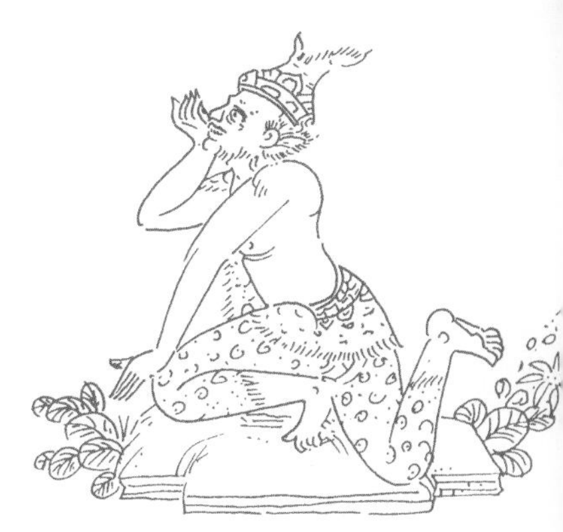

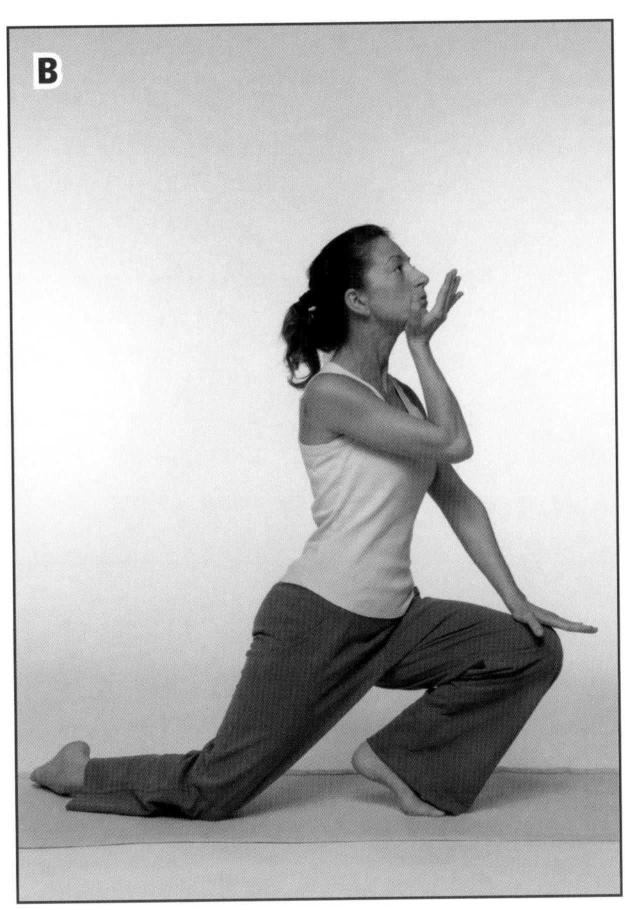

As you breathe in, lean forward as much as possible by bending your left knee and flexing your left foot, while leaning on your knee with your left hand. At the same time, push your head upward with your right hand (B).

Holding your breath, maintain this position for 3 seconds.

As you breathe out, return slowly to the starting position.

Perform the exercise 3 to 5 times. Then practice the exercise on the other side.

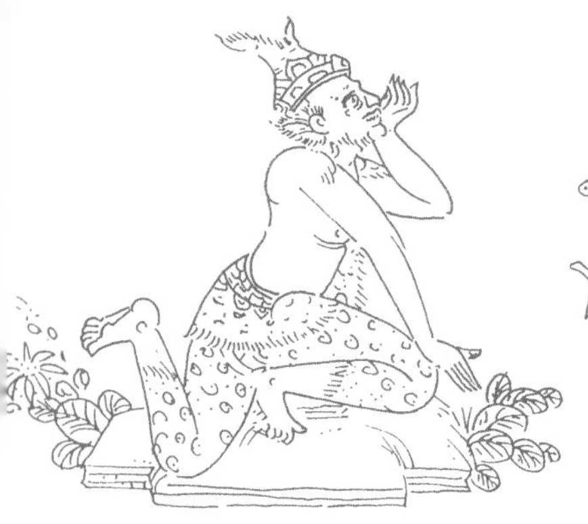

๏ พระภะรัตะดาบศโพ้น ภากเพียรนักนอ ตำหรับปะหรอดเรียน รอบรู้
โรคลมจุกเสียดเบียน บำบัดองค์เฮย นั่งคุกกดเข่าคู้ หัดถ์ค้ำคางหาย ฯ

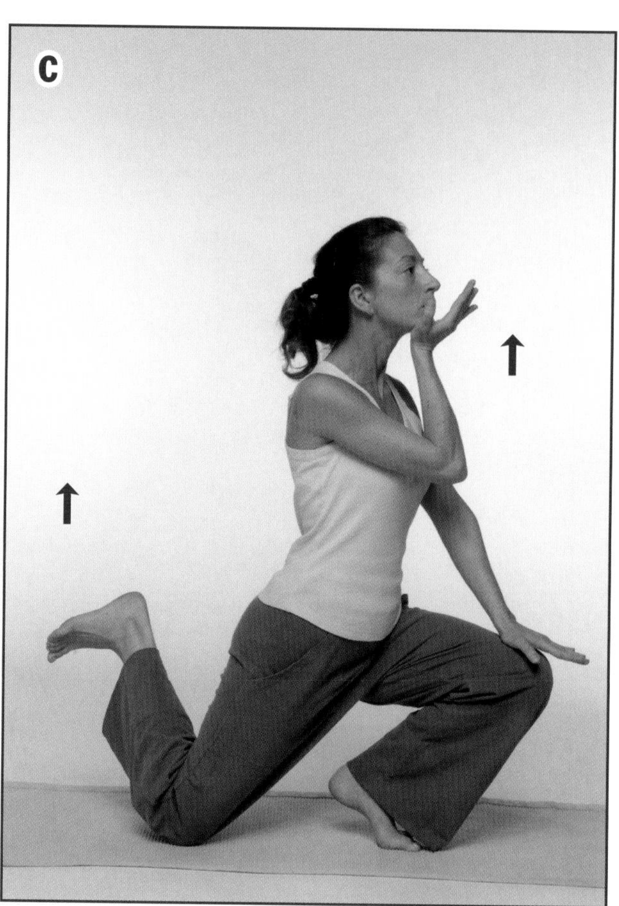

PART TWO

Perform the exercise again, this time lifting your right foot as much as possible while you are leaning forward (C).

Perform the exercise 3 to 5 times. Then practice the exercise on the other side.

24
Remedy for Abdominal Pain and Ankle Pain

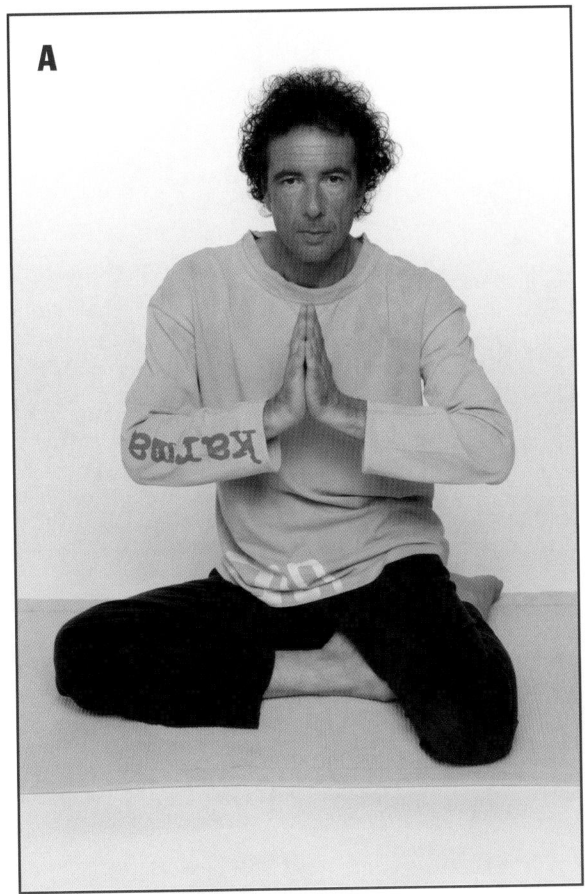
A

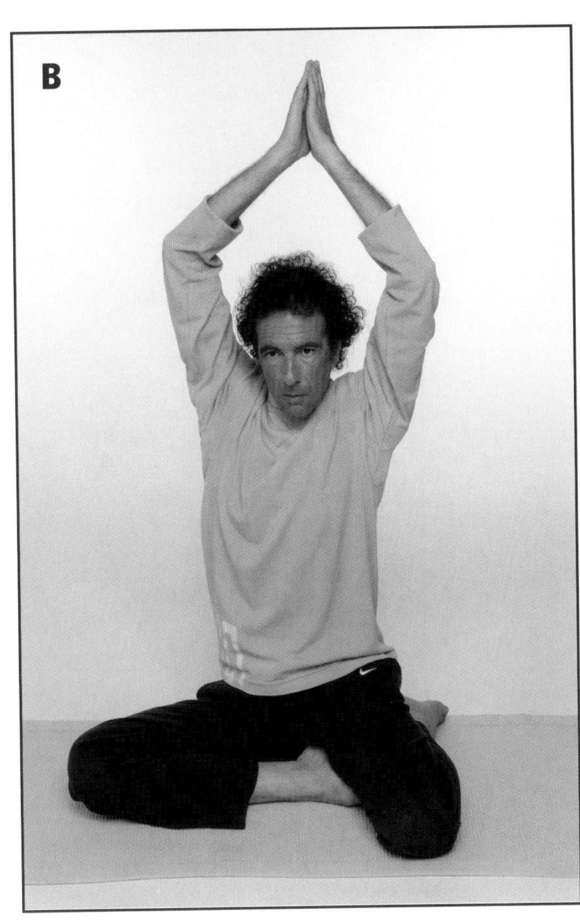
B

Sit in the Thai position, with your left leg bent to the outside and your right leg bent to the inside. Bring your palms together in front of you (A).

As you breathe in, lift your arms over your head, keeping them slightly bent, and push them backward as far as you can (B).

Holding your breath, maintain this position for 3 seconds.

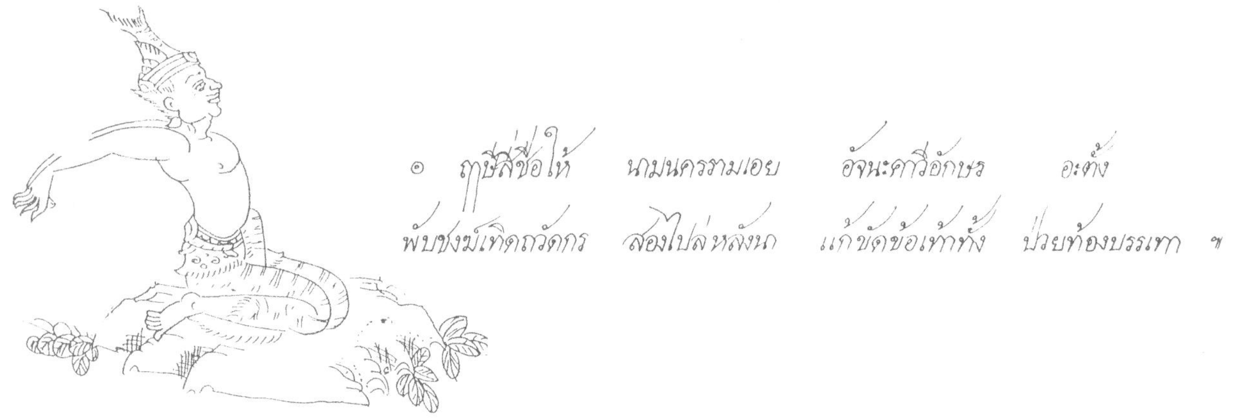

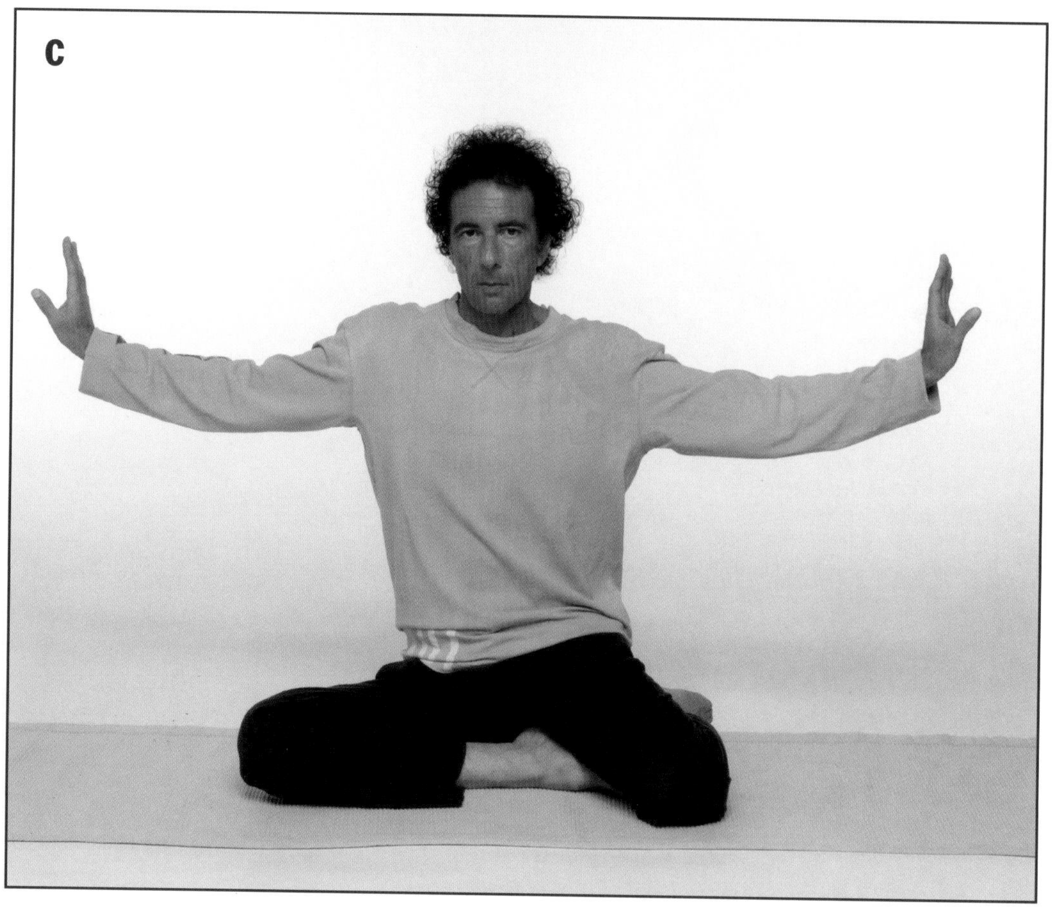

Breathing out, stretch your arms to your sides (C).

๏ ฤๅษีสี่ชื่อให้ นามนครรามเอย อัจนะคาวีอักษร อะตั้ง
พับชงฆ์เทิดถวัดกร ส่องไปล่หลังนา แก้ขัดข้อเท้าทั้ง ป่วยท้องบรรเทา ฯ

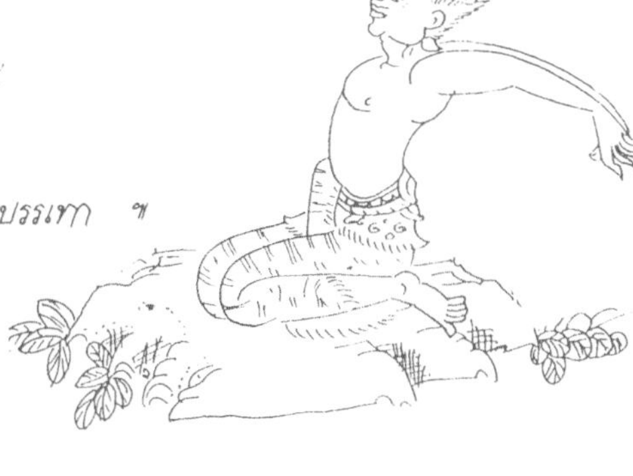

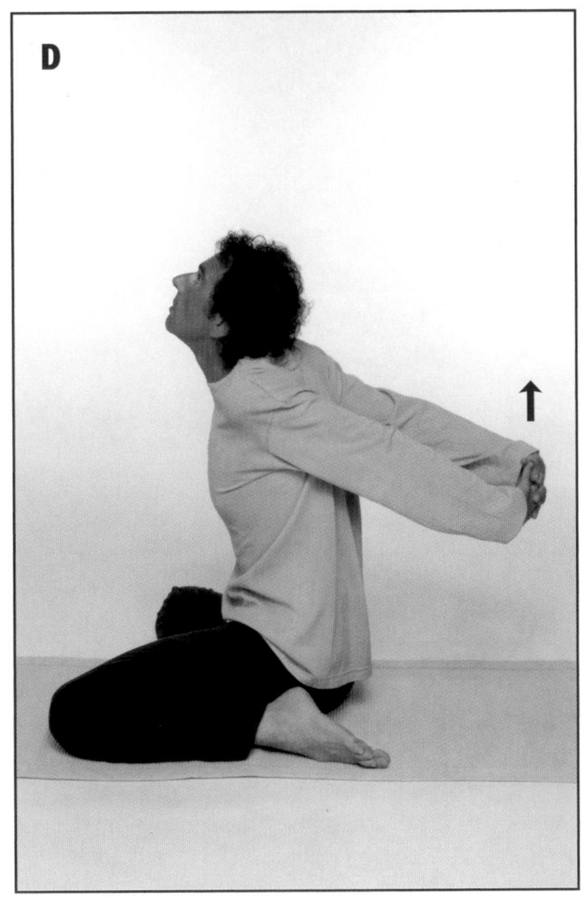

Bring your arms behind you and interlace your fingers. As you breathe in, lift your arms as much as you can, and bend your head backward (D).

Holding your breath, maintain this position for 3 seconds.

As you breathe out, return slowly to the starting position.

Perform the exercise 3 to 5 times.

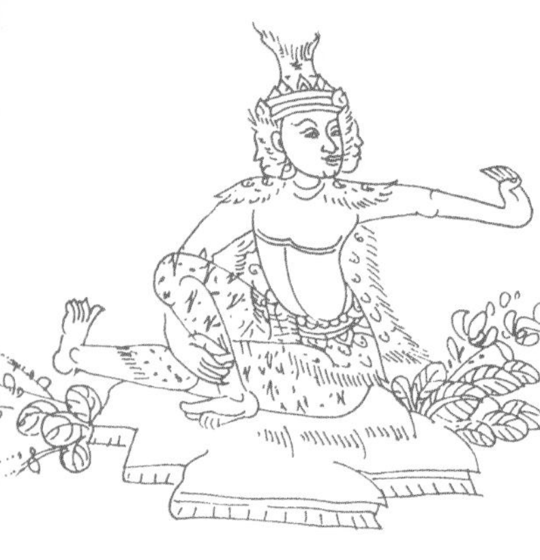

25 Remedy for Lower Back Pain

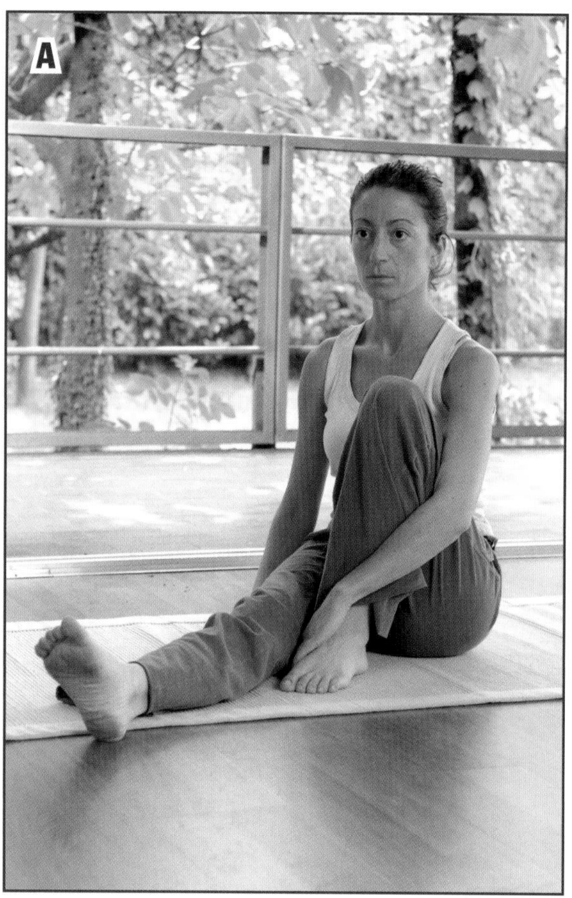

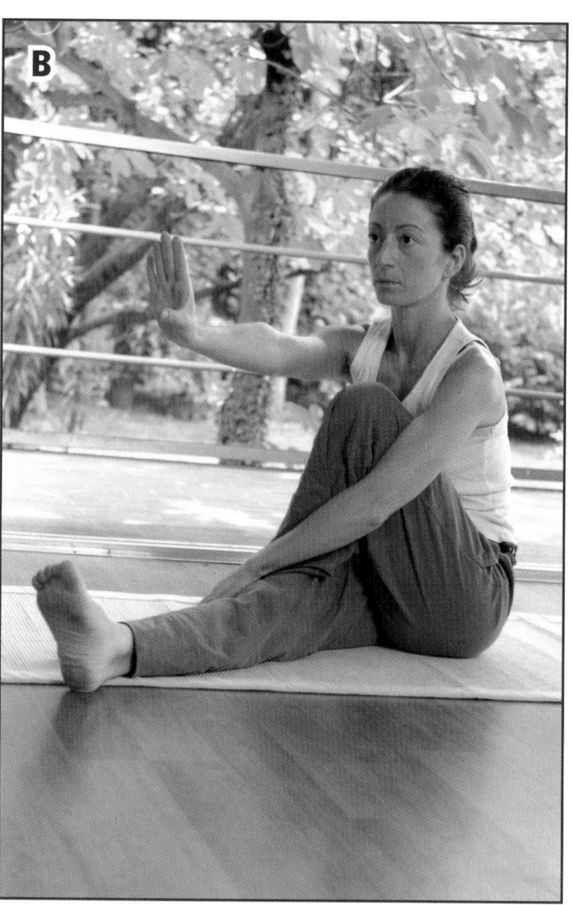

Sit with your right leg extended and your left knee bent up. Grasp the inside of your left foot with your left hand, keeping your arm outside your leg (A).

Lift your left foot and place it on the floor outside your right leg, near the knee. Extend your right arm in front of you, with your wrist flexed (B).

๑ จุลพรหมสี่ภักตรนี้ แผลงฤทธิ์ ยกเข่าเหยียดแขนอิชิค เสือกเท้า
แผนแพทย์พิดไหนดพิศ การบอกไว้ณ แก้ปัศฆาฎขึ้นเร้า อกบั้นเอวหาย

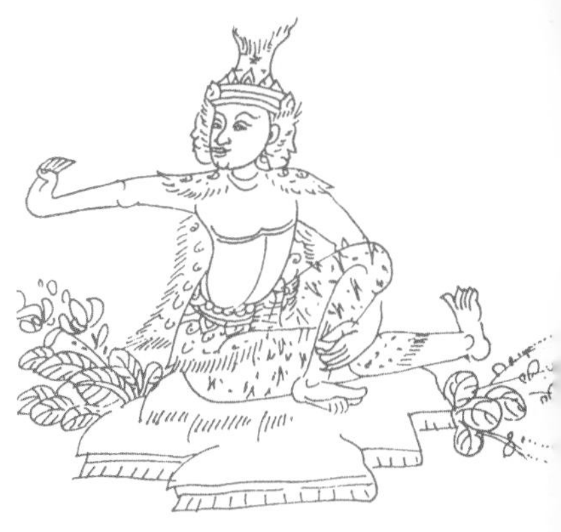

C

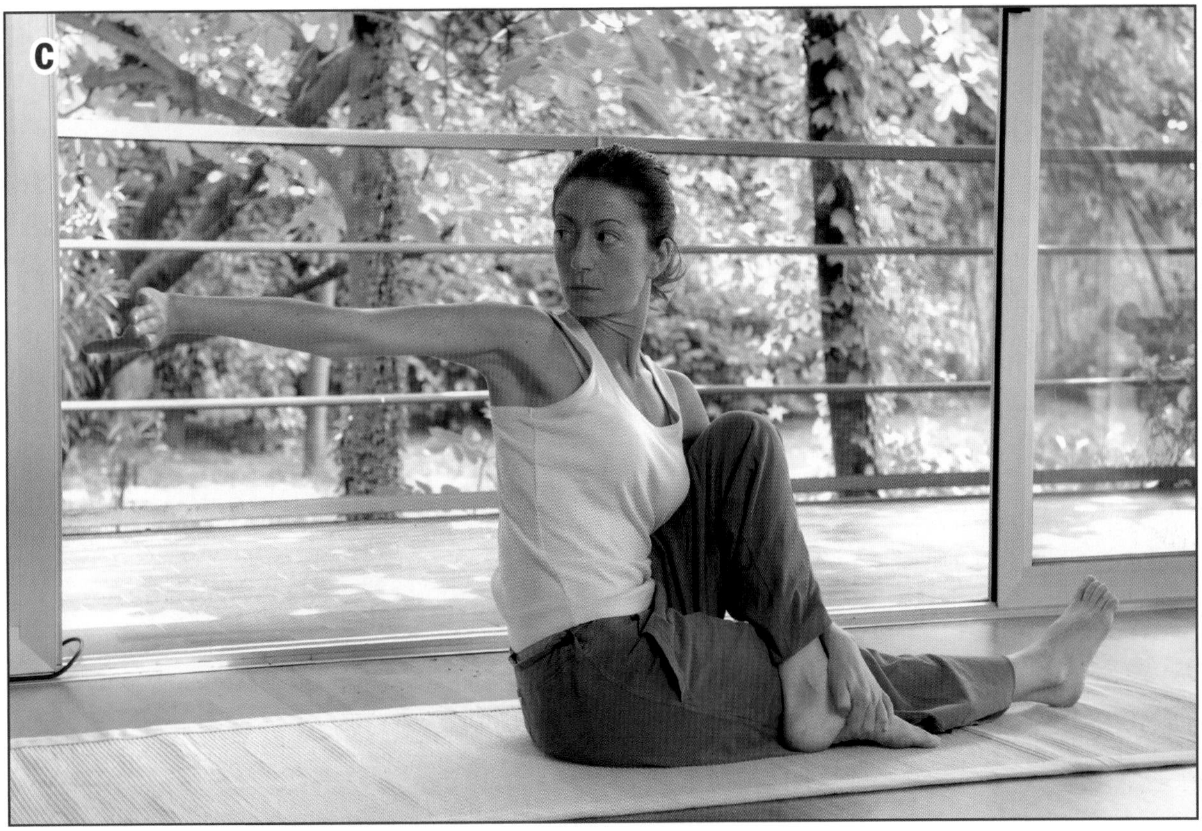

Breathing in, turn your chest and right arm to the right as far as you can. Use your right arm to pull your chest to the right, keeping the wrist well flexed and your fingers pointing to the right (C).

Holding your breath, maintain this position for 3 seconds.

Breathe out and slowly return to the starting position.

Perform the exercise 3 to 5 times on the first side. Then practice the exercise on the other side.

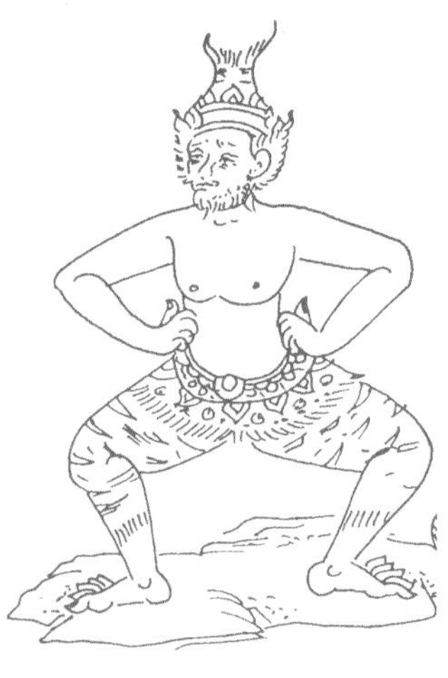

26
Remedy for Lower Back and Hip Pain

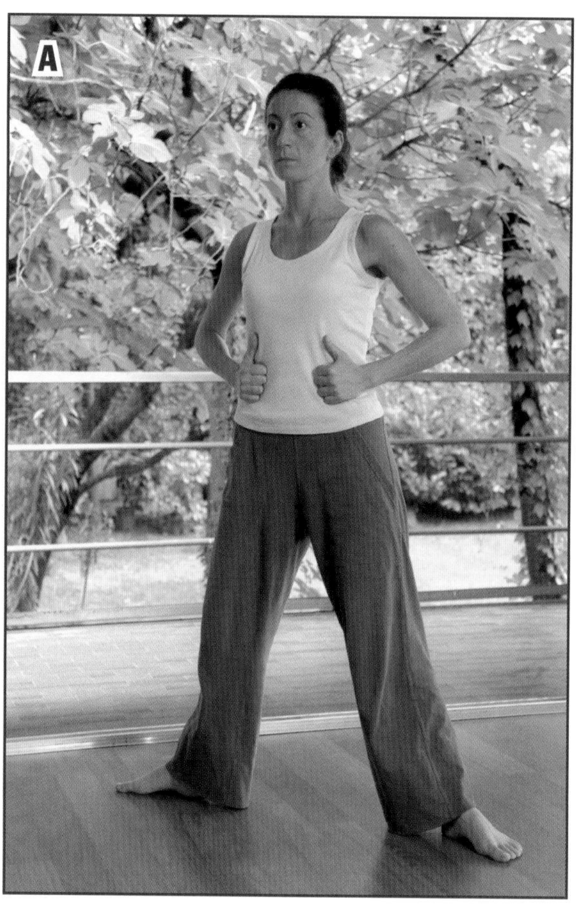

Stand with your feet 16 to 20 inches (40–50 cm) apart. Point your toes outward as much as possible while still keeping your balance, and place your fists on the outside of your abdomen, with your thumbs pointing up (A).

๏ สระภังค์ดาบศตั้ง ตนตรง ถ่างบาททั้งสองทรง แย่แต้
กำหมัดดัดกรผจง กดคู่ขนด ตะโภกสลักเพชรแม้ เมื่อยล้าขาหาย

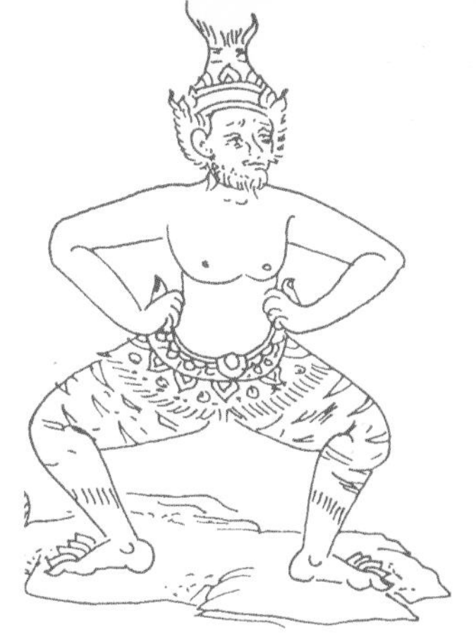

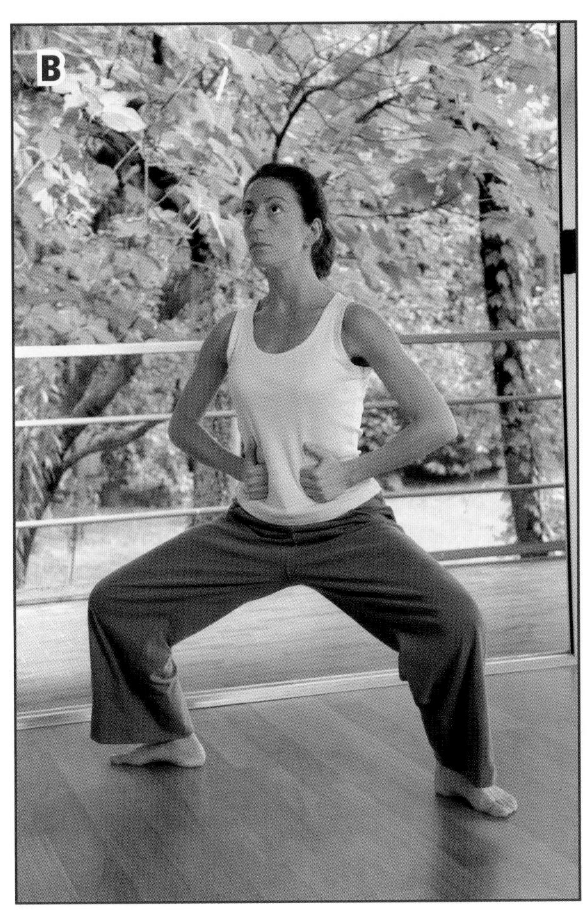

As you breathe in, lower your torso as much as possible by bending your legs outward, and at the same time push into your sides with your fists (B).

Holding your breath, maintain this position for 3 seconds.

As you breathe out, return slowly to the starting position.

Perform the exercise 3 to 5 times.

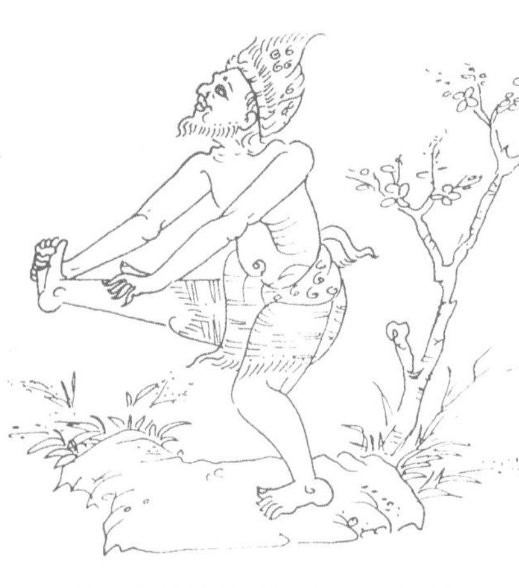

27 Remedy for Lower Back and Leg Pain

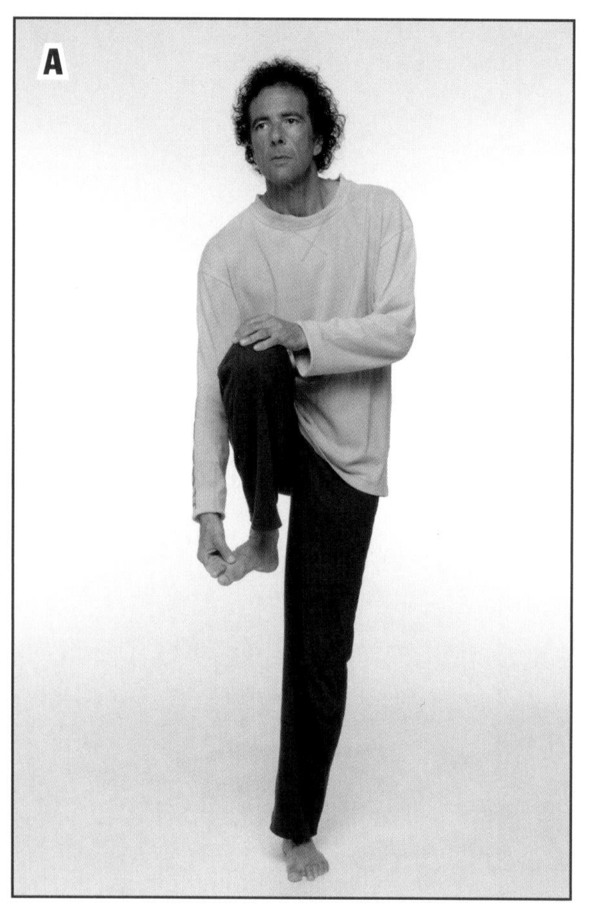

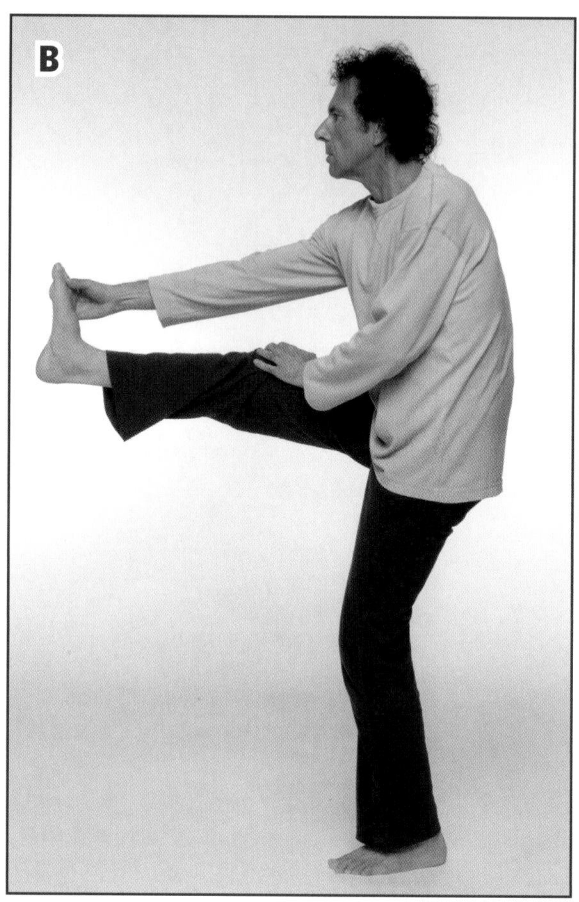

Stand with your right knee pulled up, holding your foot with your right hand and with your left hand placed on your right knee (A).

Straighten your right leg in front of you, maintaining your grip on it with your hands (B).

๏ ชฎิลดัดตนนี้นา นึกเอะใจเอย ชี้ชื่อสังปติเหนะ หง่อมง้อม
กวัดเท้าท่ามวยเตะ ตึงเมื่อย หายฮา แก้กะเอวขดค้อม เข่าคู้ไขยกไขยง

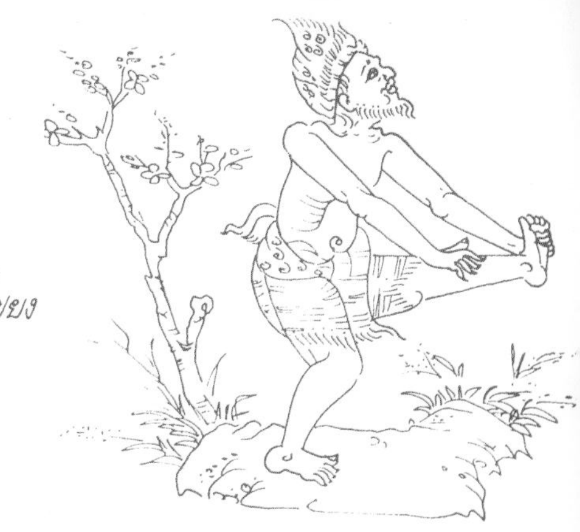

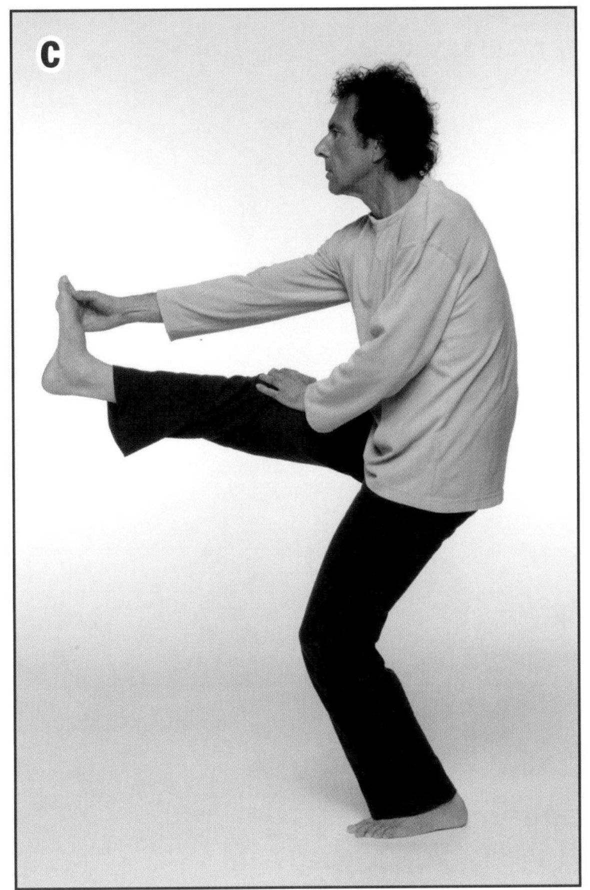

Breathe in as you bend your left knee, keeping your right leg straight (C).

Holding your breath, maintain this position for 3 seconds.

As you breathe out, return slowly to the starting position.

Perform the exercise 3 to 5 times. Then practice the exercise on the other side.

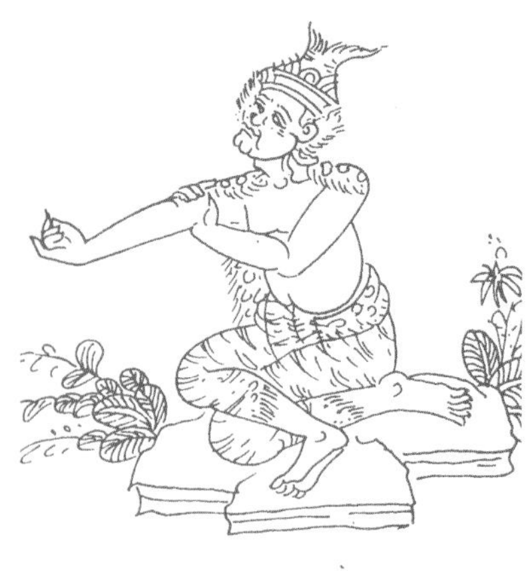

28 Remedy for Hemorrhoids

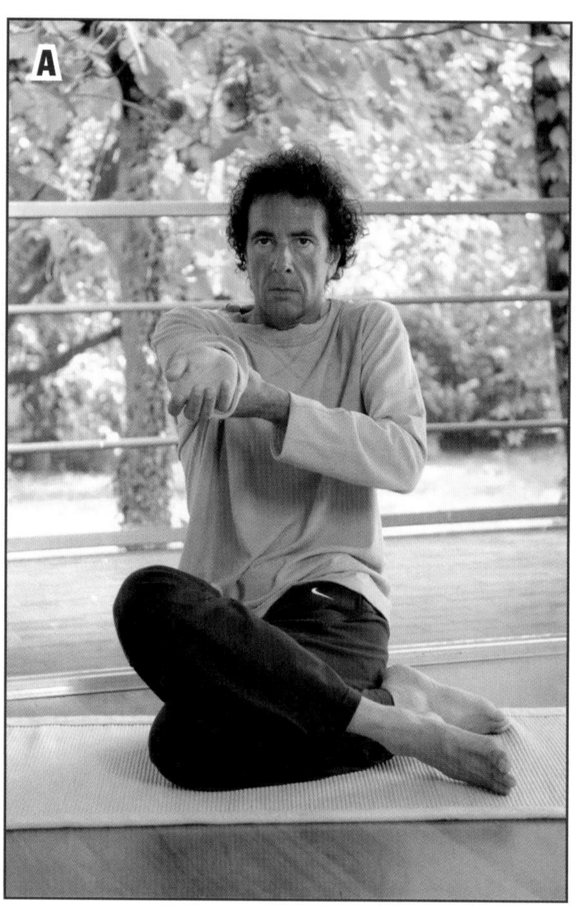

Sit with your legs folded in front of you. The left leg should fold to the inside, with the knee on the ground and pointing to the right, and the right leg should fold over the left, with the side of the right foot on the ground. Extend your right arm in front of you, and hold the right elbow with your left hand (A).

๑ อุดมนรอทรู้ กลดัดกายเฮย ทไคว่ไพล่ สนัด เท่าเข้า
เหยียดกรอ่อนเอาหัดถ์ หนึ่งส่งศอกนา ลมโรคริศดวงเร้า ชอบถ้าทำหาย

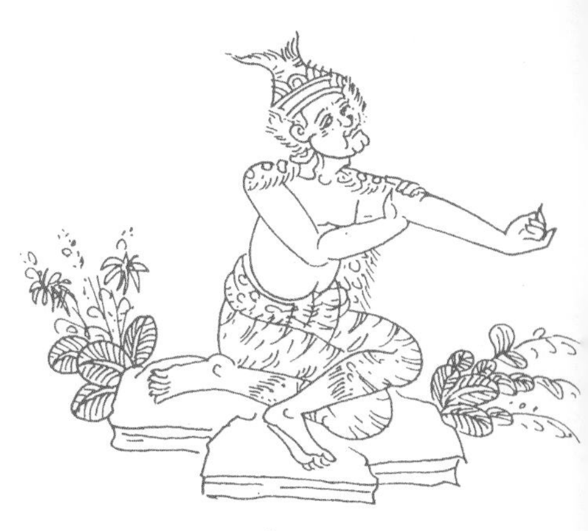

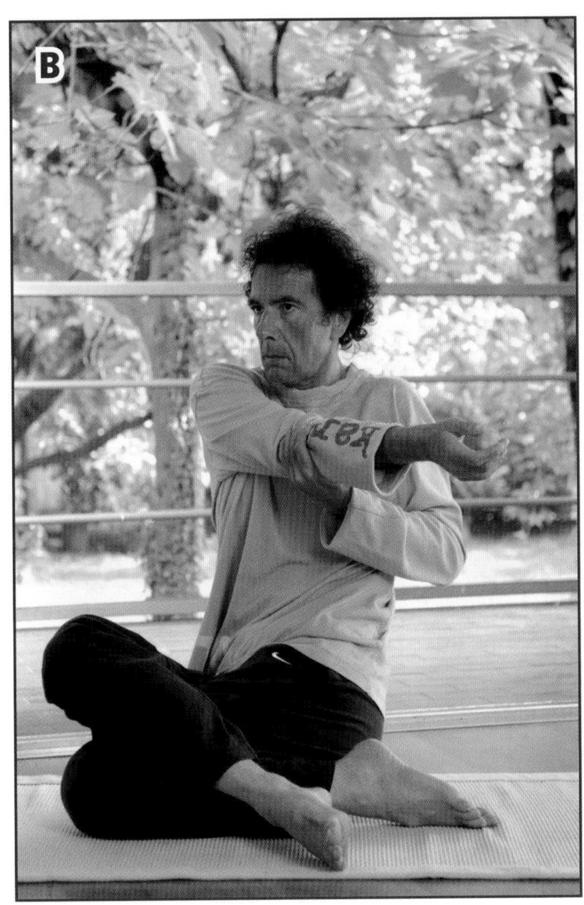

While breathing in, turn your chest to the left, pulling on the right arm with your left hand (B).

Holding your breath, maintain this position for 3 seconds.

As you breathe out, return slowly to the starting position.

Perform the exercise 3 to 5 times. Then practice the exercise on the other side.

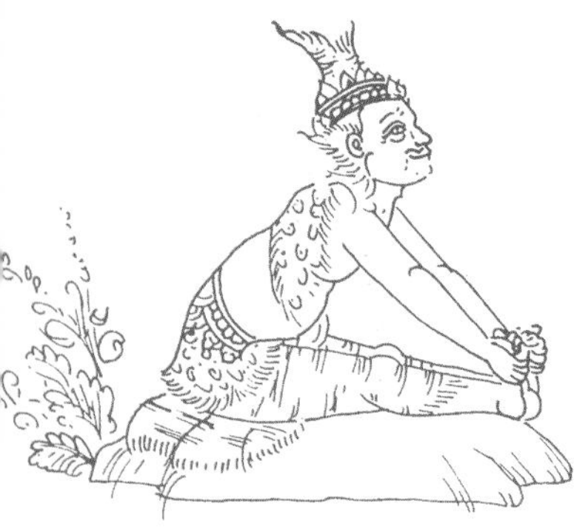

29 Remedy for Abdominal Distension and Pain in the Genital Area

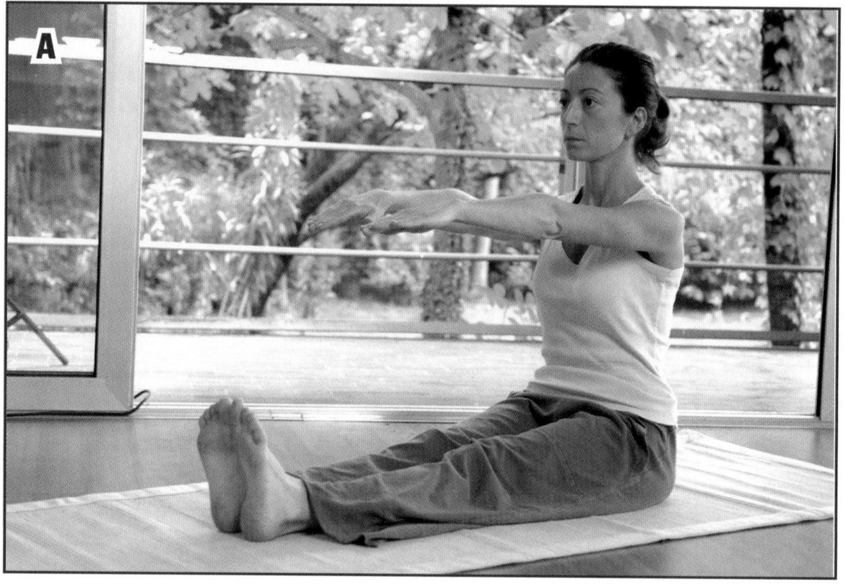

For this exercise it is important that your legs be stretched but relaxed, not tensed. Let the weight of your chest and head stretch your leg muscles; do not force the stretch.

Sit with your legs and arms extended in front of you (A).

๑ ฤาระษีพัฒนั่งน้อม โน้มกาย เท้าเหยียดมือหยิบปลาย แม่เท้า
ลมกล่อนเหือดห่างหาย เหนประจักษ์ อีกแน่นนาภีเร้า ระงับเส้นกล่อนไกษย์

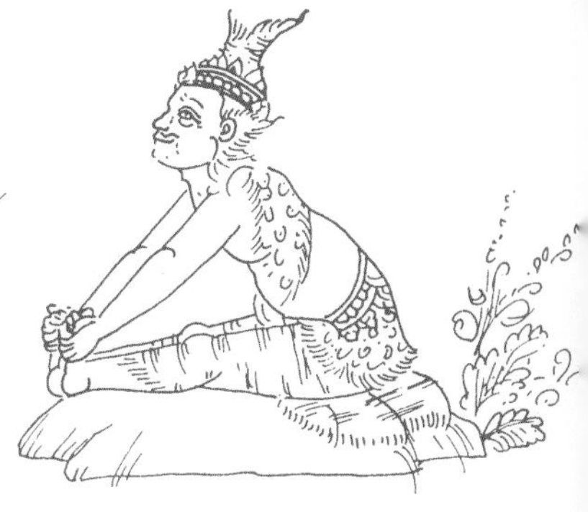

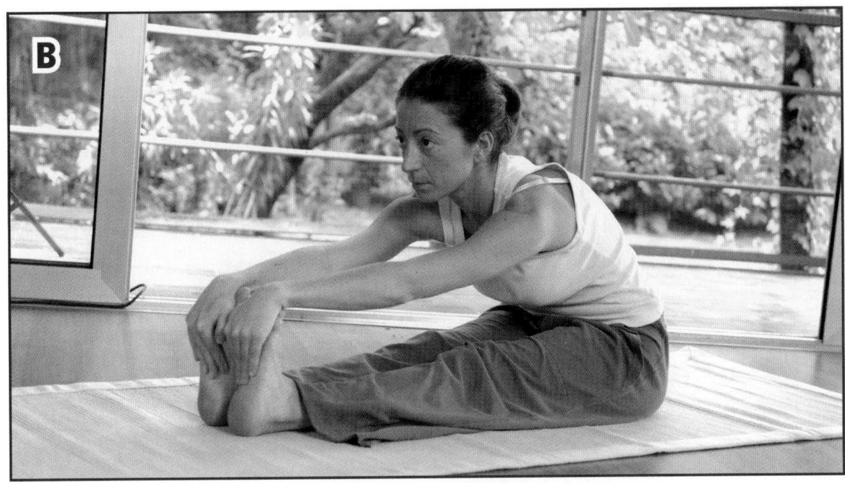

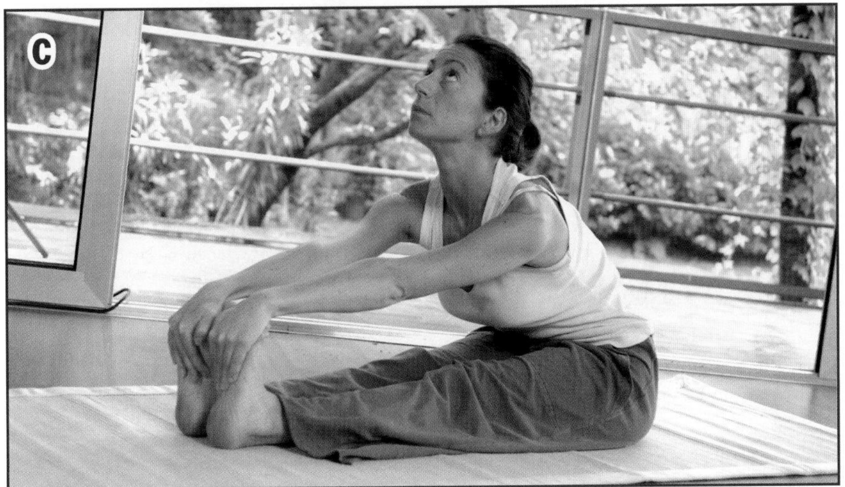

As you breathe out, bend forward, keeping your legs extended, and grab your feet with both hands (B).

Breathing in, lift your head, straightening your chest (C).

Holding your breath, maintain this position for 3 seconds.

Breathe out and slowly return to the starting position.

๑ ธาระนีพัฒนั่งน้อม โน้มกาย เท้าเหยียดมือหยิบปลาย แม่เท้า
ลมกล่อนเหือดห่างหาย เหนประจักษ อีกแน่นนาภีเร้า รงับเส้นกล่อนไกษย์

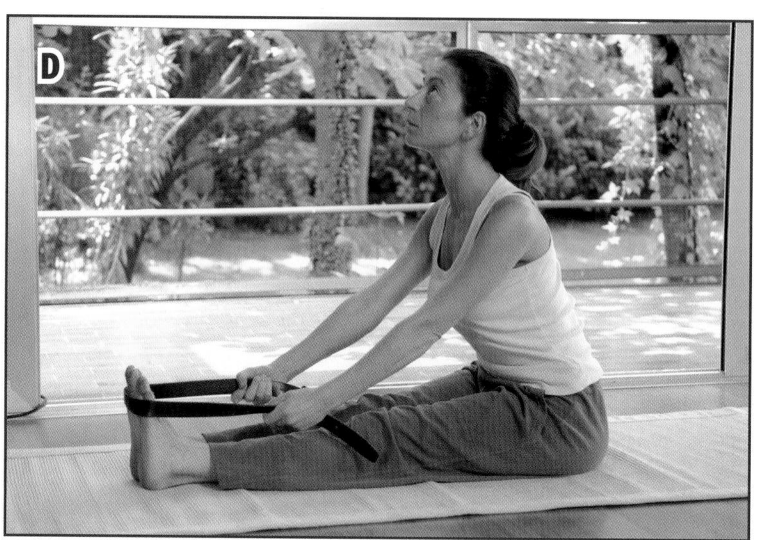

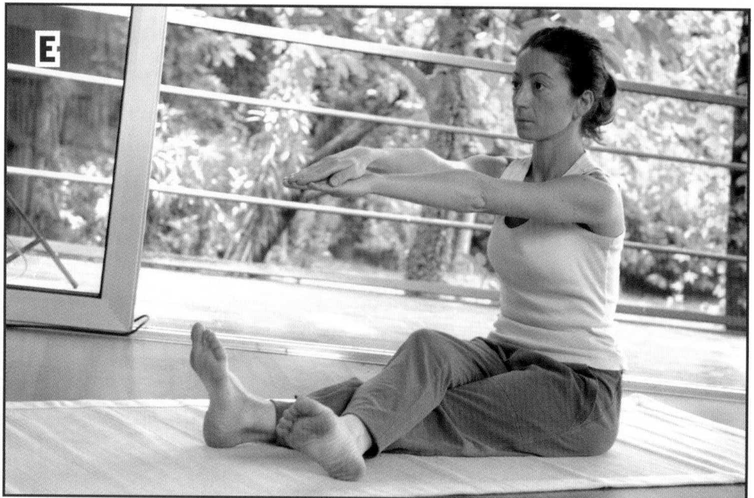

If you cannot reach your feet, you can use a belt to extend your reach (D). Then complete this part of the exercise as directed for figure C.

Place your right leg over your left leg and extend your arms in front of you, placing one hand over the other, palms down (E).

๑ ธาระนีพัฒนั่งน้อม โน้มกาย เท้าเหยียดมือหยิบปลาย แม่เท้า
ลมกล่อนเหือดห่างหาย เหนประจักษ์ อีกแน่นนถรีเว้า สงับเส้นกล่อนไกษย์

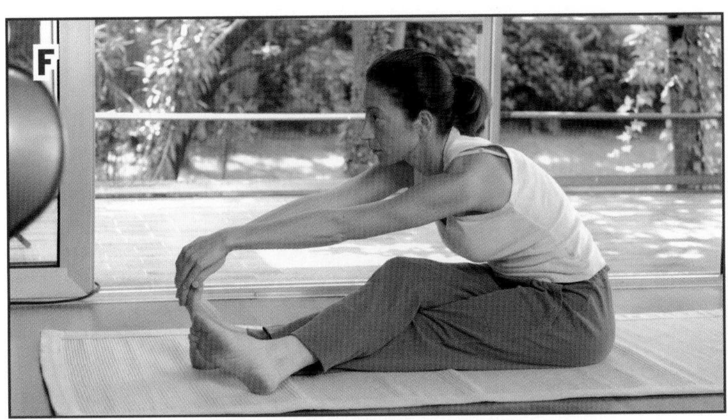

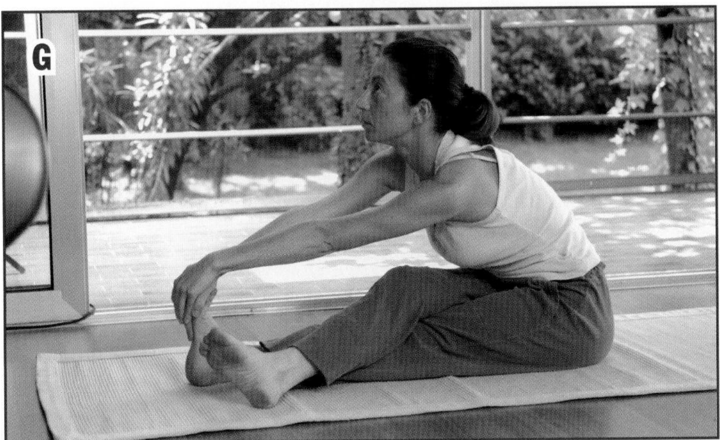

Breathe out as you bend forward, keeping your left leg extended, and grab your left foot with both hands (F).

Breathing in, lift your head, straightening your chest (G).

Holding your breath, maintain this position for 3 seconds.

As you breathe out, return slowly to the starting position.

Repeat the cross-legged stretch, now with your left leg over your right.

Perform the entire exercise sequence 3 to 5 times.

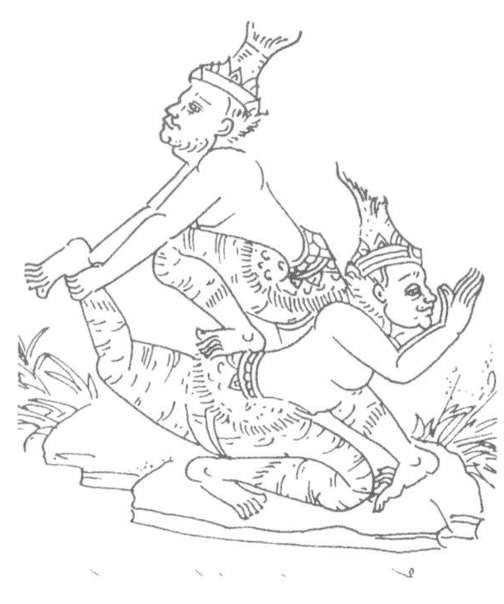

30 Remedy for Lower Abdominal Pain and Scrotal Discomfort

The original drawing of Jivaka performing this exercise shows another person assisting. The instruction we've prepared allows you to perform the exercise by yourself while remaining as faithful as possible to the original movement.

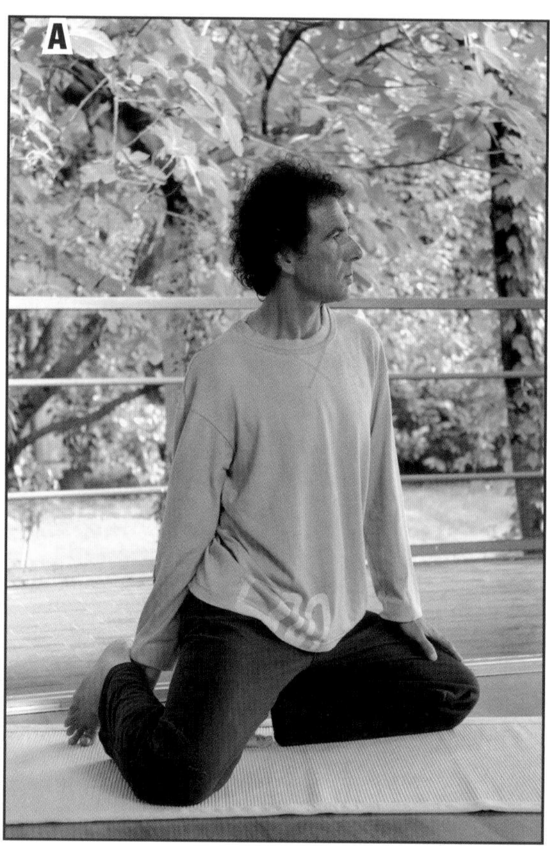

PART ONE

Kneel on your left leg, with your left foot flexed. Pull your right leg back as far as possible, and hold the inside ankle with your right hand. Place your left hand on your left thigh, keeping your arm extended (A).

๏ วาสุเทพทอดอกขว้ำ ลงกับอาศน์เอย นักสิทธิ์สุพรหมทับ ไหล่แล้
เหยียบยันจระโภกจับ ศีนเหนี่ยวนาพ่อ วาสุเทพวานแก้ กล่อนภัยเรวหาย ฯ

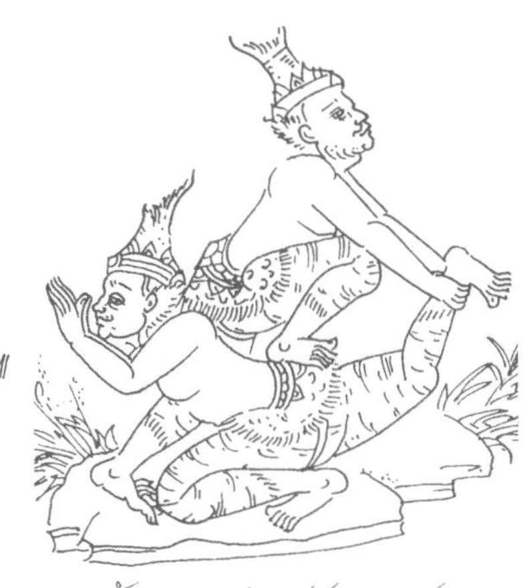

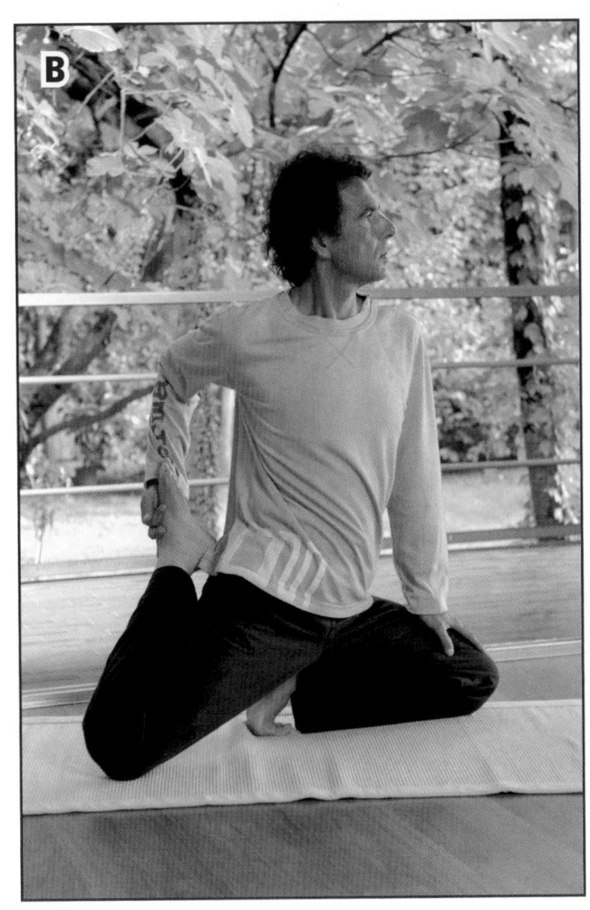

Breathe in as you pull your right foot up and forward, using your left arm to keep your chest upright (B).

Holding your breath, maintain this position for 3 seconds.

As you breathe out, return slowly to the starting position.

Perform the exercise 3 to 5 times. Then practice the exercise on the other side.

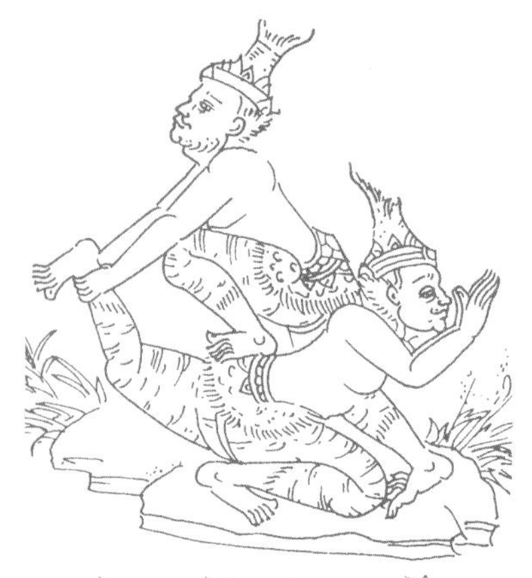

๏ วาสุเทพทอดอกขว้ำ ลงกับอาศน์เอย นักสิทธิ์สุพรหมทับ ไหล่แล้
เหยียบยันจระโภกจับ ตีนเหนี่ยวนาพ่อ วาสุเทพวานแก้ กล่อนภัยเรวหาย ฯ

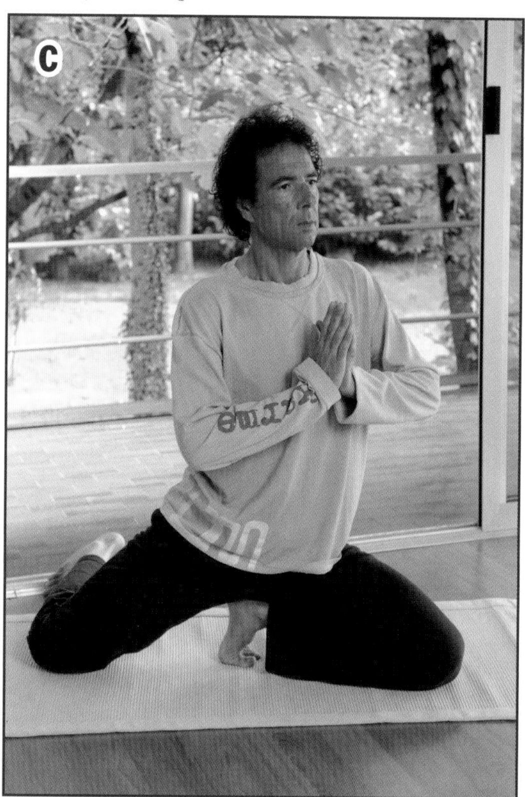

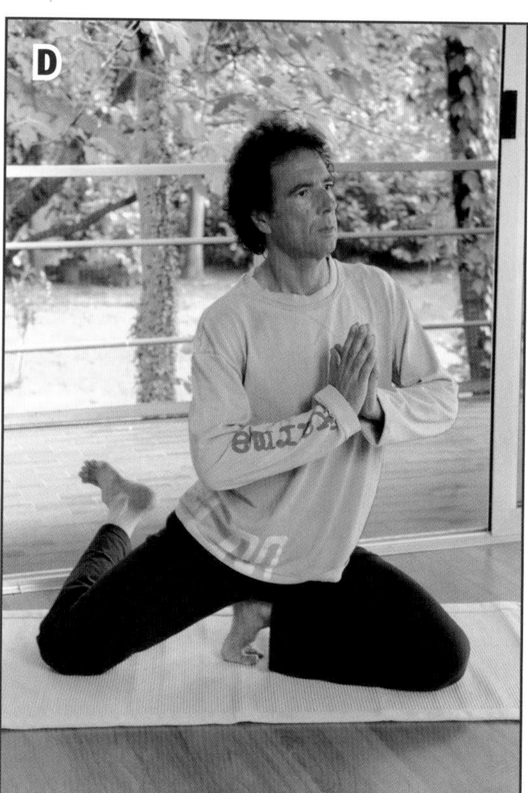

PART TWO

Kneeling in the starting position, join your palms in front of you (C).

As you breathe in, lift your right leg up and forward, holding your chest upright (D).

Holding your breath, maintain this position for 3 seconds.

As you breathe out, return slowly to the starting position.

Perform the exercise 3 to 5 times. Then practice the exercise on the other side.

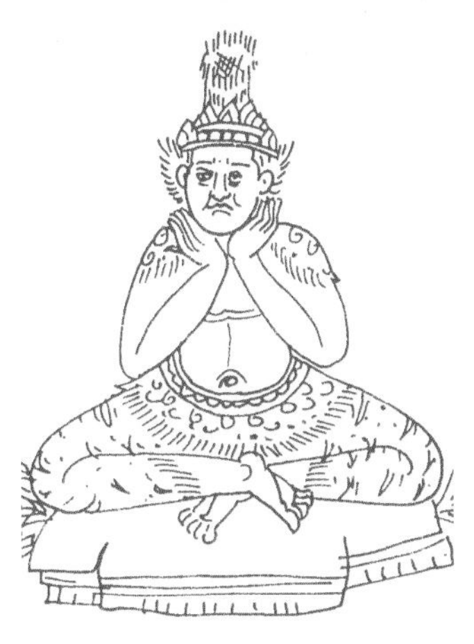

31 Remedy for Pain in the Testicles and Difficult Urination

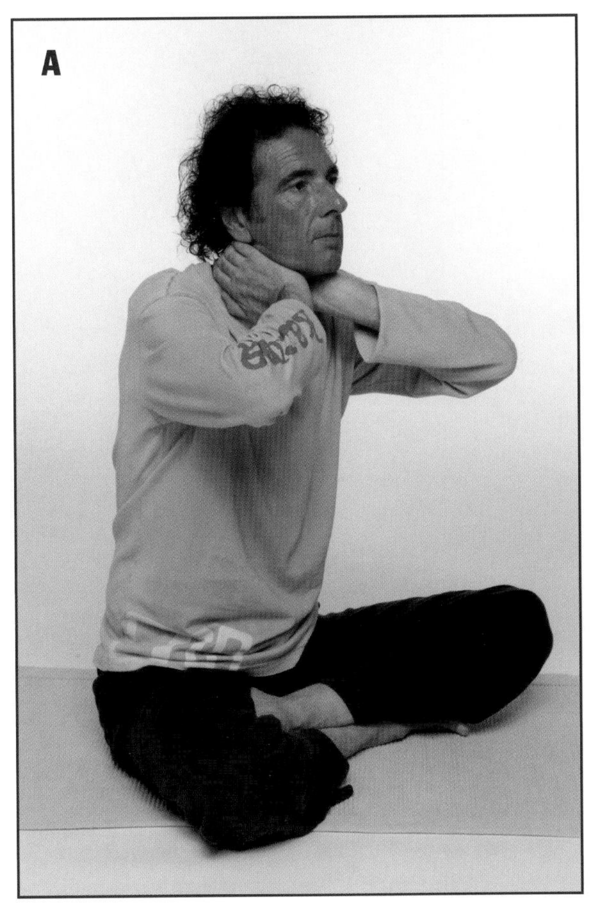
A

Sit in the half-lotus position. Place your hands against your neck, with the heels of your hands under your chin (A).

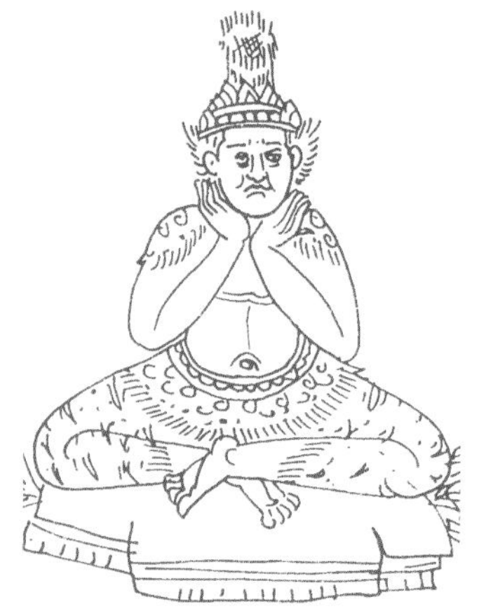

โยคีองคตกล้า สมาบัติ รู้ชาติเนาวรัตนชัด ชื่อนั้น
ก้ลมเสียดเสียวขัด ลำฝักหายแฮ นั่งสมาธิ์นวดคอคั้น ขบเขี้ยวตาขะ

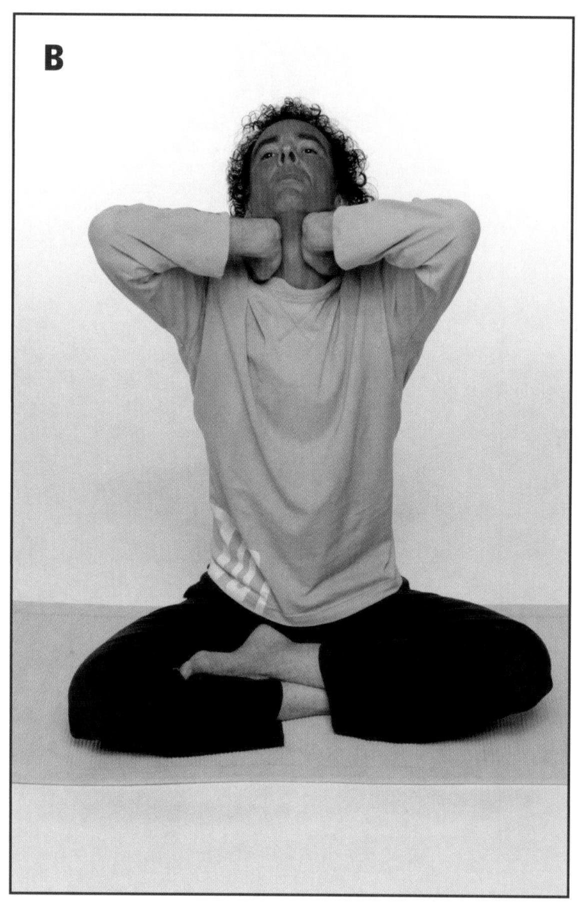

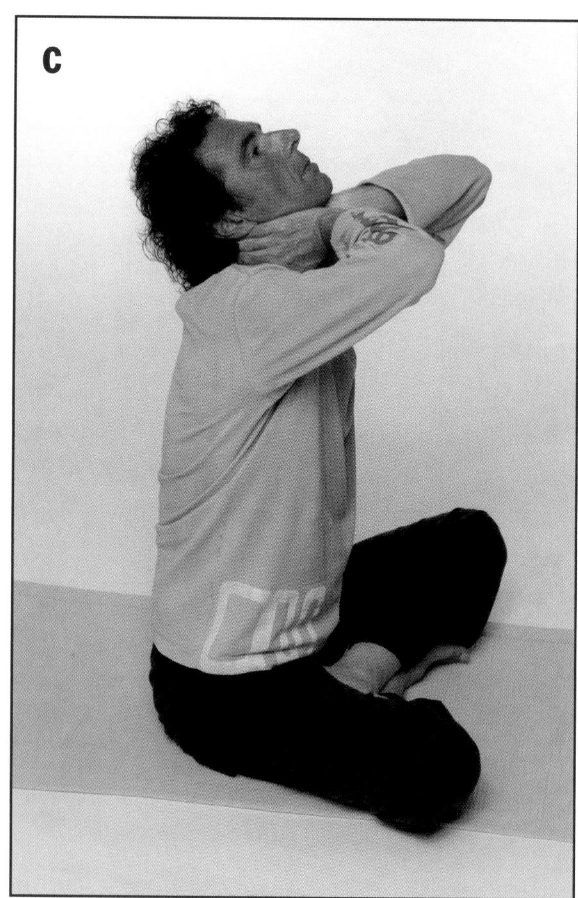

While breathing in, push your head backward as far as possible with your hands (B and C).

Holding your breath, maintain this position for 3 seconds.

As you breathe out, return slowly to the starting position.

Perform the exercise 3 to 5 times.

SIX

Postures That Benefit the Extremities

Arms, Legs, Hands, and Feet

32. Remedy for Arm Pain
33. Remedy for Arm Stiffness
34. Remedy for Joint Pain in the Arms and Hands
35. Remedy for Wrist Pain
36. Remedy for Arm and Leg Pain
37. Remedy for Hand and Foot Cramps
38. Remedy for Stiffness in the Knees
39. Remedy for Knee Pain
40. Remedy for Knee Dislocation
41. Remedy for Knee and Leg Trouble
42. Remedy for Knee, Leg, and Chest Problems
43. Remedy for Leg and Neck Pain
44. Remedy for Foot Numbness
45. Remedy for Pain in the Sole of the Foot
46. Remedy for Heel Pain

See also:

- Exercise 12, Remedy for Shoulder and Leg Stiffness
- Exercise 24, Remedy for Abdominal Pain and Ankle Pain
- Exercise 27, Remedy for Lower Back and Leg Pain

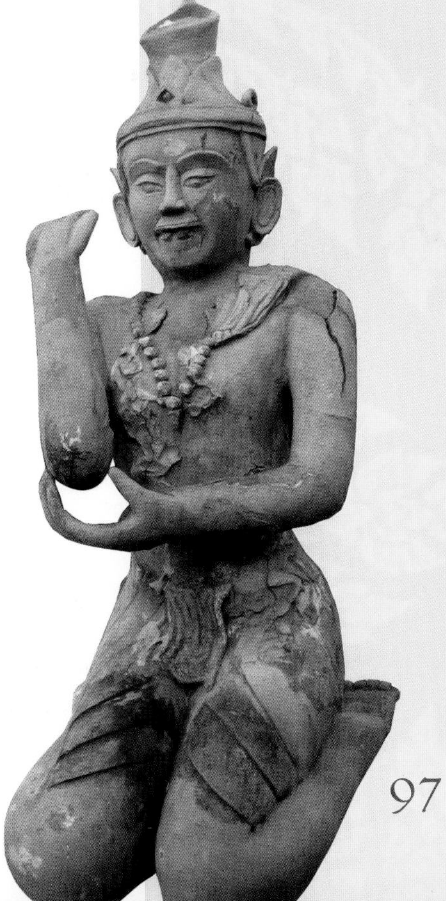

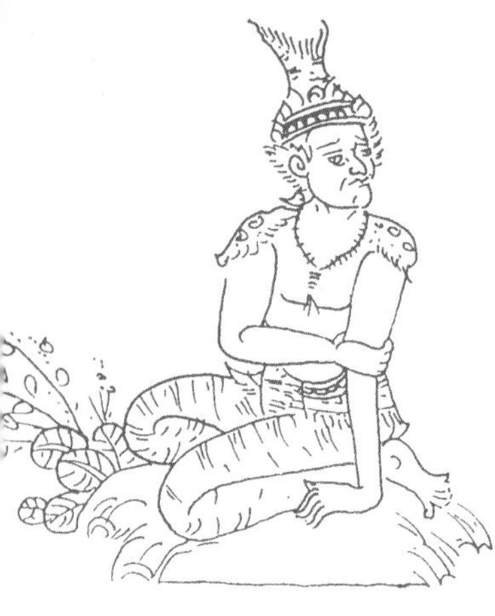

32 Remedy for Arm Pain

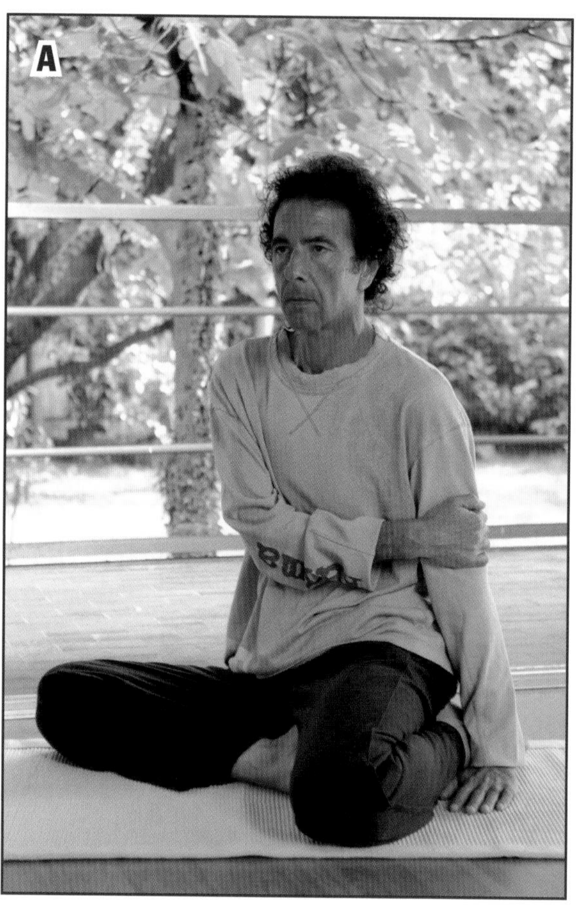

Sit in the Thai position, with your right leg bent to the inside and your left leg bent to the outside. Place your left hand on the floor next to your left ankle, with your fingers pointing forward. With your right hand, hold your left arm just above the elbow (A).

๑ ระชื่อนามโคบุตรก้อง กุณฑ์สรรค์สฤษดิ์เฮย กอดหัทไทยทศกรรฐ เก็บไว้
ท่าดัดพับเพียบผัน ภักตร์น่อยณแฮ แขนได่ขัดท้าวให้ หัดกั๊ปไข้นวดแขน ฯ

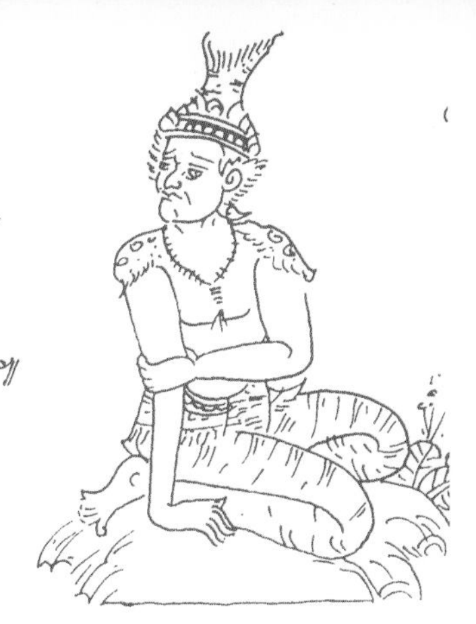

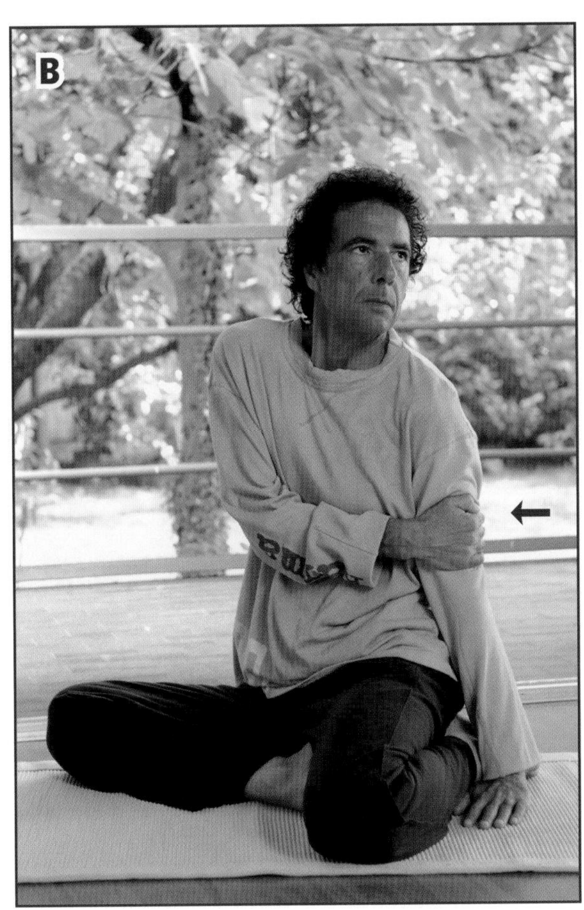

Breathing in, with your left hand still on the floor, pull your left arm toward your body and turn your head to the left (B).

Holding your breath, maintain this position for 3 seconds.

As you breathe out, return slowly to the starting position.

> Perform the exercise 3 to 5 times. Then practice the exercise on the other side.

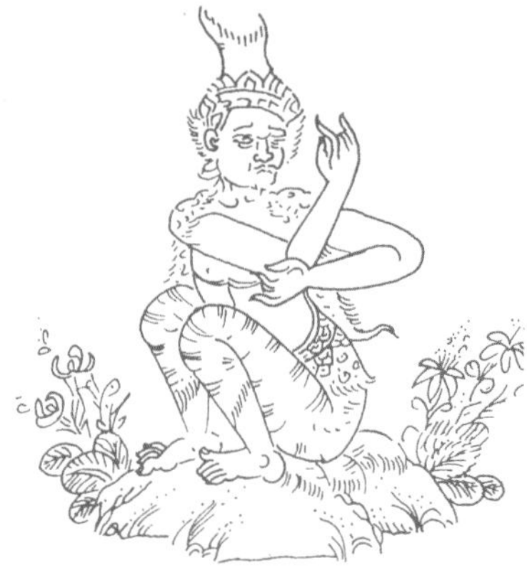

33 Remedy for Arm Stiffness

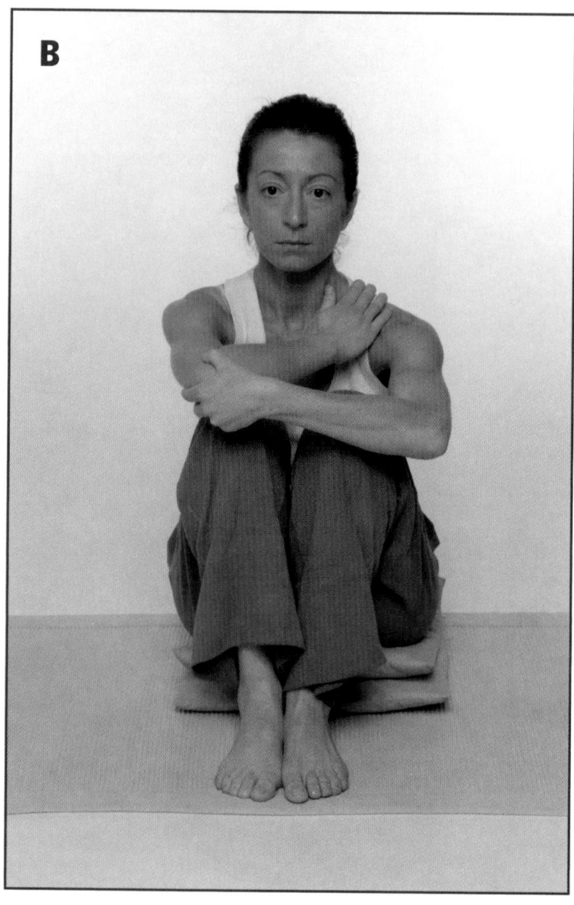

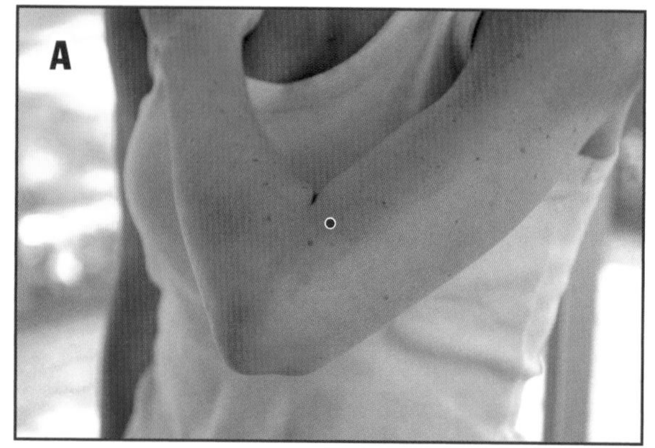

This technique requires finger pressure on a point located just above the elbow on the outside arm (A). To find it exactly, touch the area until you find the most sensitive point.

Sit on a cushion with your legs folded as closely as possible to your chest. Bend your right arm in front of you, with your right hand on your left shoulder. Hold your right elbow with your left hand, placing your thumb on the pressure point (B).

๏ พระโสณะสันโดษฐ์ก้าว คงคริม ภูตโขมดไมยครหึม กู่ก้อง
ล้มไข้ขบเศียรซึม ยอกขัดแขนนา ยกศอกขึ้นเข่าจ้อง จรดซ้ายเปลี่ยนขวา ฯ

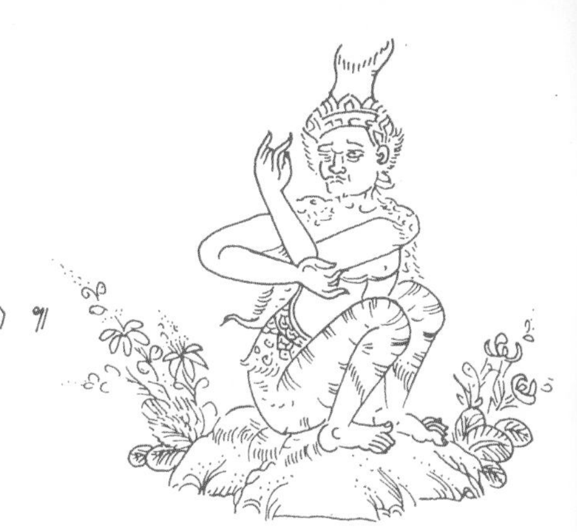

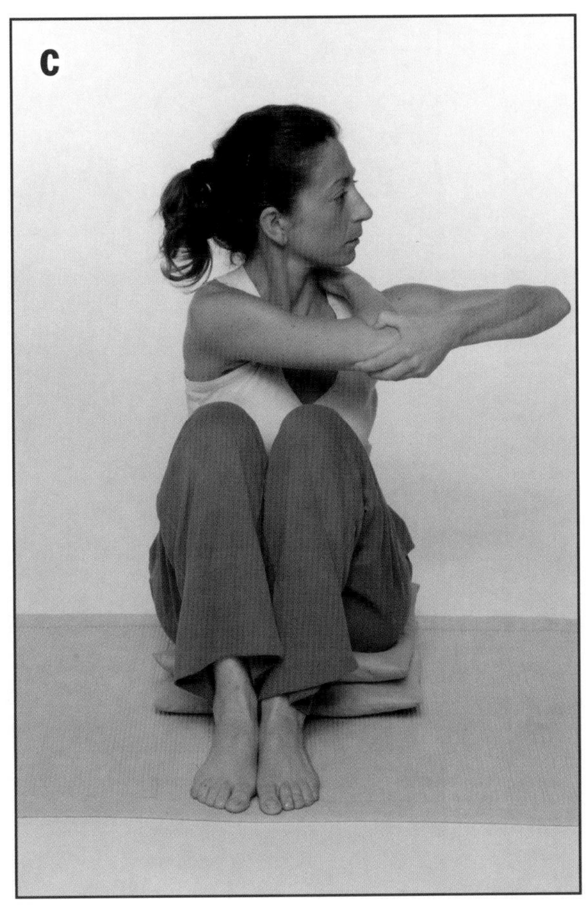

As you breathe in, pull your right arm to the left, turn your head in the same direction, and push with your thumb on the pressure point (C).

Holding your breath, maintain this position for 3 seconds.

As you breathe out, return slowly to the starting position.

Perform the exercise 3 to 5 times. Then practice the exercise on the other side.

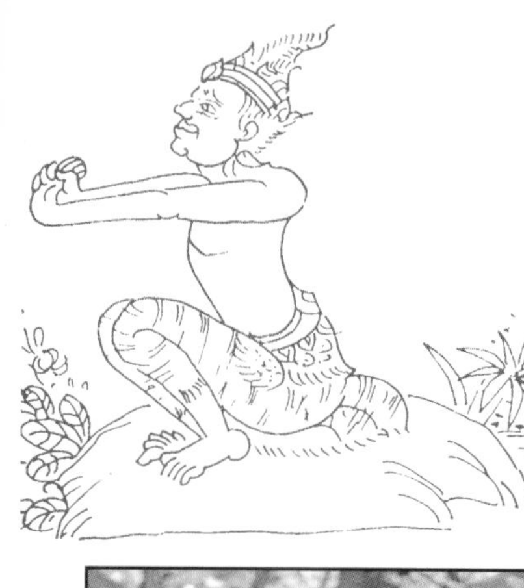

34
Remedy for Joint Pain in the Arms and Hands

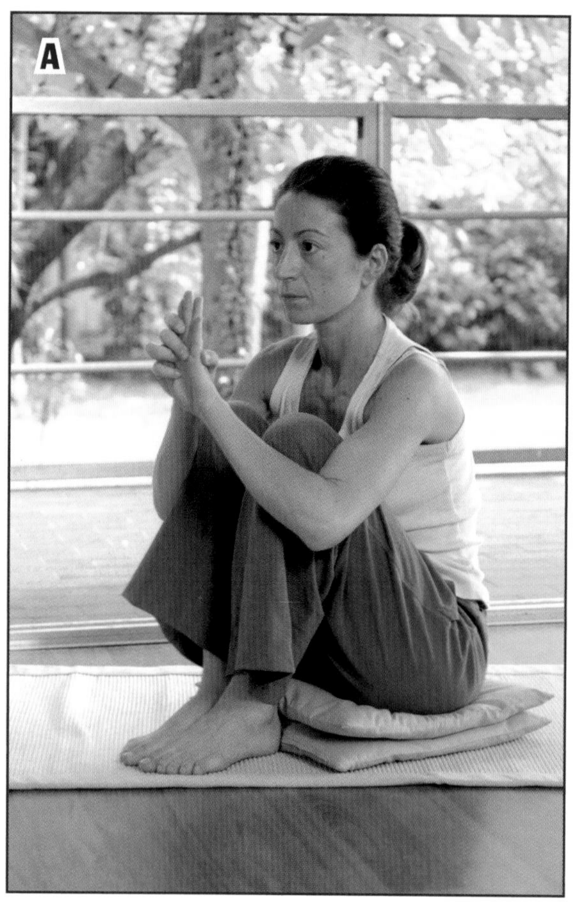

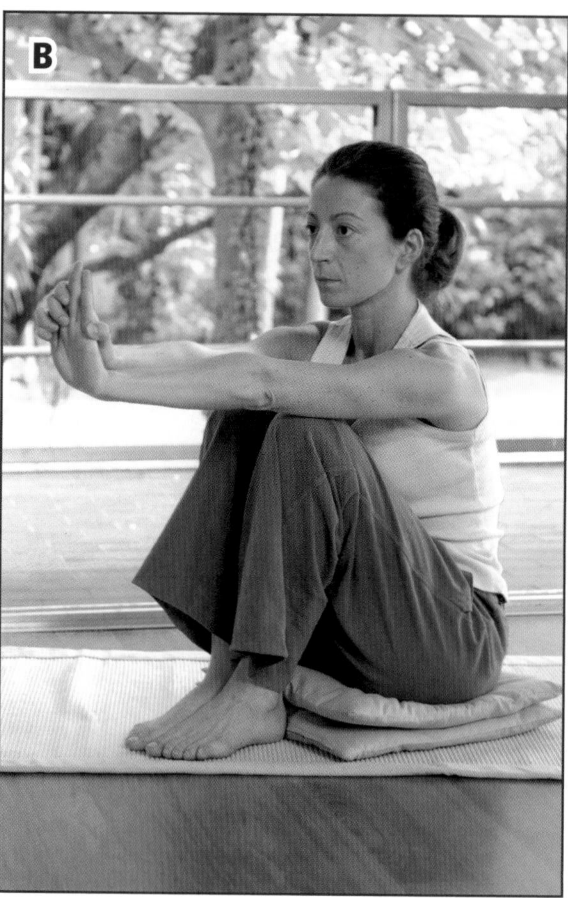

Sit on a cushion with your legs folded up to your chest. With your right hand, hold the fingers of your left hand so that they face away from you, pointing up (A).

Breathing out, stretch the right arm in front of you, and pull the fingers on your right hand, flexing your right wrist (B).

๏ เหยียดหัดถ์ดัดนิ้วนั่ง ชันเพลา แก้เมื่อยขัดแขนเบา โทษได้
ยาคะรุปนี้เอา ยาชื่อใส่เฮย ผสมสิ่นักสิทธิให้ ชื่ออ้างอยุทธยา

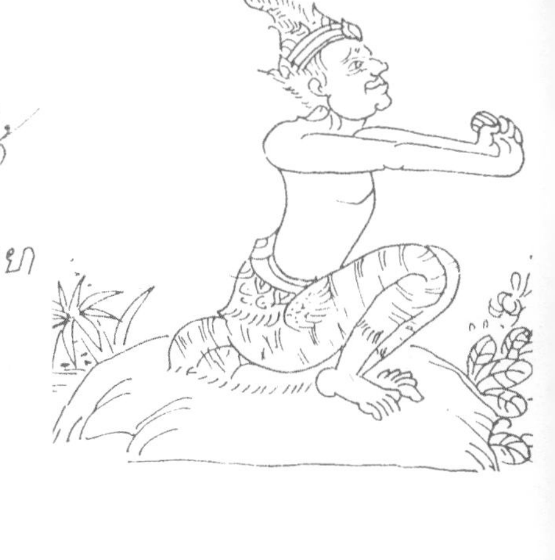

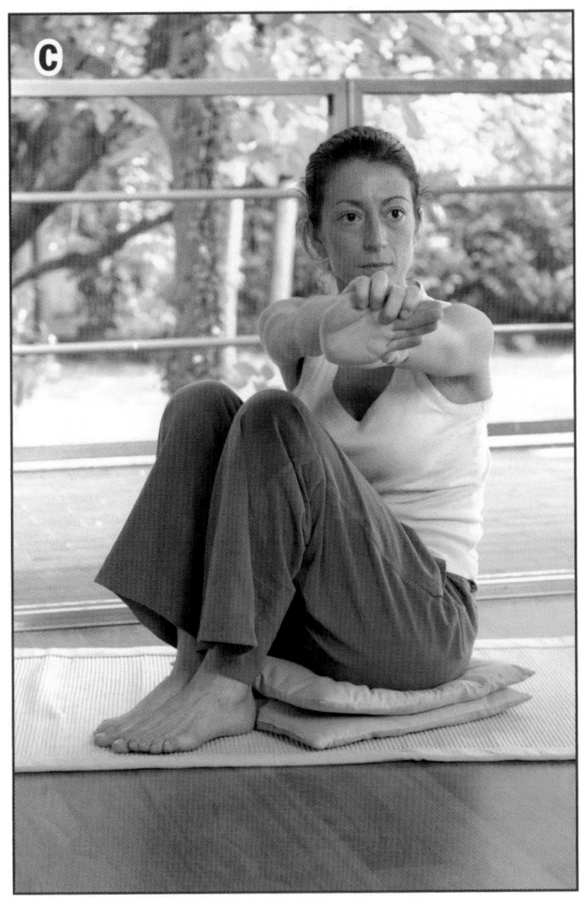

As you breathe in, point your fingers to the left and turn your head and your arm to the left, increasing the pull on your wrist (C).

Holding your breath, maintain this position for 3 seconds.

As you breathe out, return slowly to the starting position.

Perform the exercise 3 to 5 times. Then practice the exercise on the other side.

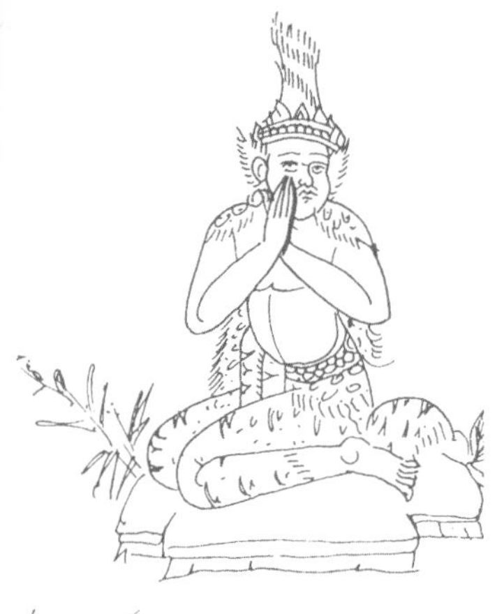

35
Remedy for Wrist Pain

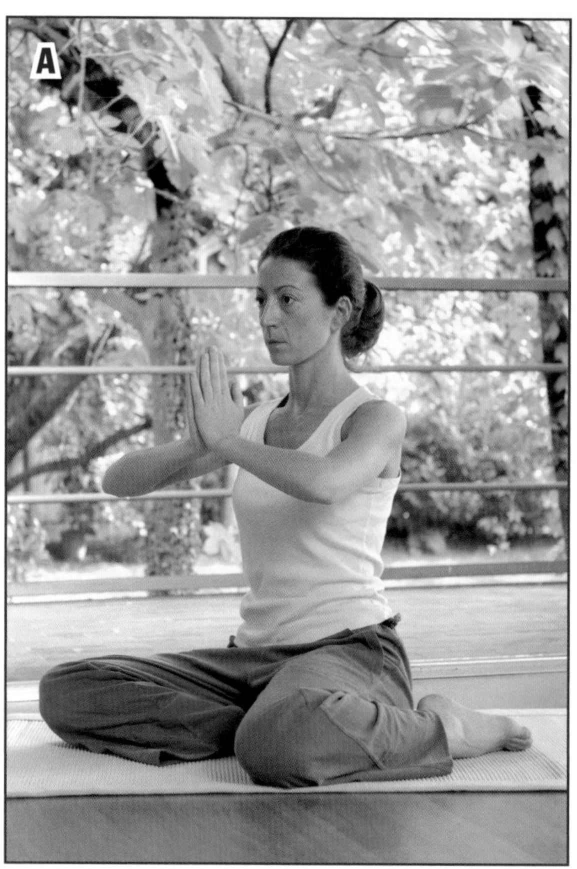

Sit in Thai position, with your left leg bent to the outside and your right leg to the inside.

Bring your palms together in front of you (A).

๑ อนิตถิคันธ์ท่านนิ่วหน้า ตากลิ้ง ลมเสียดสองหัตถ์ตึง ปวดติ้ว

พับเข่านั่งคำนึง นึกดัดดั่งฤๅ กายขดชระดัดนิ้ว นบถ้าเทพนม ฯ

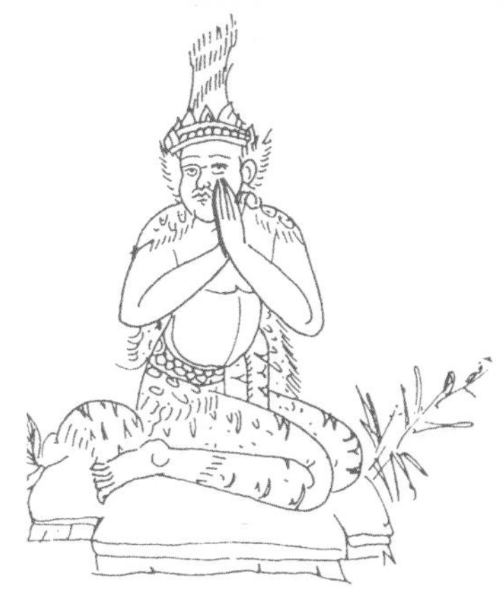

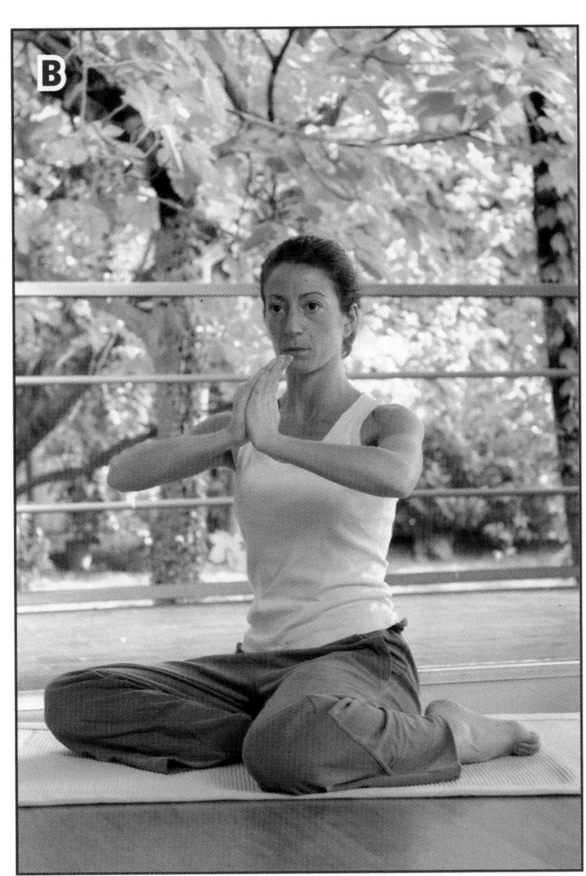

While breathing in, push the fingers of your right hand against those of your left hand, forcing them back. At the same time, turn your chest a little to the left (B).

Holding your breath, maintain this position for 3 seconds.

As you breathe out, straighten your fingers.

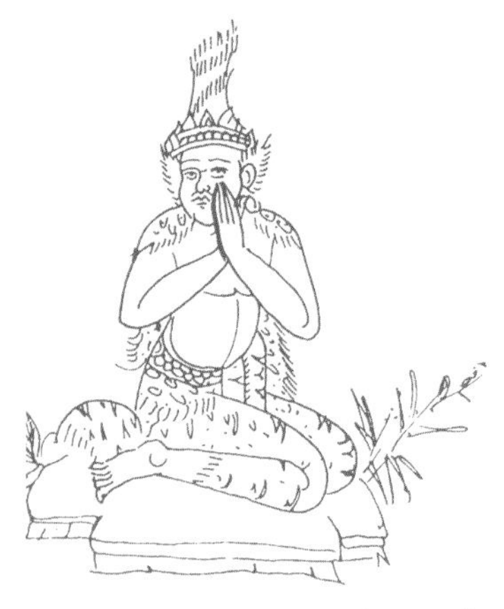

๏ อนิดถิคันธ์ท่านนิ่วหน้า ฑากลึ้ง ลมเสียดสองหัตถ์ตึง ปวดติ้ว
พับเข่านั่งคำนึง นึกดัดดั่งฤๅ กายขดชระดัดนิ้ว นบถ้าเทพนม 

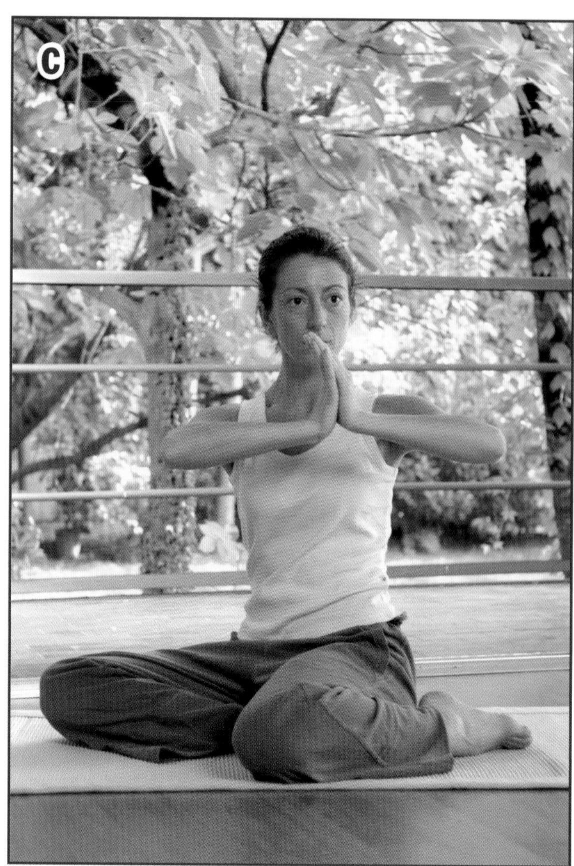

Breathing in, push the fingers of your left hand against those of the right hand, forcing the right-hand fingers back. At the same time, turn your chest a little more to the left (C).

Holding your breath, maintain this position for 3 seconds.

As you breathe out, straighten your fingers.

๏ อนิดถิคันธ์ท่านนิ่วหน้า ตากลิ้ง ลมเสียดสองหัตถ์ถึง ปวดตั้ว

พับเข่านั่งคำนึง นึกดัดดั่งฤๅ กายขดชระดัดนิ้ว นบถ้าเทพนม ฯ

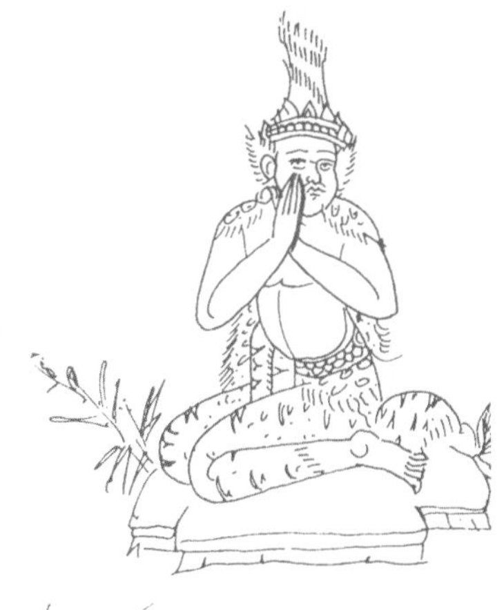

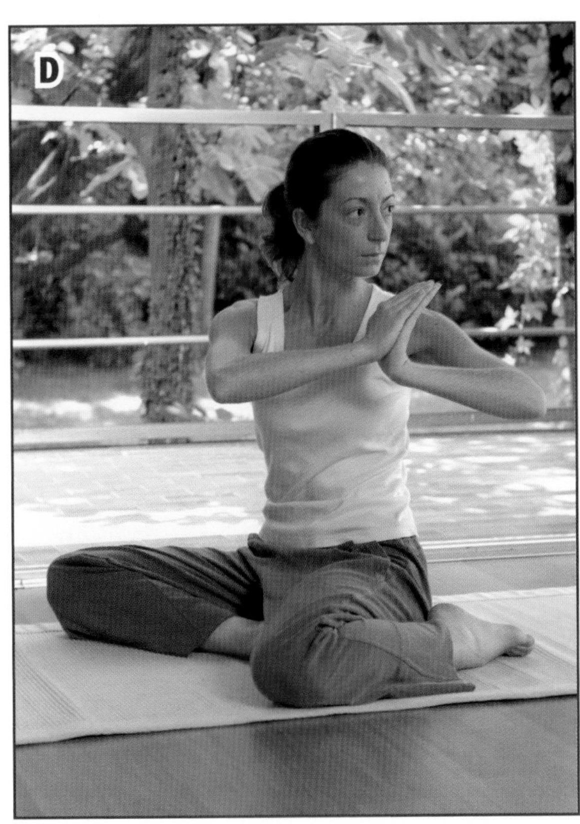

Breathing in, push the fingers of your right hand against those of the left hand, forcing the left-hand fingers back. At the same time, turn your chest to the left as far as possible (D).

Holding your breath, maintain this position for 3 seconds.

As you breathe out, return slowly to the starting position.

Perform the exercise 3 to 5 times. Then practice the exercise on the other side, reversing the direction in which you bend your fingers, so that you bend them first to the right, then to the left, and then again to the right.

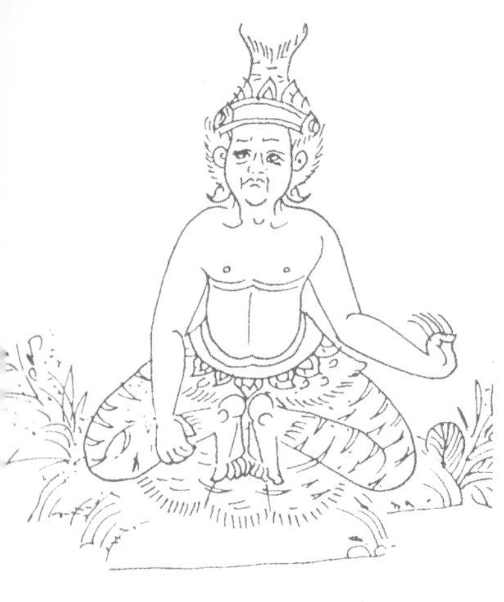

36 Remedy for Arm and Leg Pain

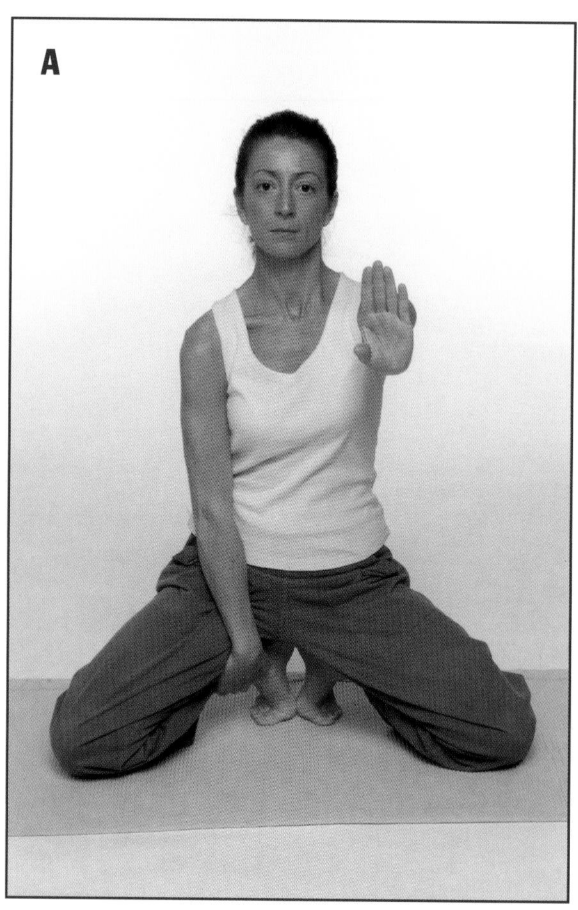

Kneel with your feet flexed, resting your buttocks on your heels and opening your legs as widely as you can. Grasp your right ankle with your right hand. Extend your left arm out in front of you, keeping your wrist well flexed (A).

๏ พระสุทัศน์สถิตย์ถ้ำ เถื่อนระหง ครองเครื่องนักสิทธิ์ทรง ห่อเกล้
ลมคั่งคอหัดถ์ชงฆ์ หัดถ์ช่วยดัดเอว นั่งกระหย่งยุดเท้า หัดถ์ช้อยเช่นรำ

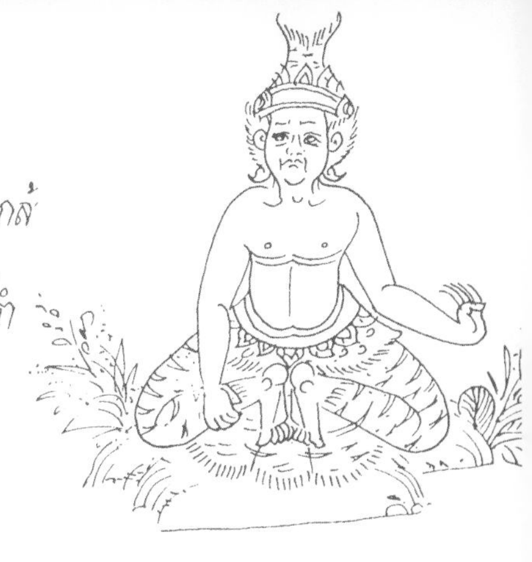

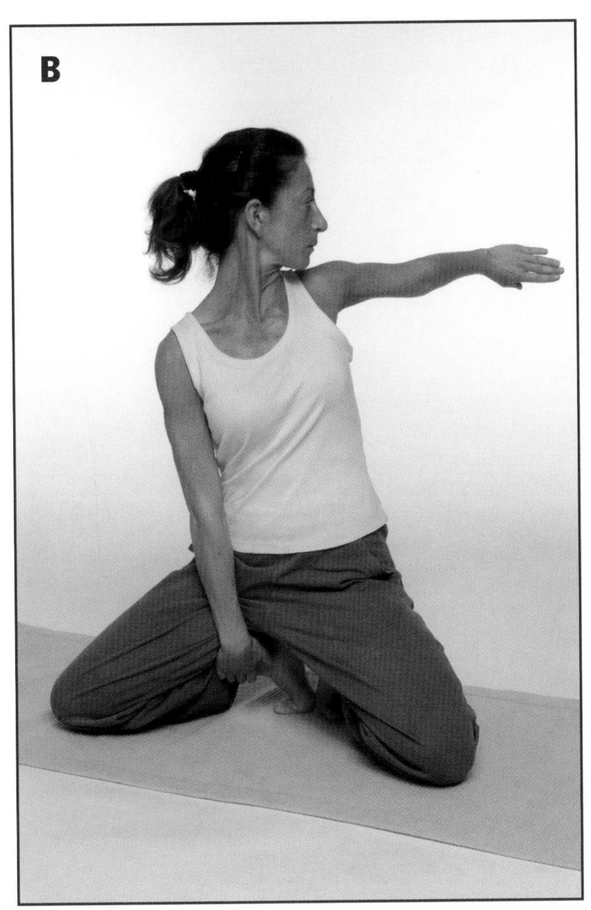

While breathing in, turn your chest to the left as far as you can, extending the turn by pulling with your left arm and keeping your legs anchored (B).

Holding your breath, maintain this position for 3 seconds.

As you breathe out, return slowly to the starting position.

Perform the exercise 3 to 5 times. Then practice the exercise on the other side.

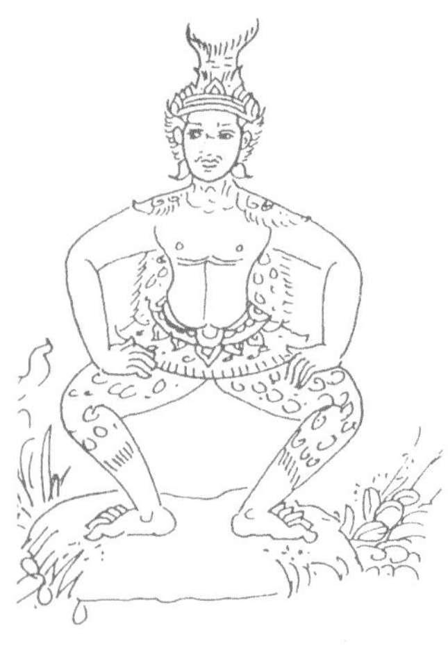

37 Remedy for Hand and Foot Cramps

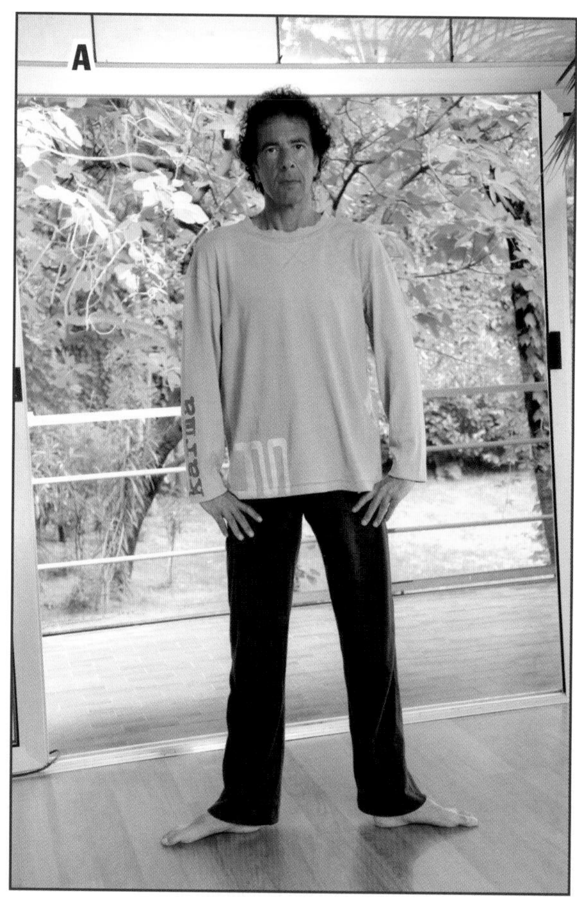

Stand with your feet 10 to 12 inches (25–30 cm) apart. Point your toes outward as much as possible while still maintaining your balance. Place your hands on your thighs, with your fingers pointing to the inside (A).

๏ อัคนีเนตร์นี้อัค ศิโขนเนตรฤๅ ยืนแย่หย่งยักษ์โขน ออกเค้น
กางกรกดสองโคน ขานิ่ดเน้นนอ แก้ตะคริวริ้วเส้น แต่แข้งตลอดเขน ฯ

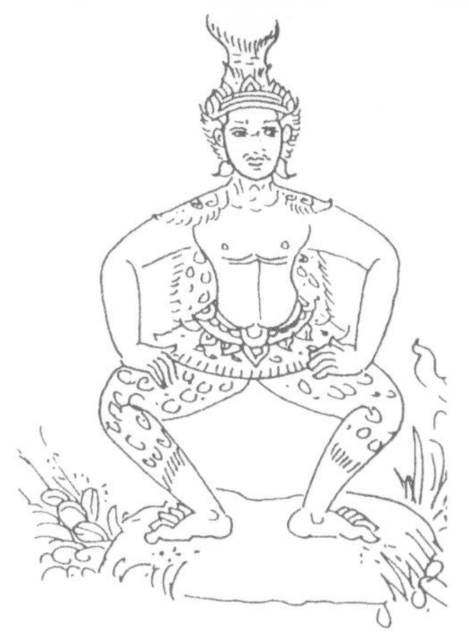

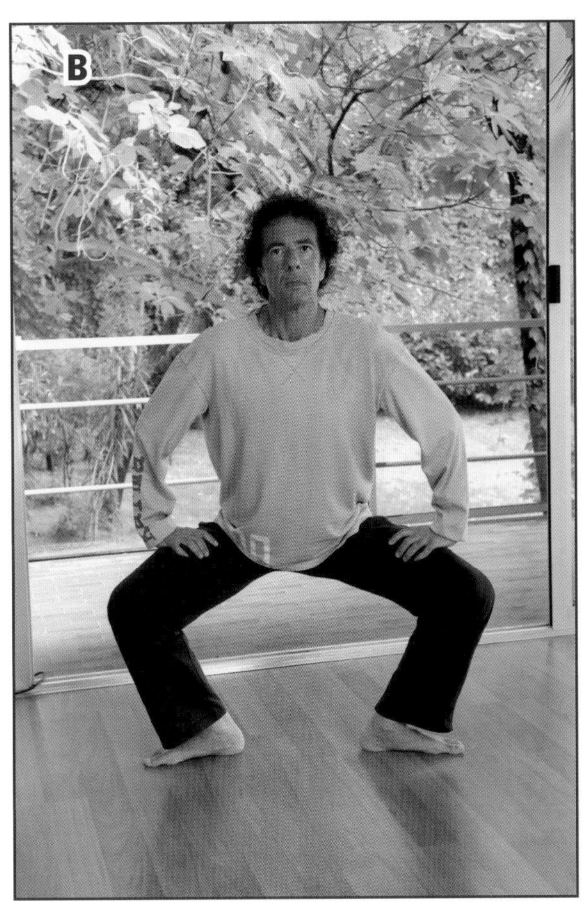

As you breathe in, lower your torso as much as possible by bending your knees outward (B).

Holding your breath, maintain this position for 3 seconds.

As you breathe out, return slowly to the starting position.

Perform the exercise 3 to 5 times.

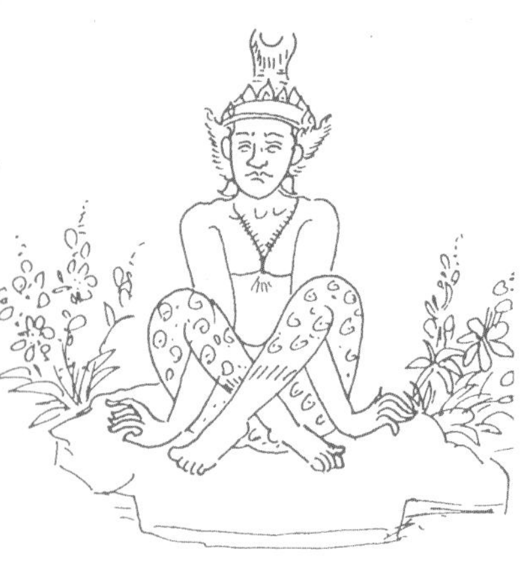

38 Remedy for Stiffness in the Knees

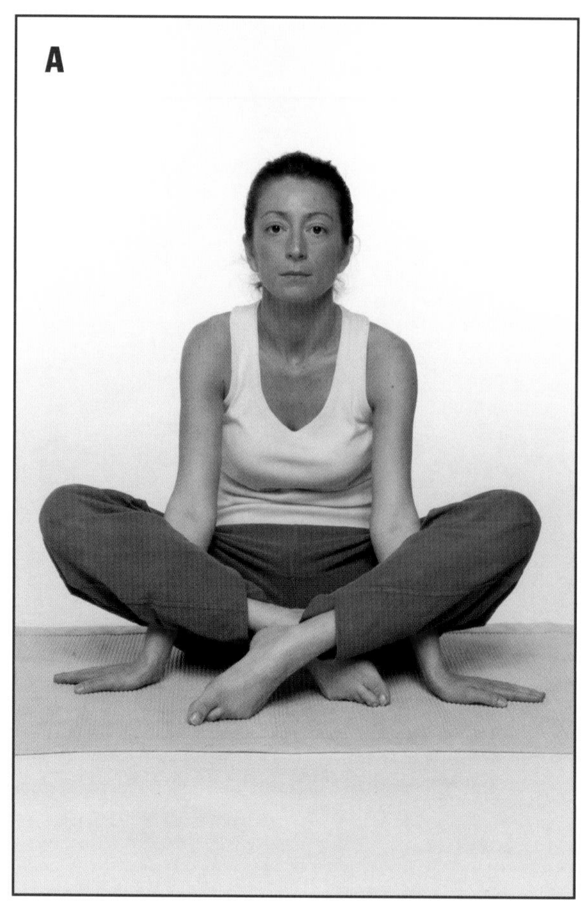

Sit cross-legged with the tips of your toes on the floor and your legs lifted. Place your arms inside your legs, where the thighs and calves meet, and place your hands flat on the floor, with your fingers pointing outward (A).

๏ ฤๅษีวะชิระรู้สาตร์ สฤษดิกายกบแฮ ชื่อเทพมณีโทษาย มากชู้ ๑๐
แก้ลมเข่าขทาย สิ่งเมื่อยมึนเอย ท้าวหัตถ์ชันเข่าคู้ ท่าแม้นลม้ายสิงห์

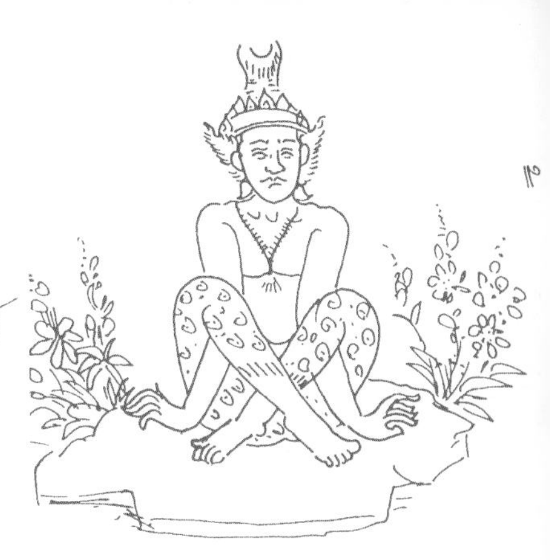

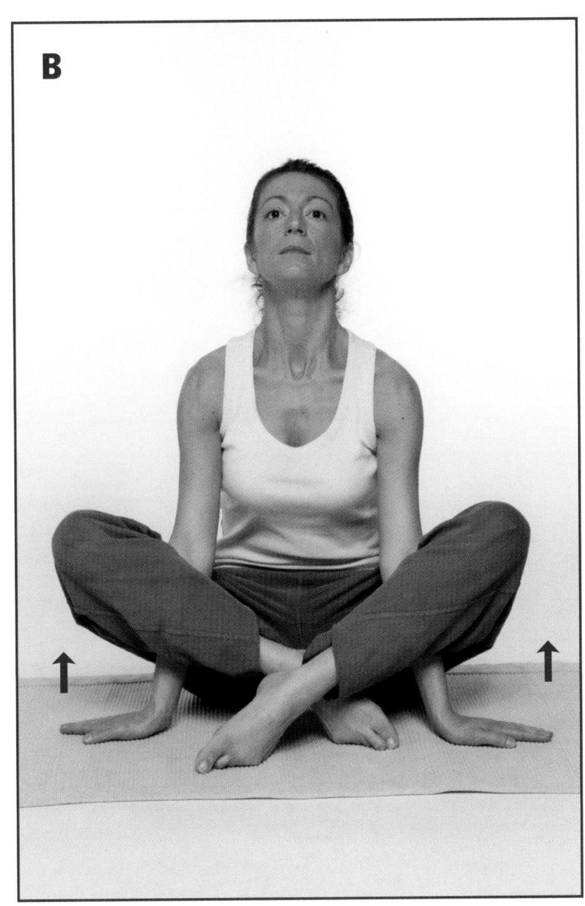

While breathing in, pull your legs in, as if you wanted to fold them more tightly. At the same time press your hands against the floor in order to hold your legs in place, so that your legs push against your arms (B).

Holding your breath, maintain this position for 3 seconds.

As you breathe out, return slowly to the starting position.

Perform the exercise 3 to 5 times.

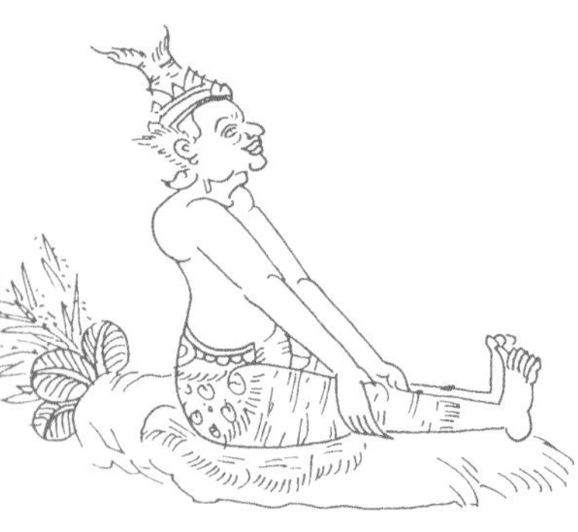

39
Remedy for Knee Pain

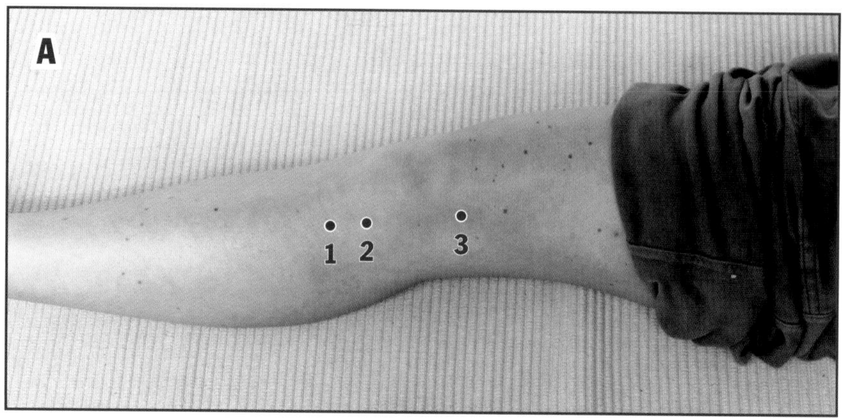

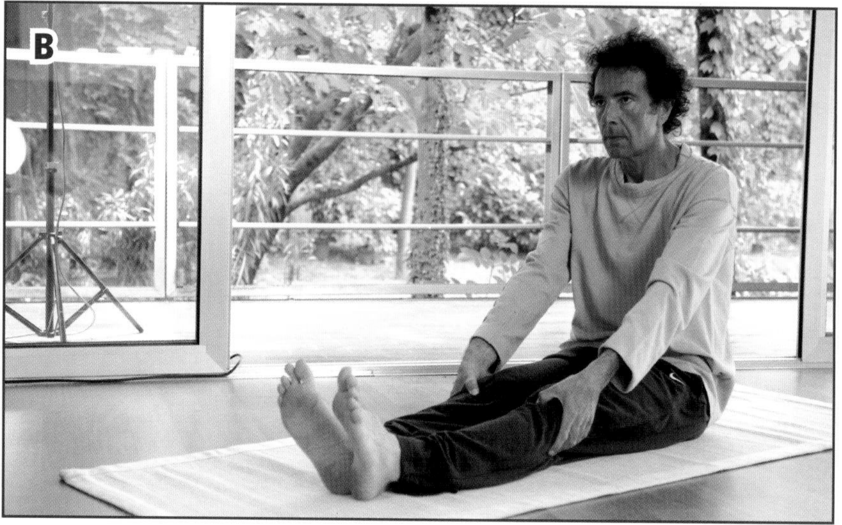

This exercises requires finger pressure on three points: point 1 is located just below and to the outside of the knee cap; point 2 is located on the lower outside corner of the knee cap; and point 3 is located on the inner thigh, two fingers' width from the knee cap (A).

Sit with your legs extended in front of you. Hold your knees with your hands, keeping your fingers on the outside of your legs and your thumbs on point 1 on each leg (B).

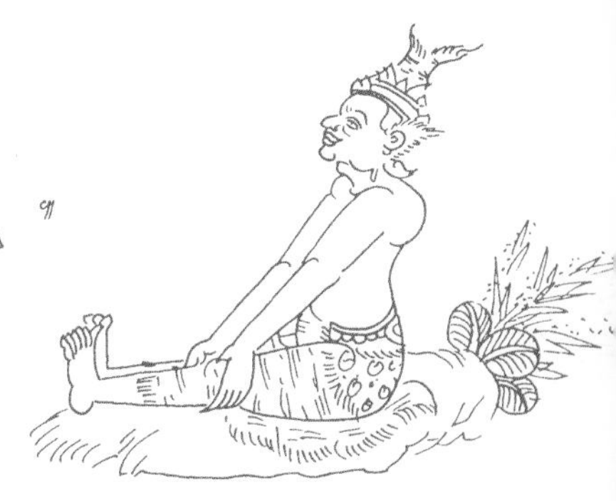

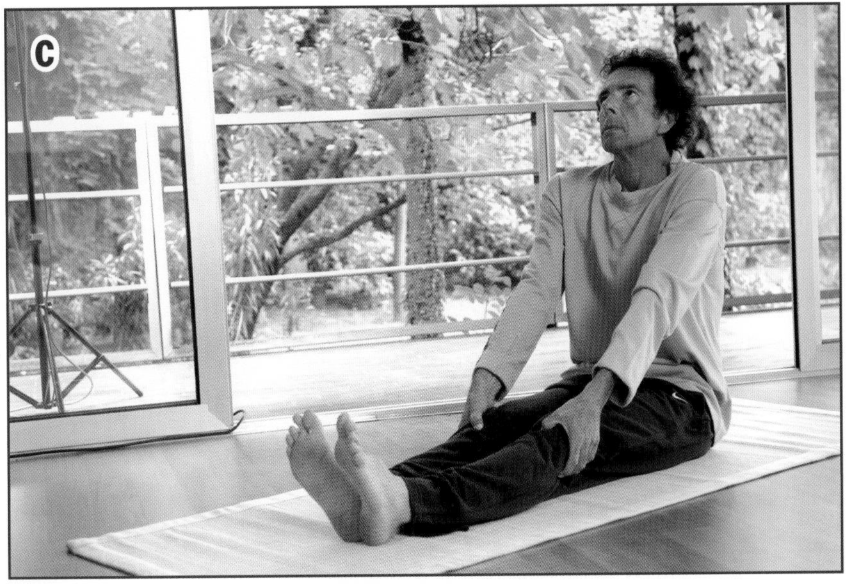

As you breathe in, slightly lift your head, stretching your chest, while pressing your thumbs on point 1 on each leg (C).

Holding your breath, maintain this position for 3 seconds.

As you breathe out, return slowly to the starting position.

Perform the exercise pressing first point 1, then point 2, and then point 3. Go back to point 1 and repeat until each point has been pressed 3 to 5 times.

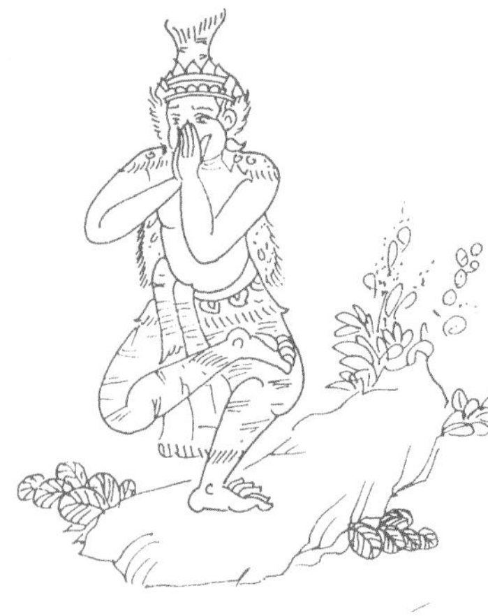

40
Remedy for Knee Dislocation

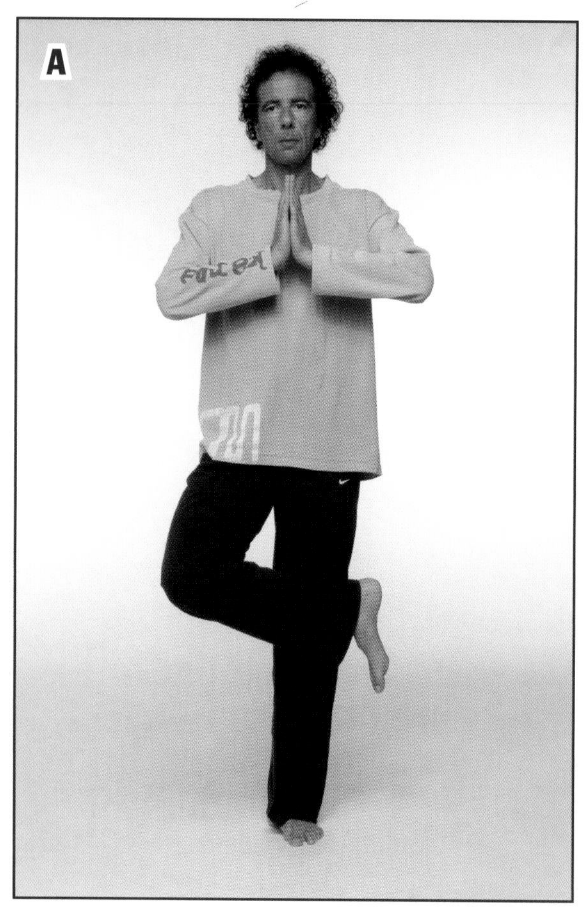

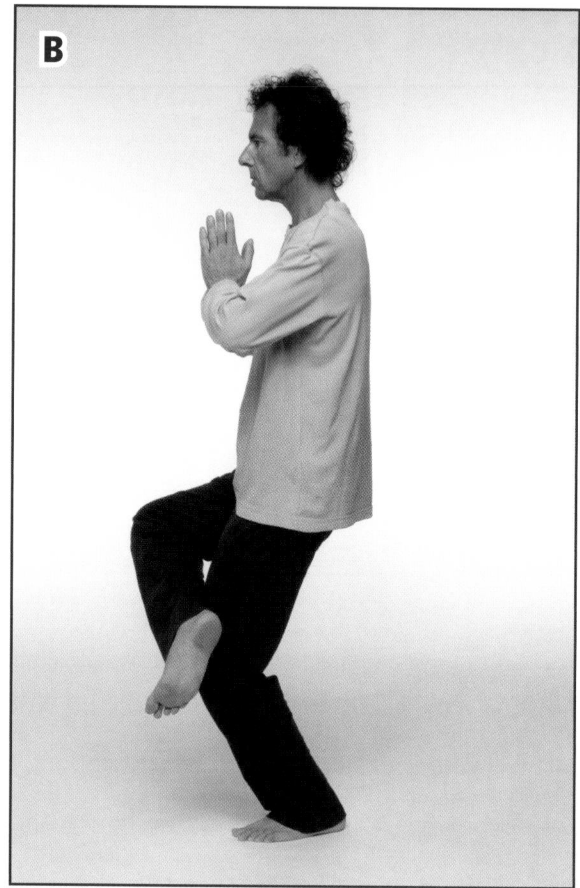

PART ONE

Stand on your left leg with your right leg bent over the left. Bring your palms together in front of you (A).

As you breathe in, slightly bend your left knee (B).

Holding your breath, maintain this position for 1 second.

๏ ชฎิลดาบศเบื้อง แบบฉบับ ยืนยกชาขวาทับ เข่าซ้าย
ประนมหัตถ์ดัดกายกลับ เบือนบิดตนแฮ ลมขัดคอเข่าร้าย เร่งร้างห่างสูญ :

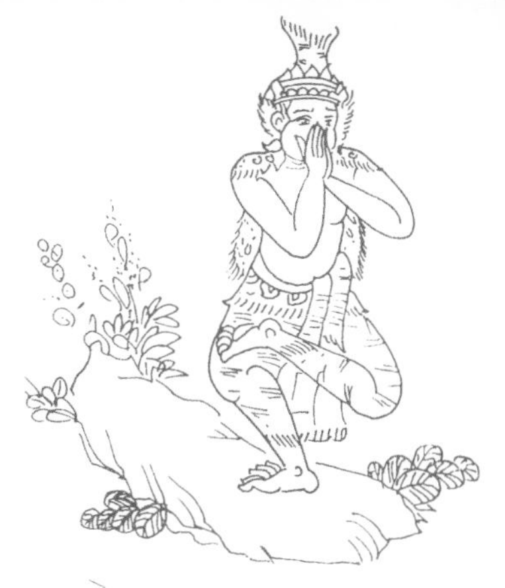

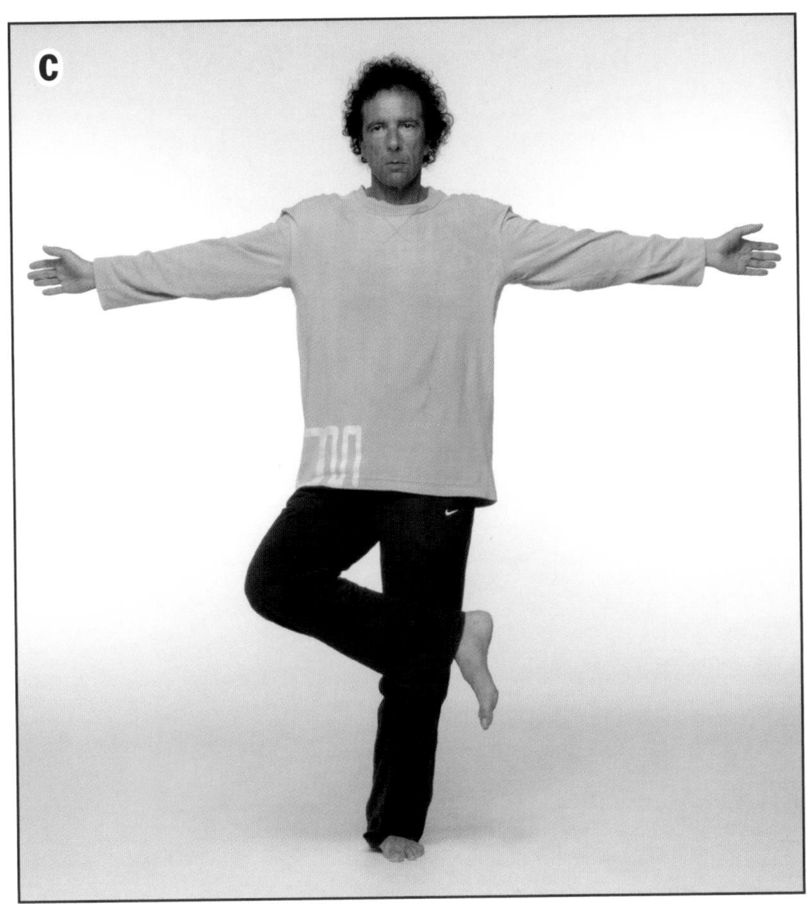

Continuing to hold your breath, extend your arms to your sides (C), and maintain this position for 1 second.

Continuing to hold your breath, again bring your palms together in front of you (B), and maintain this position for 1 second.

As you breathe out, return slowly to the starting position.

Perform the exercise 3 to 5 times. Then practice the exercise on the other side.

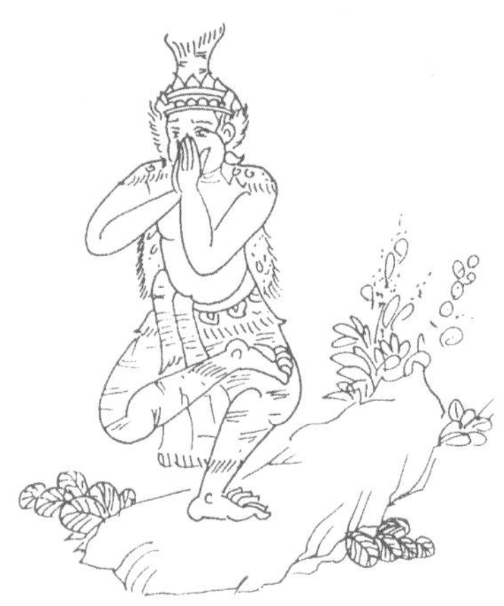

๏ ชฎิลดาบศเบื้อง แบบฉบับ ยืนยกชาขวาทับ เข่าซ้าย
ประนมหัตถ์ดัดกายกลับ เบือนบิดตนแฮ ลมขัดคอเข่าร้าย เร่งร้างห่างสูญ ฯ

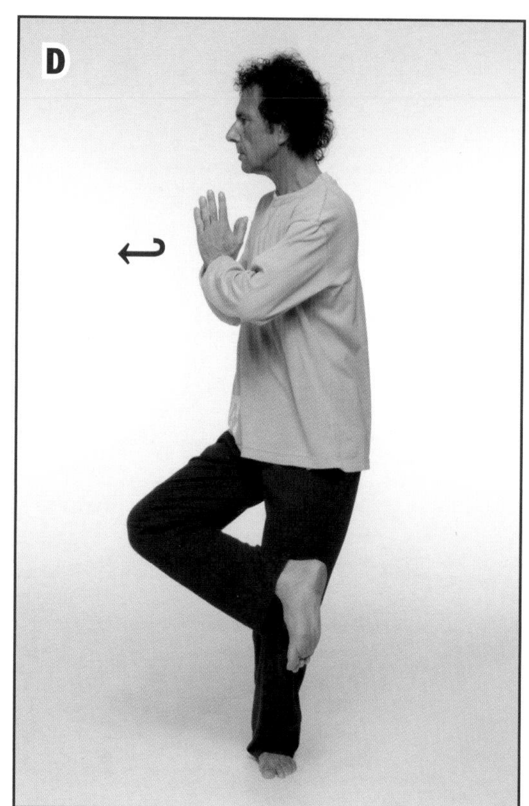

PART TWO

Return to the starting position (A).

Breathing out, bend your left knee (B).

As you breathe in, turn your chest as far to the right as you can while still keeping your balance (D).

Holding your breath, maintain this position for 3 seconds.

As you breathe out, return slowly to the starting position.

After taking a breath, breathe out while bending your left knee again (B).

๏ ชฎิลดาบศเบื้อง แบบฉบับ ยืนยกขาขวาทับ เข่าซ้าย
ประนมหัตถ์ดัดกายกลับ เบือนบิดตนแฮ ลมขัดคอเข่าร้าย เร่งร้างห่างสูญ :

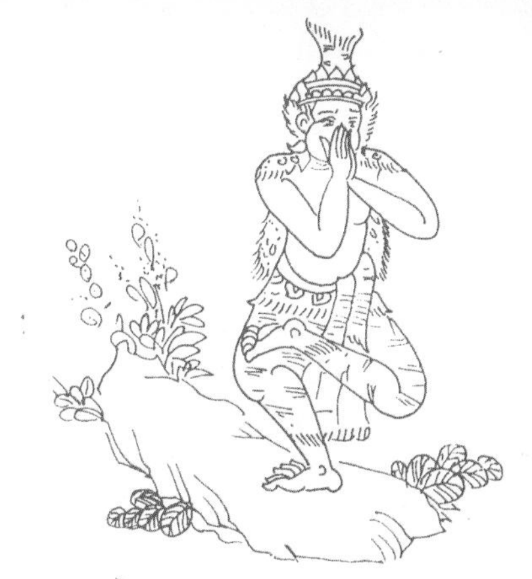

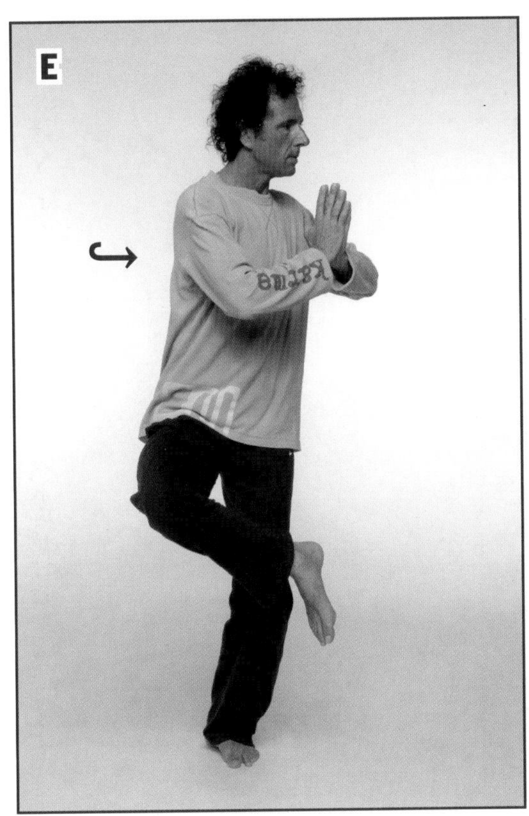

As you breathe in, turn your chest as far to the left as you can while still keeping your balance (E).

Holding your breath, maintain this position for 3 seconds.

As you breathe out, return slowly to the starting position.

Perform the exercise twice. Then practice the exercise on the other side. Note: If you suffer from knee pain, do not exceed the suggested number of repetitions while balanced on the ailing leg.

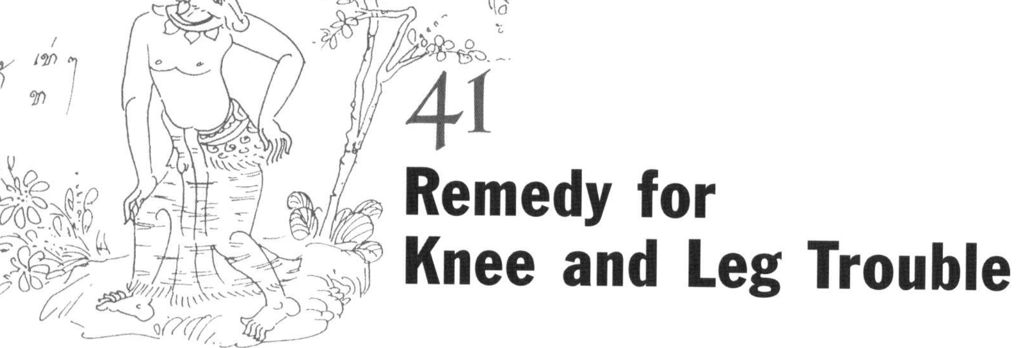

41
Remedy for Knee and Leg Trouble

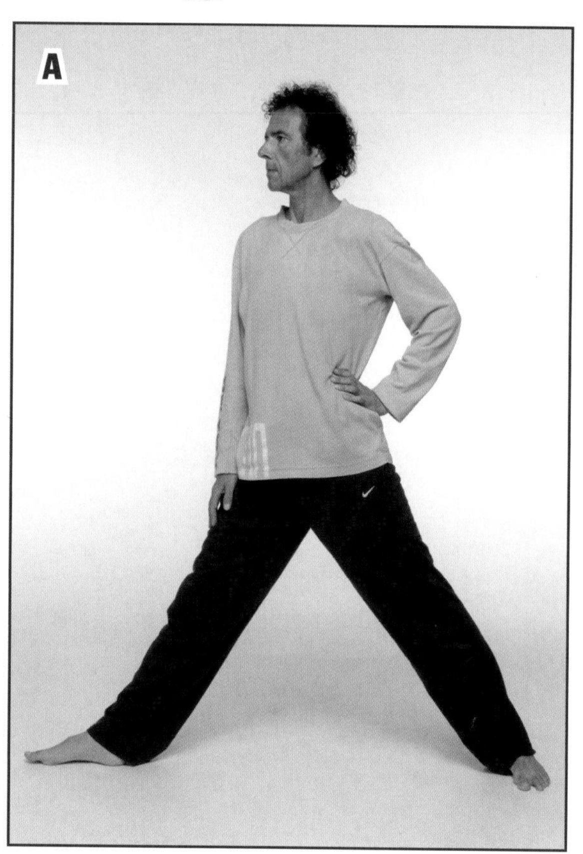

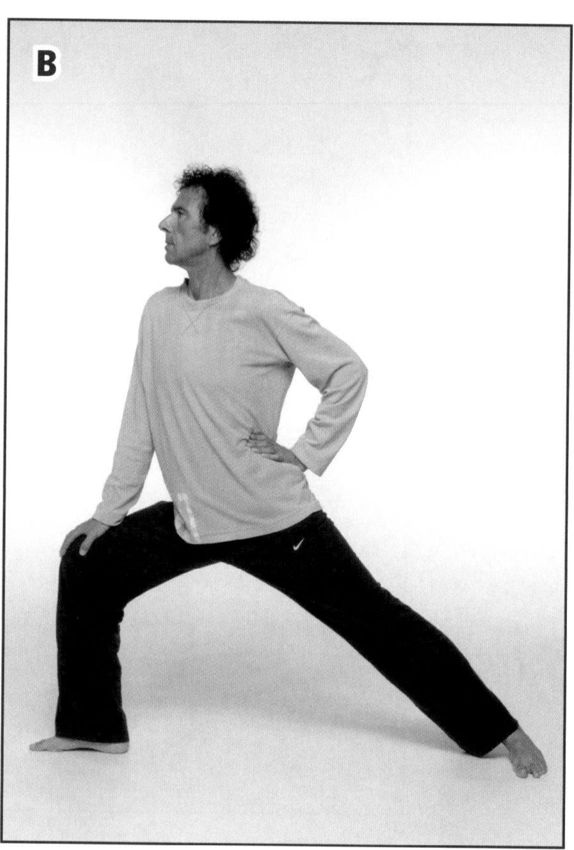

Stand with your legs apart. Pull your left leg back and point your right foot forward, so that your heels are aligned and your feet are perpendicular to each other. Place your left hand on your side and your right hand on your right leg (A).

Breathing out, bend your right leg to a 90-degree angle, stretching your left leg (B).

๏ อิษีสิงค์หน้ามฤค ฌาณมอศม้ายแฮ สลบเพื่อนางฟ้ากอด ท่านนั้น
ฟื้นองค์ครั่นครางออด ทำไหล่ขัดเอย ยืนย่อบาทบีบคั้น เข่าทั้งโคนขา ฯ

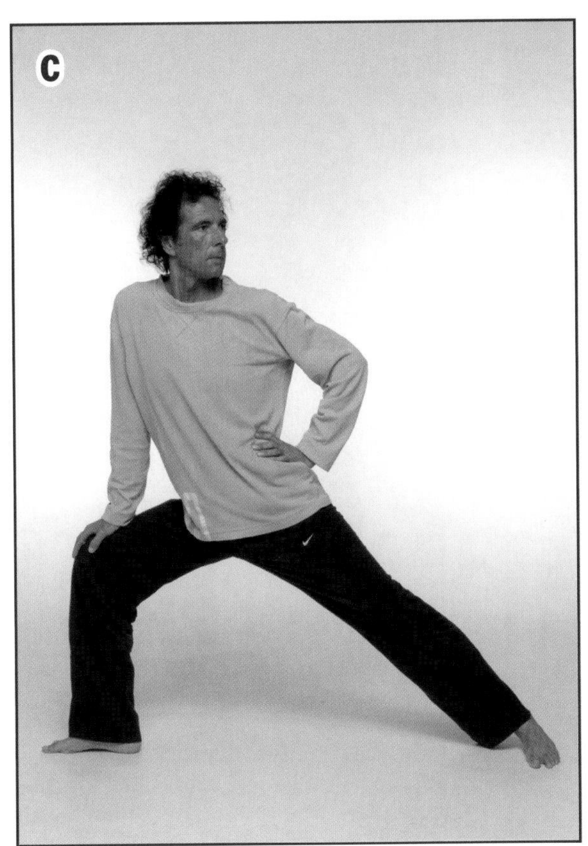

As you breathe in, turn your head to the left as far as you can (C).

Holding your breath, maintain this position for 3 seconds.

As you breathe out, return slowly to the starting position.

Perform the exercise 3 to 5 times. Then practice the exercise on the other side.

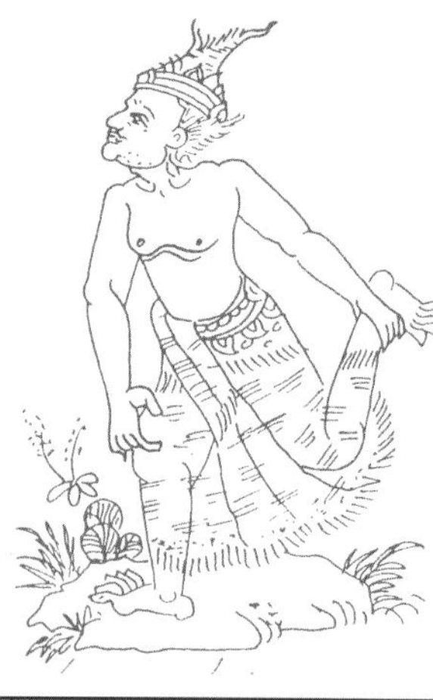

42
Remedy for Knee, Leg, and Chest Problems

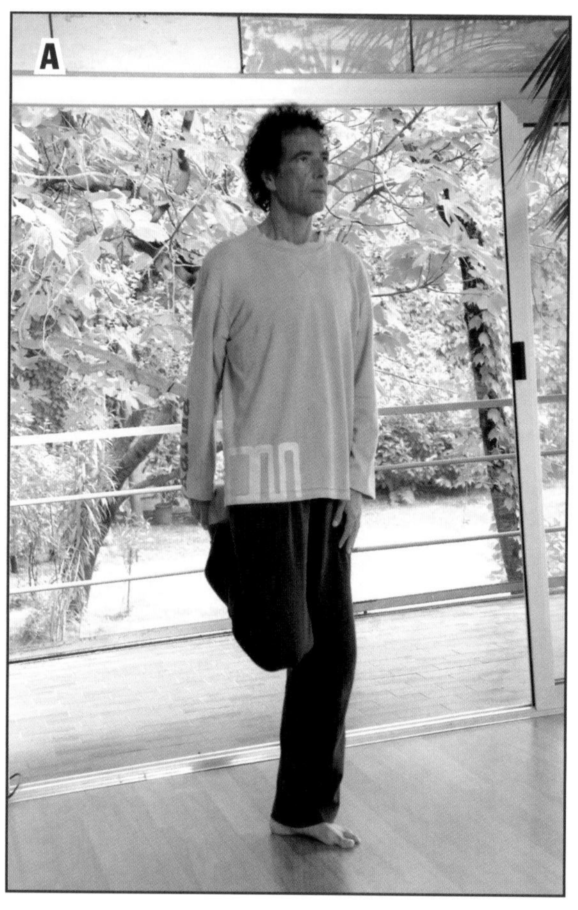

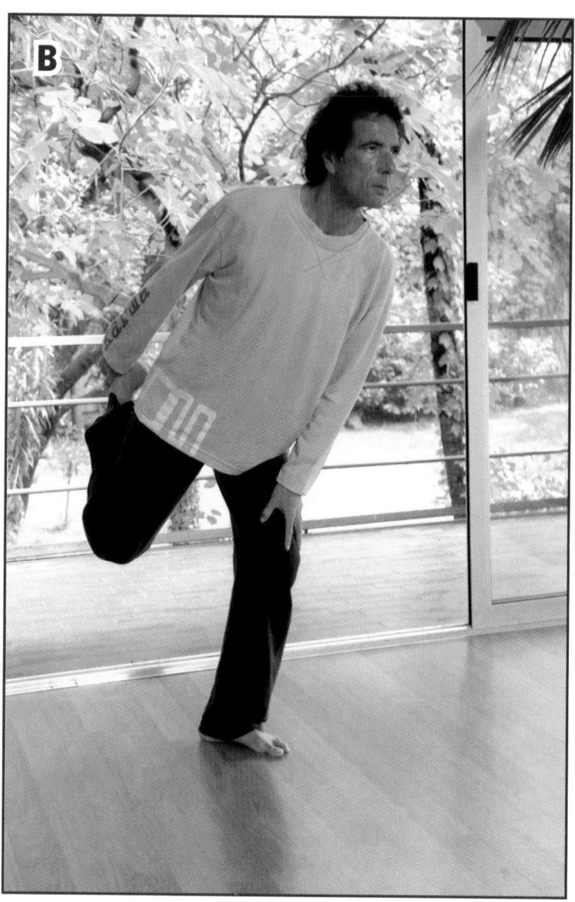

Stand with your right leg bent back, holding the ankle with your right hand. Place your left hand on your left thigh (A).

While breathing out, slightly bend your left knee, keeping your hand on your thigh (B).

๏ พระนารอทวายุเร้า ทรงรั้นทำนา ขัดเข่าขาและจันท ฎาฎร้าย
ฉวยเท้าท่ายืนหัน เหอรเยี่ยงเหาะแฮ มือหนึ่งคั้นเข่าซ้าย เสื่อมสิ้นสิ่ลม ฯ

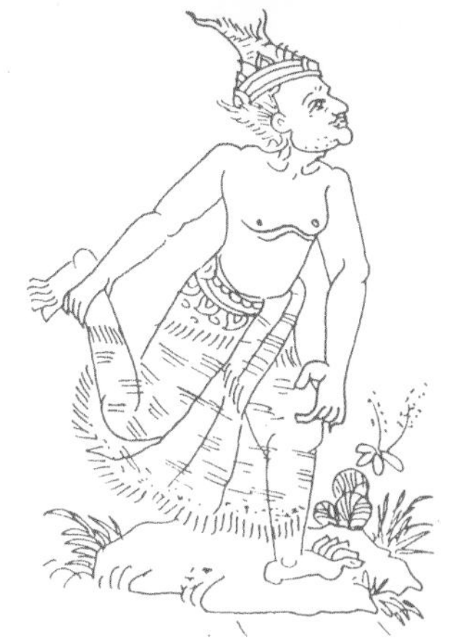

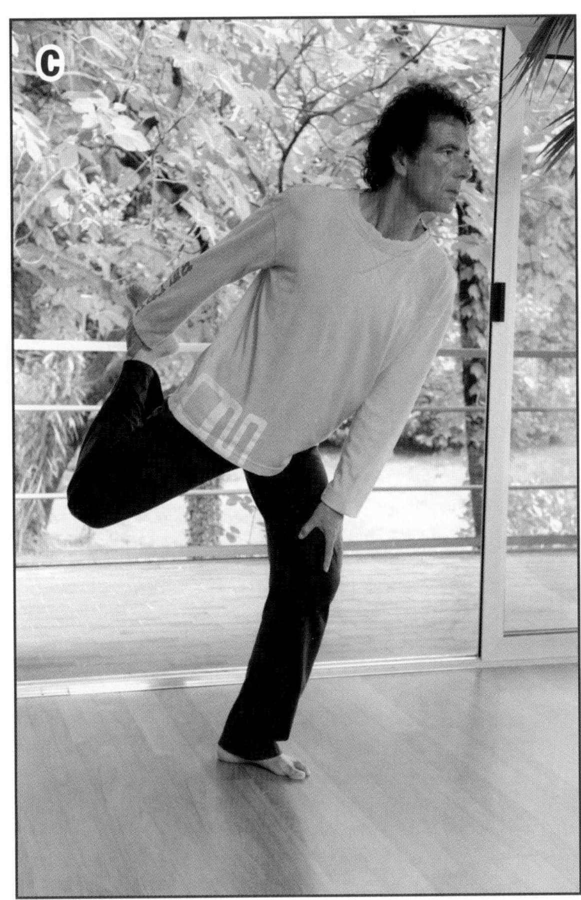

As you breathe in, extend your right leg until your right arm has straightened, letting your chest turn to the right (C).

Holding your breath, maintain this position for 3 seconds.

As you breathe out, return slowly to the starting position.

After taking a breath, slightly bend your left knee again while breathing out (B).

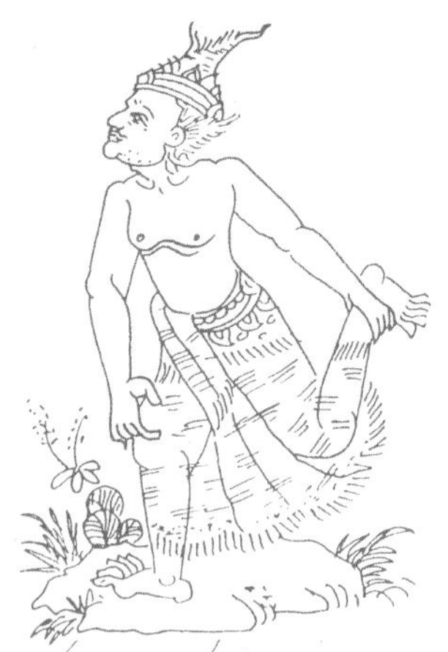

๏ พระนารอทวายุเร้า ทรงรั้นทำนา ขัดเข่าขาและจันท มฎฎร้าย
ฉวยเท้าท่ายืนหั่น เหอรเยี่ยงเหาะแฮ มือหนึ่งค้นเข่าซ้าย เสื่อมสิ้นสี่ลม ฯ

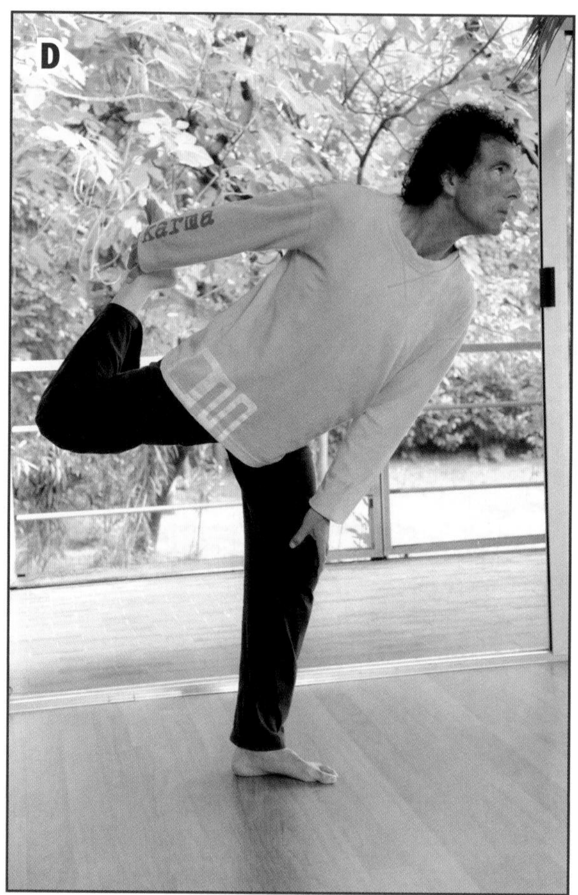

As you breathe in, lift and extend your right leg as much as possible, at the same time leaning your chest forward and lifting your head (D).

Holding your breath, maintain this position for 3 seconds.

As you breathe out, return slowly to the starting position.

Perform this exercise sequence 3 to 5 times. Then practice the exercise on the other side.

43 Remedy for Leg and Neck Pain

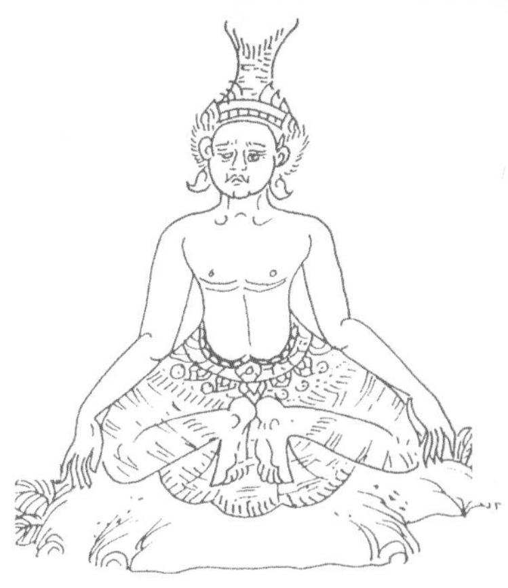

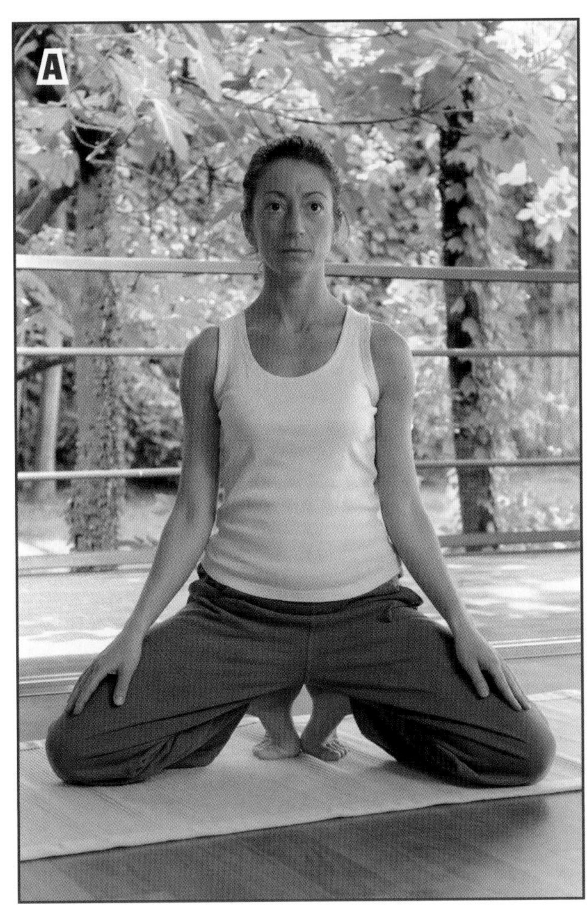

Kneel with your feet flexed, resting your buttocks on your heels and opening your legs as widely as you can. Place your hands on your thighs, letting your arms hang at your sides so that your shoulders remain relaxed (A).

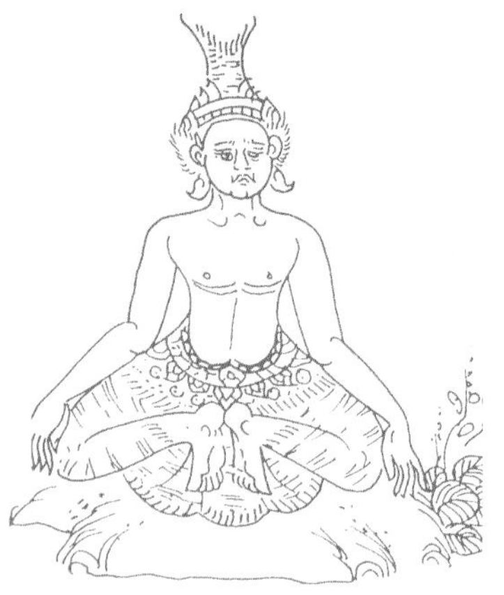

๑ แยกขายืนเข่าตั้ง ตนตรง แขนแนบหนีบสเอวองค์ แน่นแฟ้น
ฅาวินทร์ธดำง กายดัดนี้ฤๅ แก้กล่อนปัศฆาฎแม้น แพทย์แก้มวยมิ้น

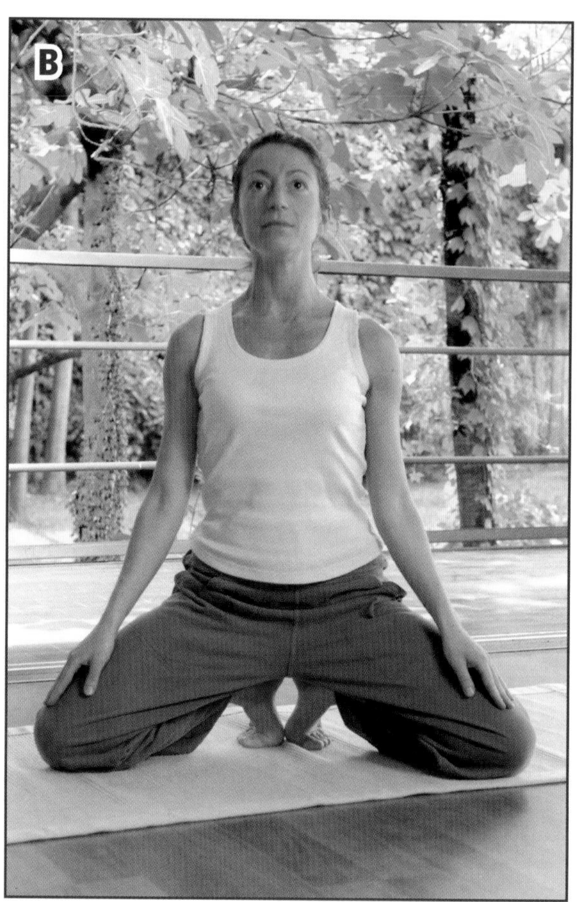

Breathing in, extend and lift your torso, and slightly lift your head (B).

Holding your breath, maintain this position for 3 seconds.

As you breathe out, return slowly to the starting position.

คุกเข่าซ่นติดเช้า เข่าขยาย มือประทับกับเพลาหมาย มุ่งฟ้า
ก้มขาขัดคอหาย ห่างเมื่อยลงแฮ โรมสิงค์สิทธิศักดิ์กล้า กล่าวนี้นามขนาน ฯ

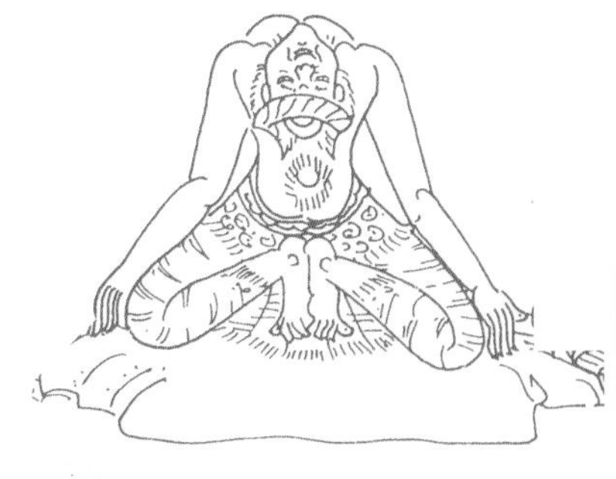

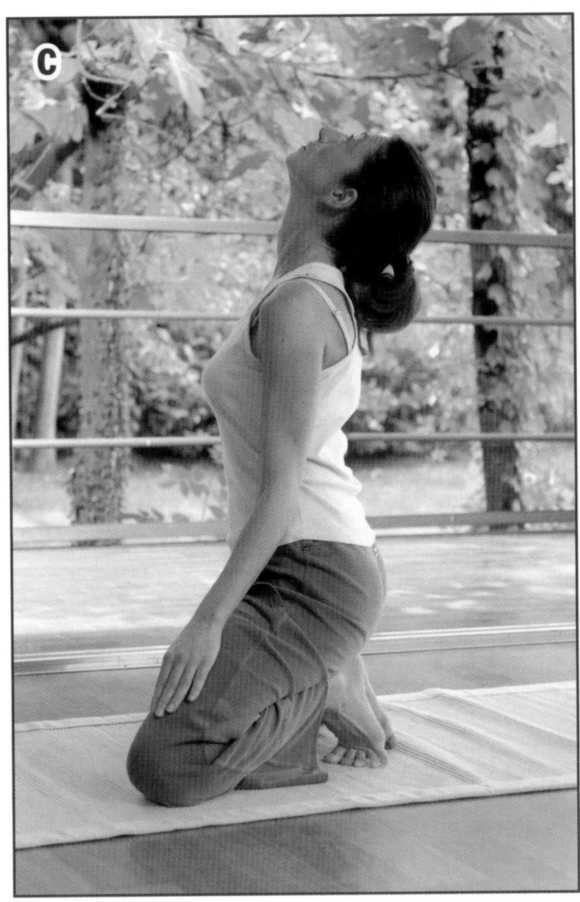

Breathing in again, let your head fall back. Keep your neck and shoulders relaxed, and avoid letting your chest lean backward (C).

Holding your breath, maintain this position for 3 seconds.

As you breathe out, return slowly to the starting position.

Perform the exercise 3 to 5 times.

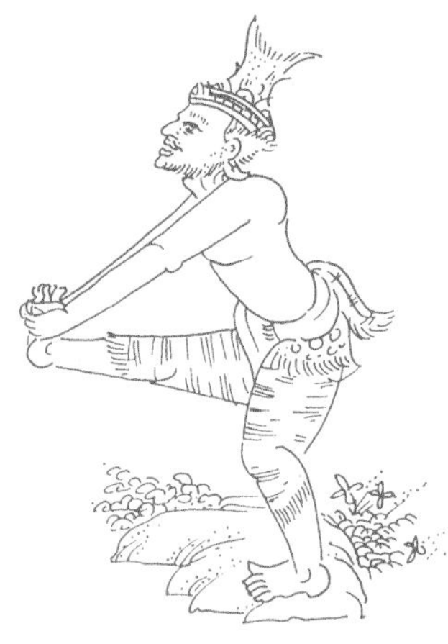

44
Remedy for Foot Numbness

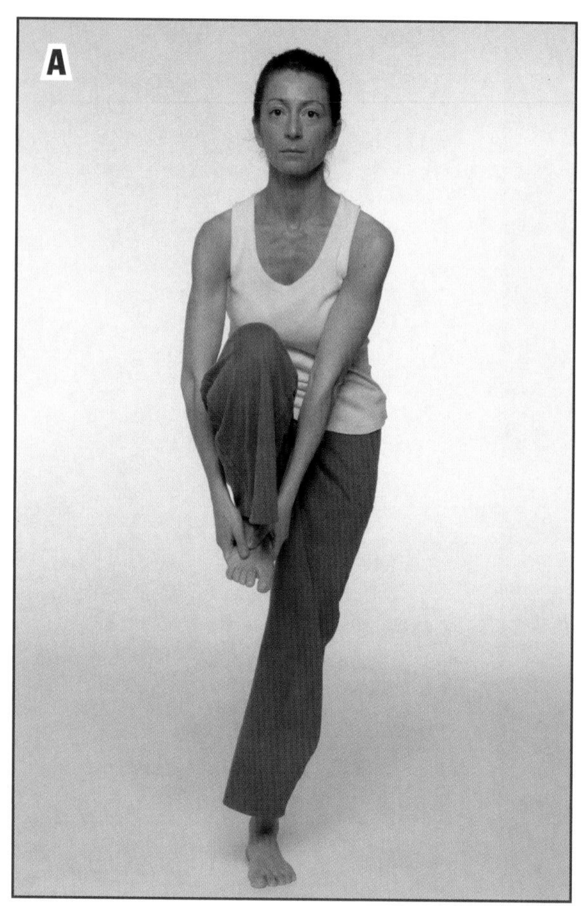

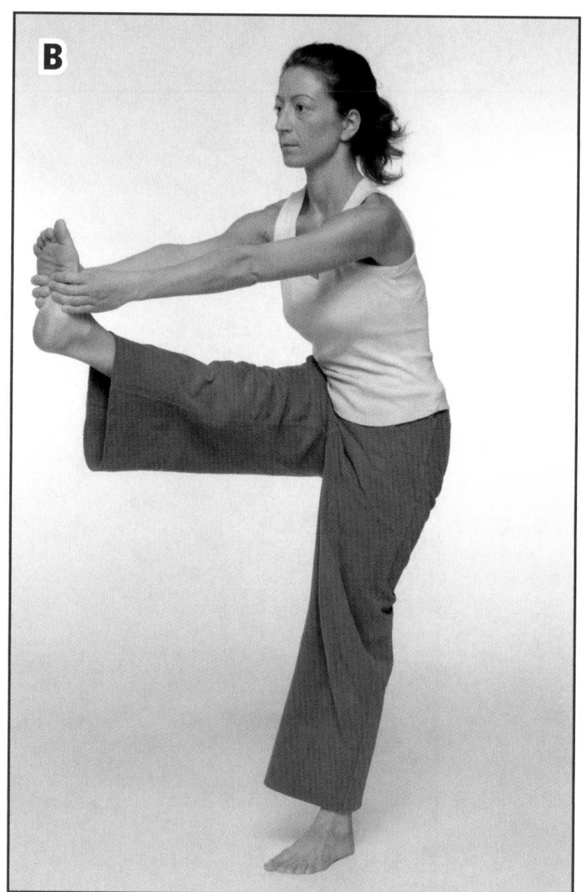

Bend your right knee up to your chest and hold your foot with both hands (A).

Extend your right leg in front of you (B).

๏ เหนทุกข์เหนเท้าโทษ เบญขันธ์ คือพระมาฆะนักธรรม์ สถิตยถ้ำ
มือยุดฝ่าเท้ายัน ยืนย่อตัวนา เท้าเหน็บเยนยิ่งน้ำ เหนี่ยวแก้เหน็บหาย ฯ

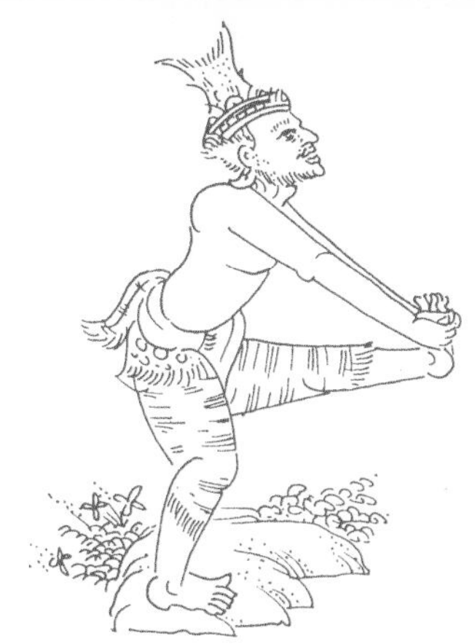

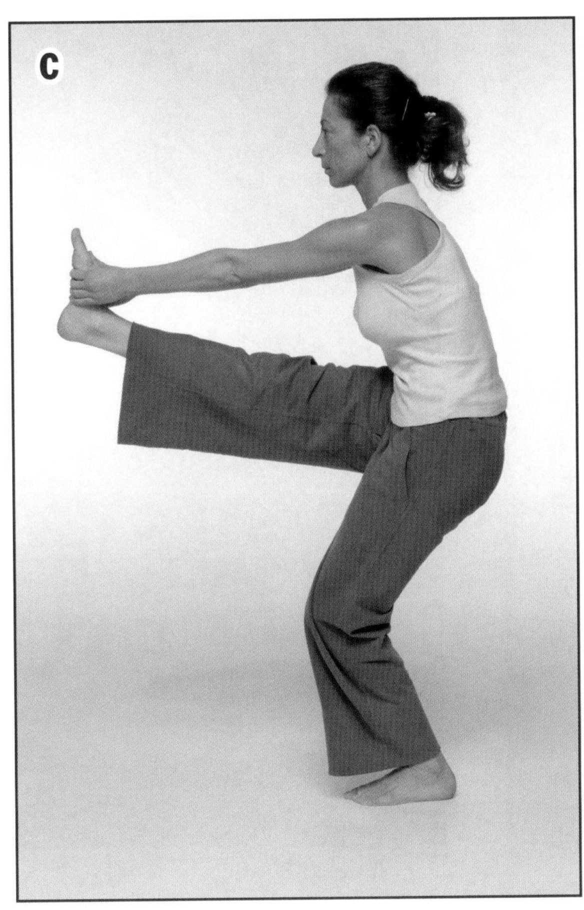

As you breathe in, bend your left knee, keeping your right leg extended (C).

Holding your breath, maintain this position for 3 seconds.

As you breathe out, return slowly to the starting position.

Perform the exercise 3 to 5 times. Then practice the exercise on the other side.

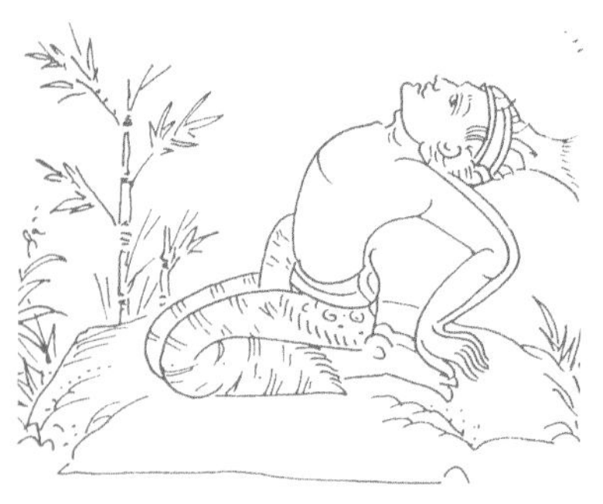

45
Remedy for Pain in the Sole of the Foot

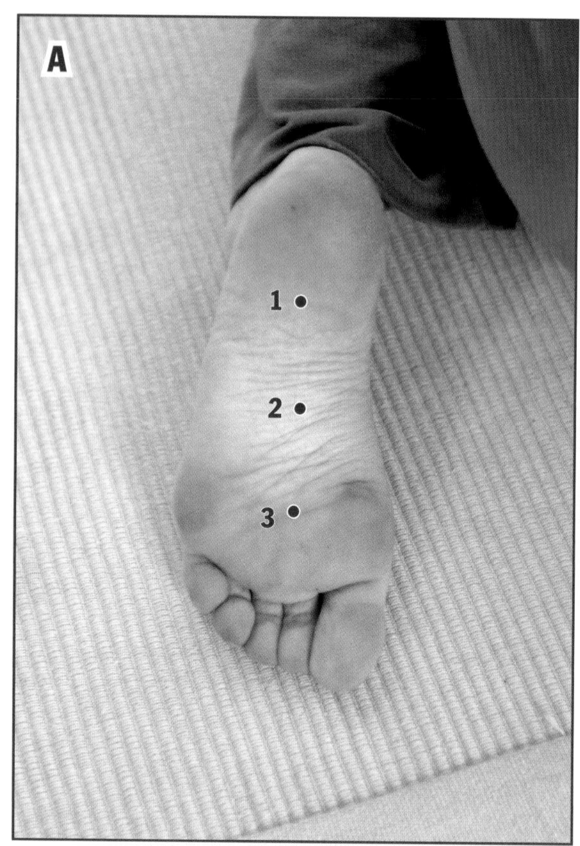

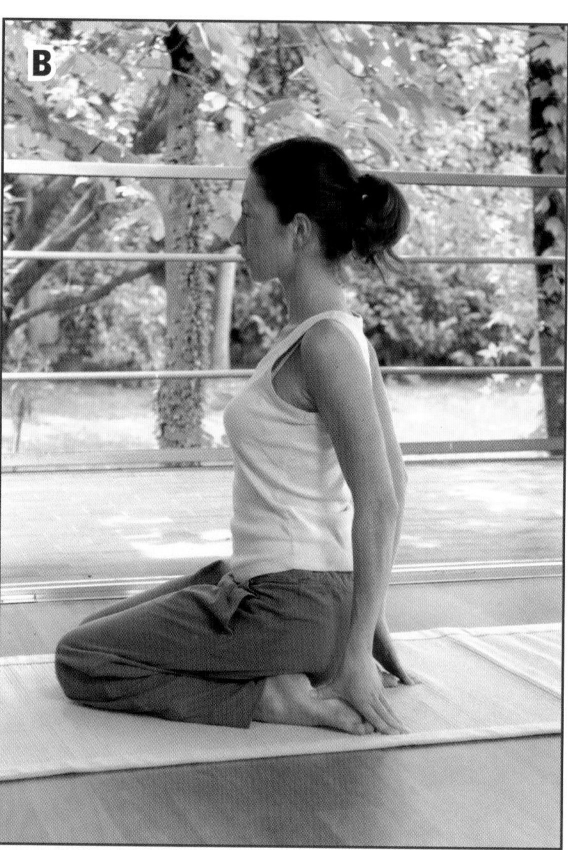

This exercise calls for applying pressure to three points on the soles of the feet (A).

Kneel with the soles of your feet facing up. Place your thumbs on point 1 on each foot (B).

๏ เอนกายกรกดเท้า ภักตร์เหิน หาวแฮ หายที่ขั้นลมเดิน ขัดข้อง -
หมอฤๅษีคุชวัฒน์เจริญ ฌานเกิด ไพ่ฤๅ โลกเรียกชีคุขพ้อง ชื่อผู้เจริญฌาน

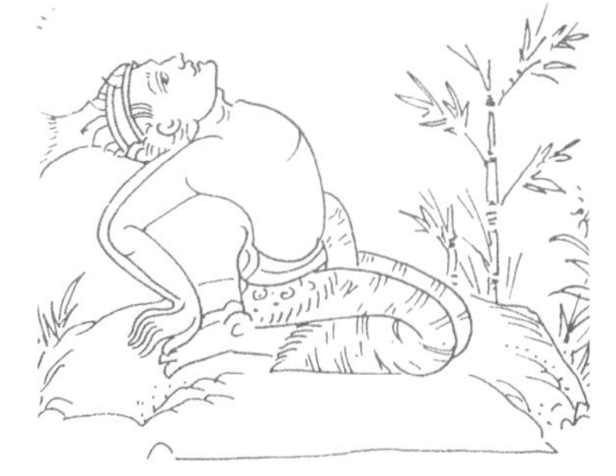

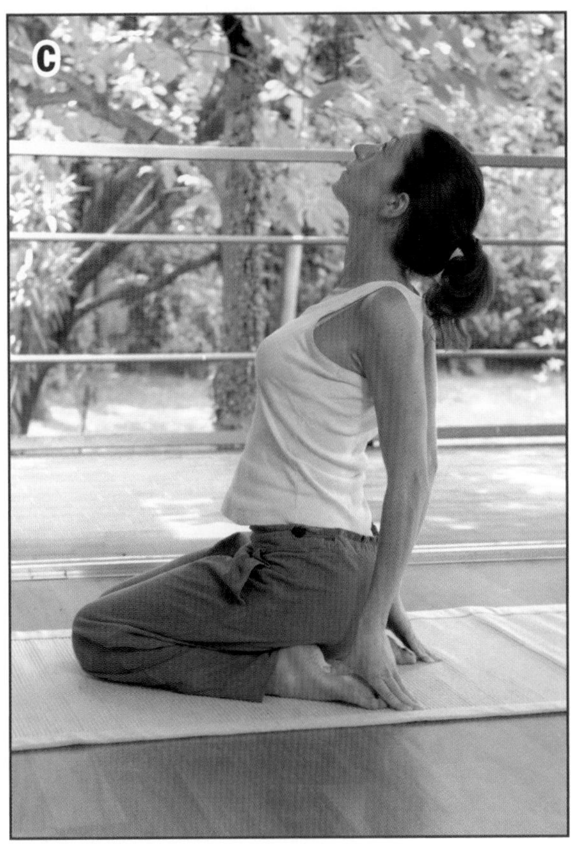

While breathing in, press down on point 1 with your thumbs, allowing the force of your thumbs to bend your head and shoulders backward (C). Avoid moving your chest backward.

Holding your breath, maintain this position for 3 seconds.

As you breathe out, return slowly to the starting position.

Perform the exercise pressing first point 1, then point 2, and then point 3. Go back to point 1 and repeat until each point has been pressed 3 to 5 times.

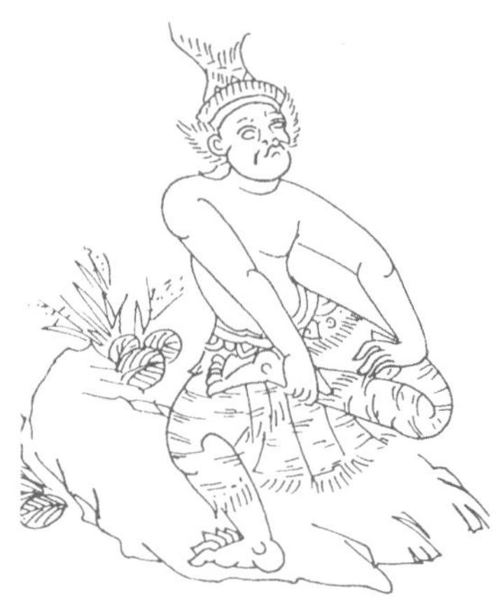

46 Remedy for Heel Pain

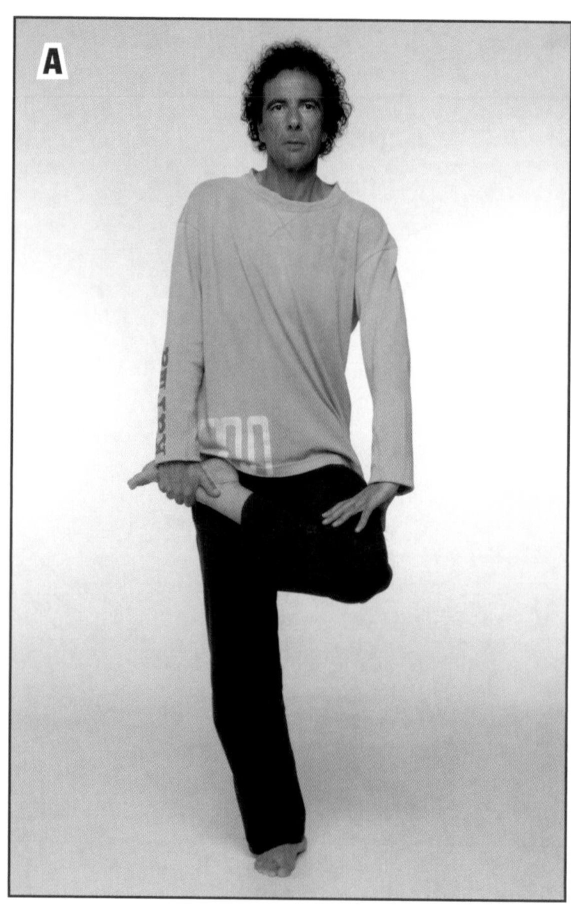

Stand with your left leg bent in front of you, with your left foot on your right hip. Hold your foot with your right hand, and place your left hand on your left thigh, pointing your fingers inward (A).

๏ นักไลยไกรเกรอกฟ้า ดินขาม หมู่แพทย์พึงนับนาม ท่านไหว้
บาทาธึกกะทกตาม ตาตุ่มแลพ่อ กดเข่าเหนี่ยวแค่งให้ ชั่นเท้ามะละลม

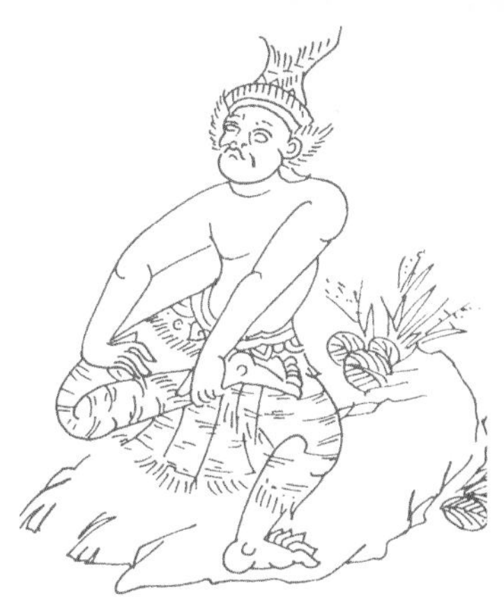

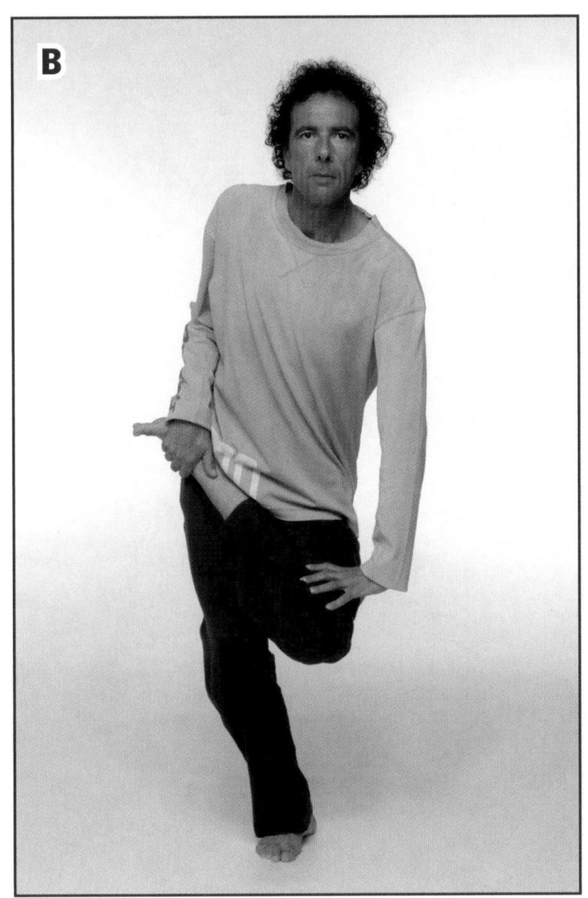

As you breathe in, bend your right knee, and at the same time push your left thigh down and lift your left foot as much as possible (B).

Holding your breath, maintain this position for 3 seconds.

As you breathe out, return slowly to the starting position.

Perform the exercise 3 to 5 times. Then practice the exercise on the other side.

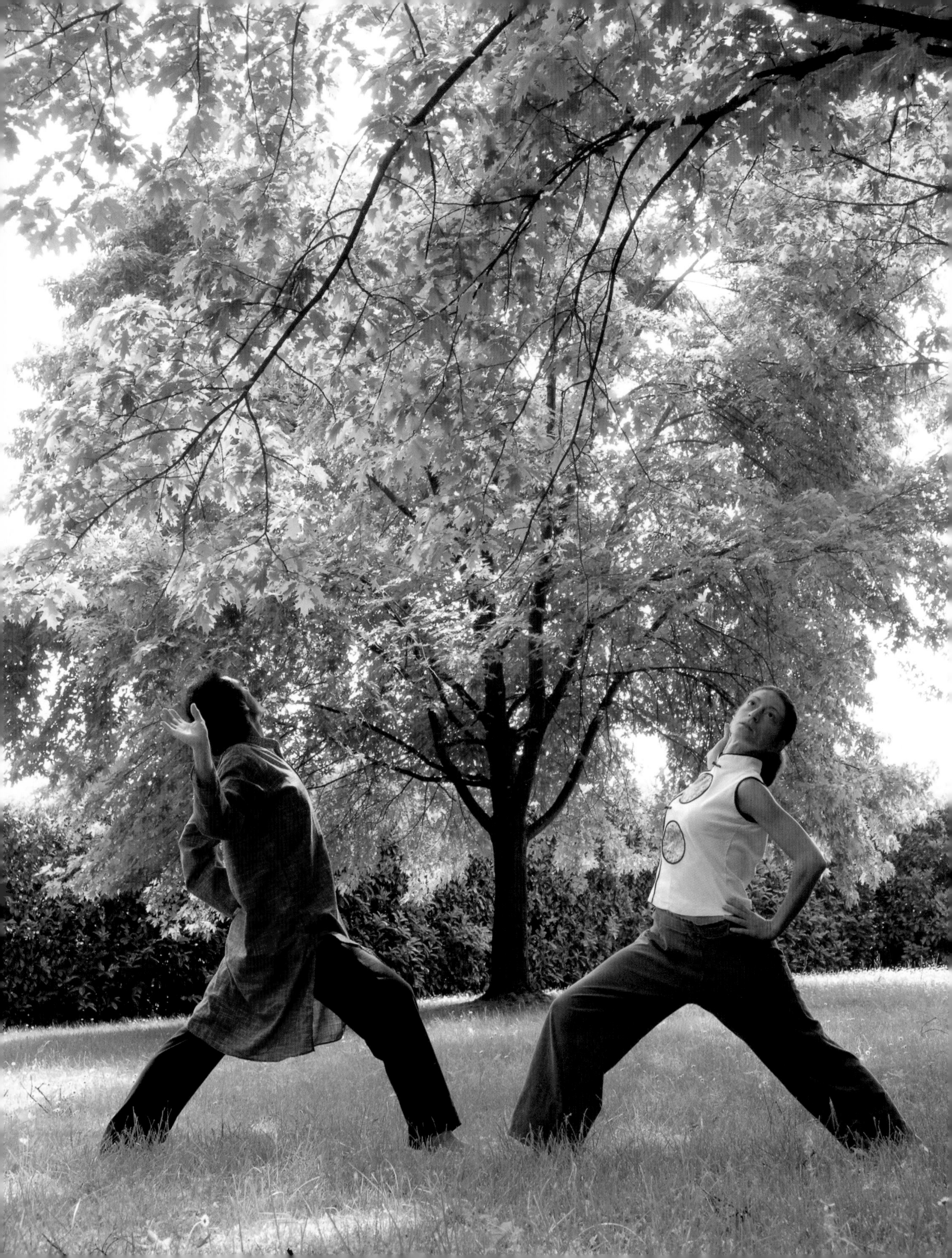

SEVEN

Postures That Remedy Overall Physical or Emotional Health Problems

47. Remedy for Overall Uneasiness
48. Remedy for a Lack of Motivation
49. Remedy for a State of Drowsiness
50. Remedy for a Feeling of Suffocation
51. Remedy for Shortness of Breath
52. Remedy for Feeling Faint
53. Remedy for Nausea and Dizziness
54. Remedy for Vertigo 1
55. Remedy for Vertigo 2
56. Remedy for Chronic Muscular Discomfort
57. Remedy for Painful Muscle Cramps
58. Remedy for Muscle Cramps
59. Remedy for Hemiplegia
60. Posture for Enhancing Longevity

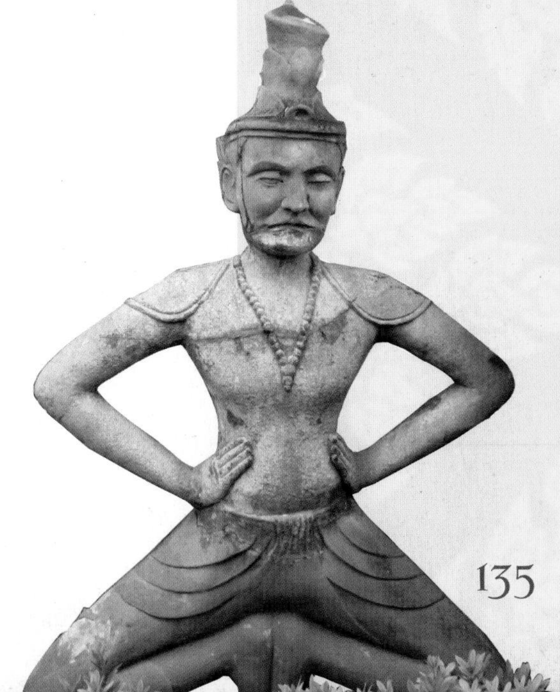

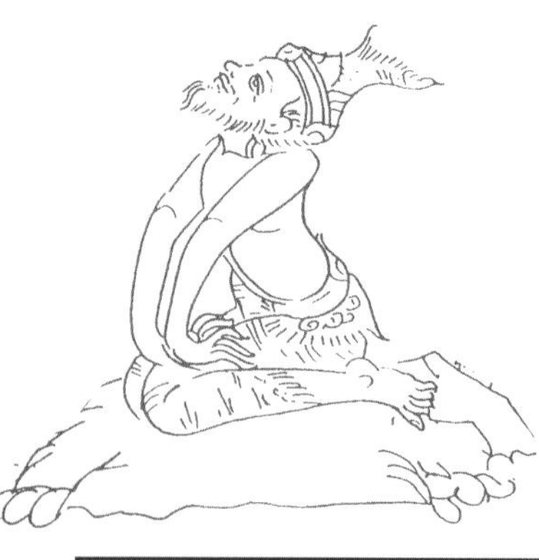

47
Remedy for Overall Uneasiness

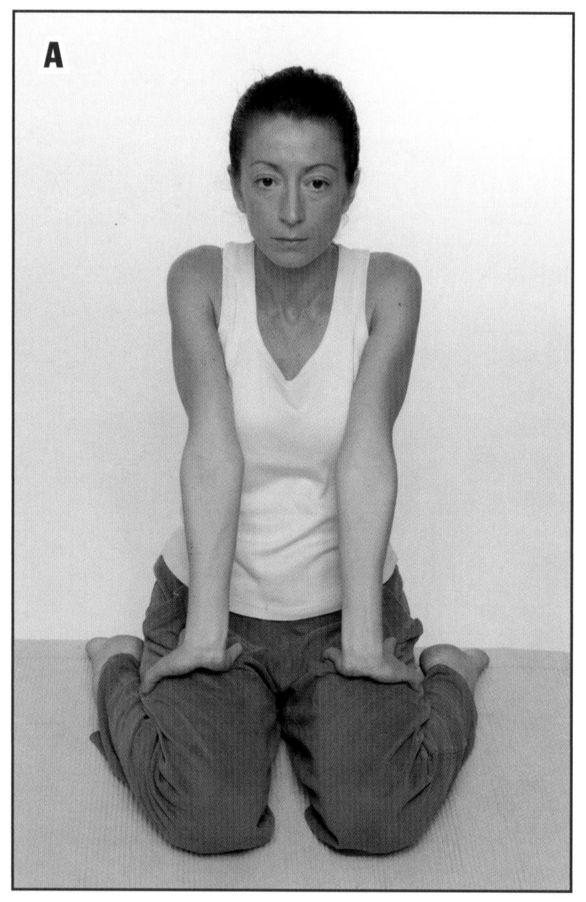
A

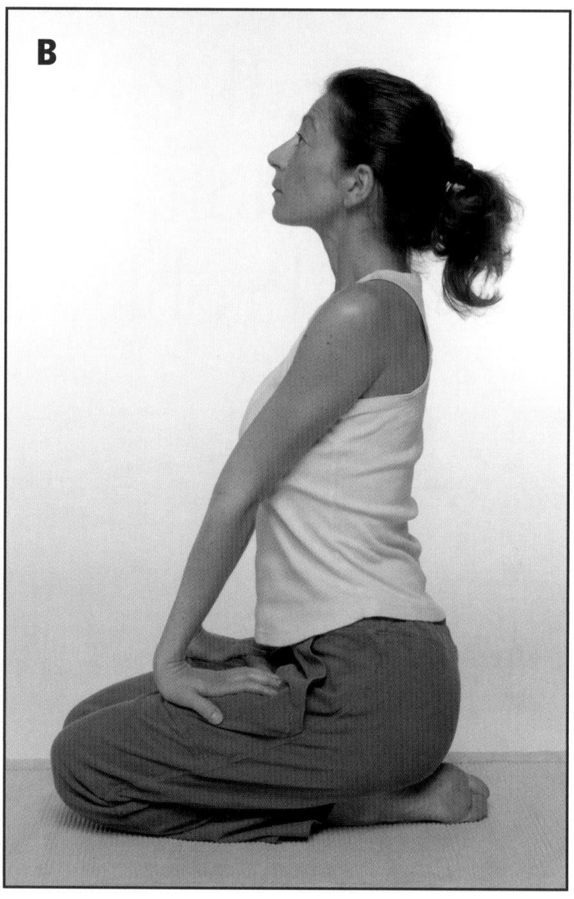
B

Kneel with your legs bent outward and your buttocks on the floor. Turn your arms and place your hands on your legs near your hips, so that your fingers point toward your torso (A). If you cannot achieve this position, you can bring your legs closer together and sit on your feet (B).

๏ เสลขกามนฤมิวิสุทธิก้อง ไตรภพ องค์แอ่นแหงนภักตร์ขบ ขะเม่นฟ้า
กลับแขนกดขทาบ เน้นนิ่งอยู่นา ลมเสียดสารพางค์กล้ำ ดับด้วยดัดเอง

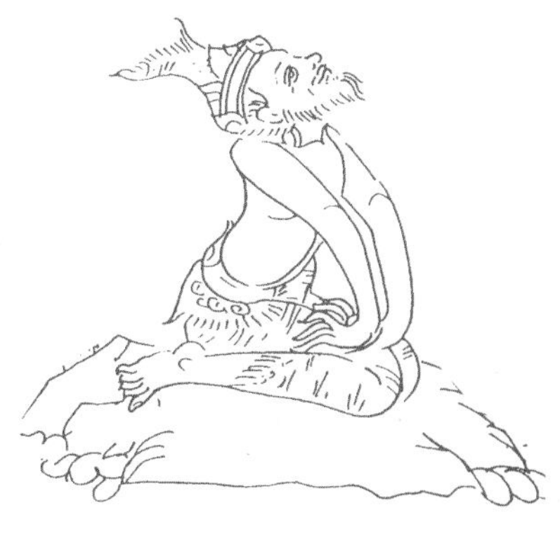

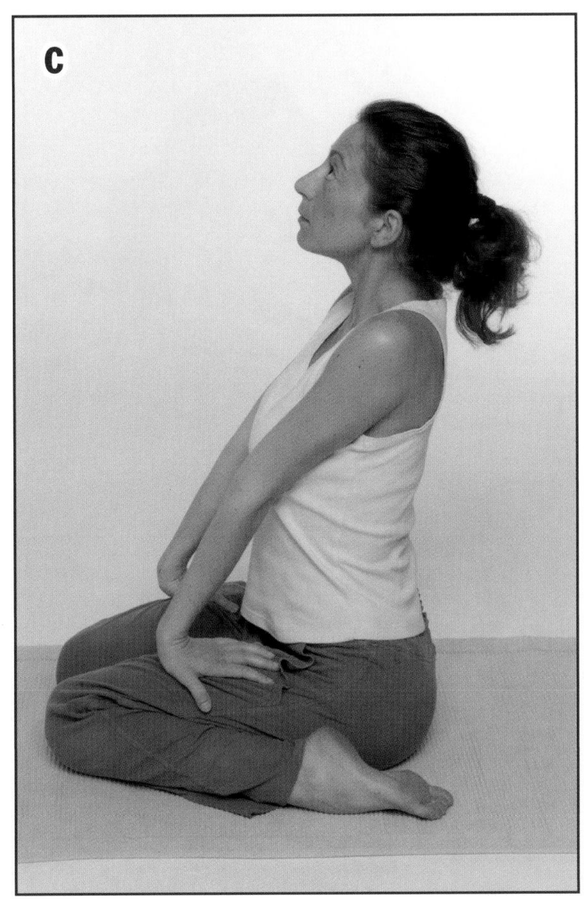

While breathing in, extend your chest, and slightly lift your head backward (C). This movement will further increase the flexion of the wrists.

Holding your breath, maintain this position for 3 seconds.

As you breathe out, return slowly to the starting position.

Perform the exercise 3 to 5 times.

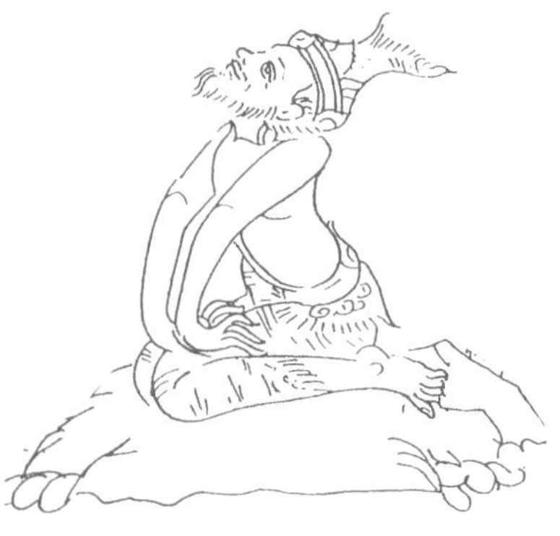

เสลขกามนฤมิวิสุทธิก้อง ไตรภพ องค์แอ่นแหงนภักตร์ขบ ขะเม่นฟ้า

จับแขนกดขาทบ เน้นนิ่งอยู่นา ลมเสียดสารพางค์กล้า ดับด้วยดัดเอง

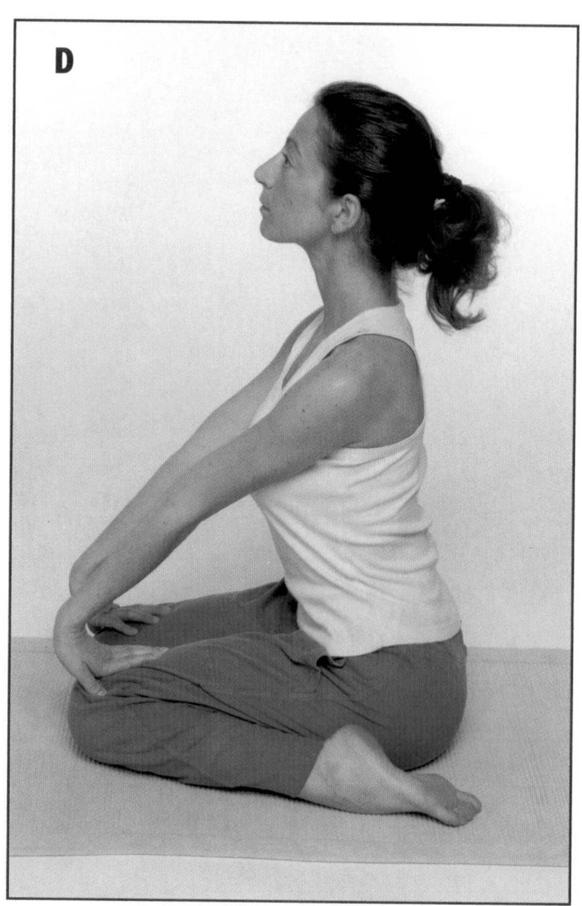

If flexing your wrists so close to your torso is difficult, you can place your hands farther away, near your knees (D). Then complete the exercise as directed for figure C.

48

Remedy for a Lack of Motivation

(Due More to Physical than to Psychological Causes)

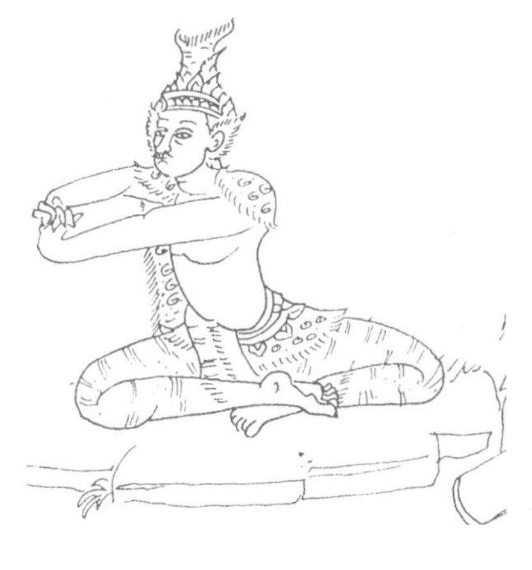

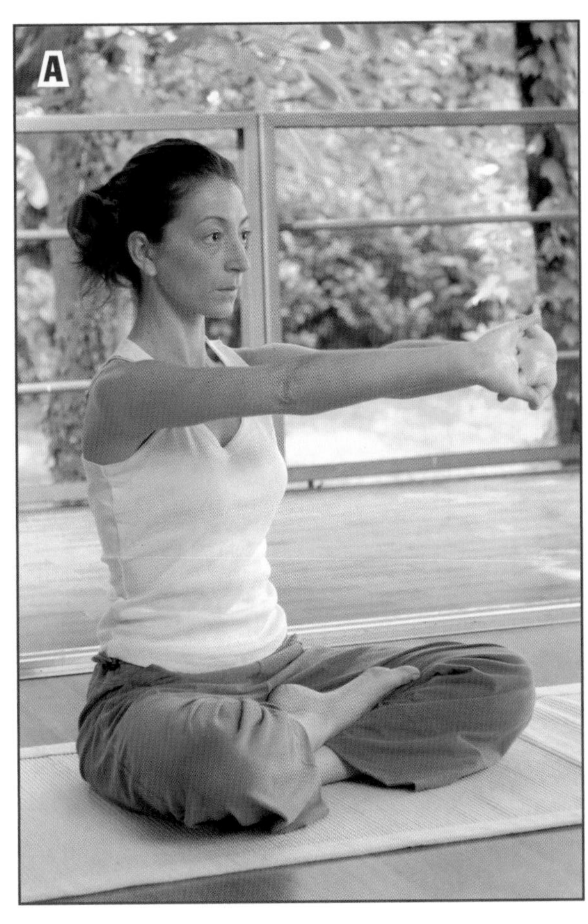

Sit in the half-lotus position with your right leg over your left. Intertwine your fingers and stretch your arms out in front of you, with your palms facing away from you (A).

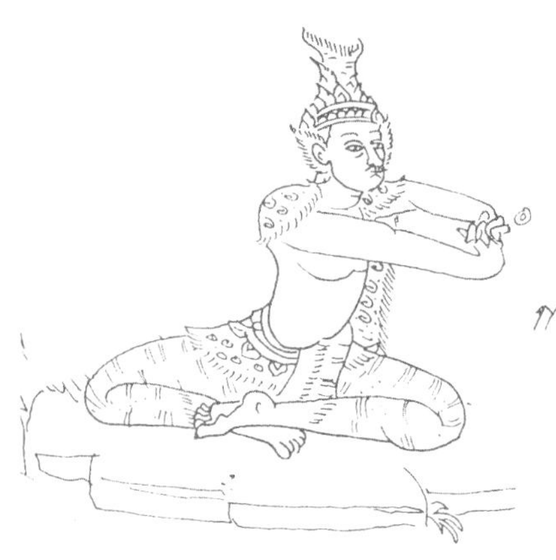

๑ สังกะสีดีบุกเช้า ระคนเจือ หล่อคณะนั่งหนังเสือ สถิตไว้
กามันตะกี่เชื่อ ข่อยหนุ่ม นักหนอ เหยียดยืดหัตถ์ดัดได้ แต่แก้เกียจกาย 

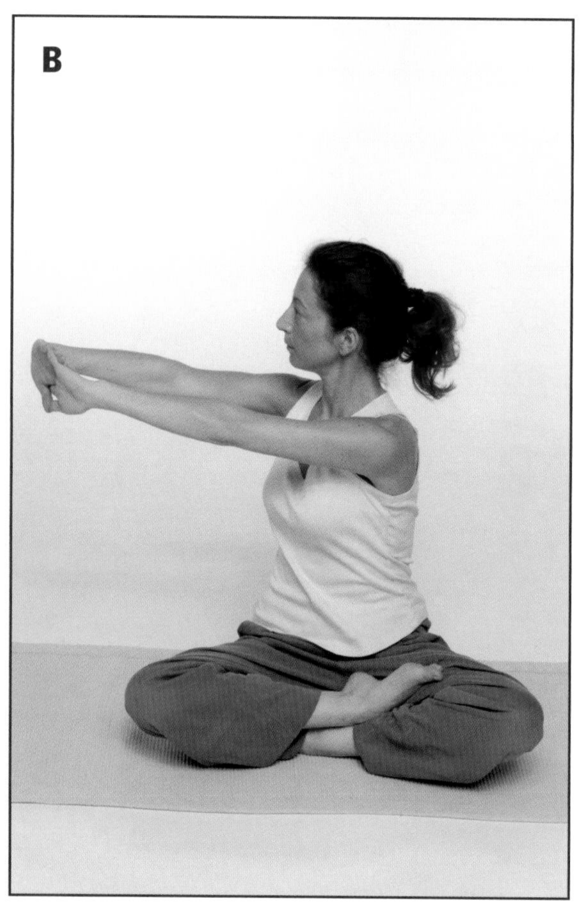

B

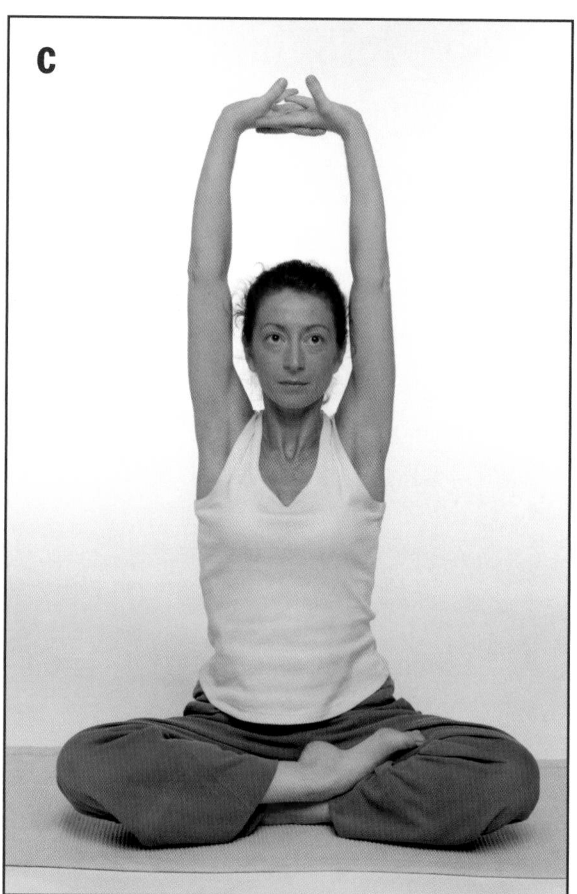

C

Breathing in, turn your body to the right as far as you can, using your arms to extend the turn (B).

Holding your breath, maintain this position for 3 seconds.

As you breathe out, return slowly to the starting position.

Keeping your fingers intertwined, lift your arms over your head (C).

๑ สังกะสีดีบุกเข้า ระคนเจือ หล่อคณะนั่งหนังเสือ สถิตไว้
กามันตะกีเชื่อ ข้อยหนุ่ม นักนอ เหยียดยืดหัตถ์ดัดได้ แต่แก้เกียจกาย ฯ

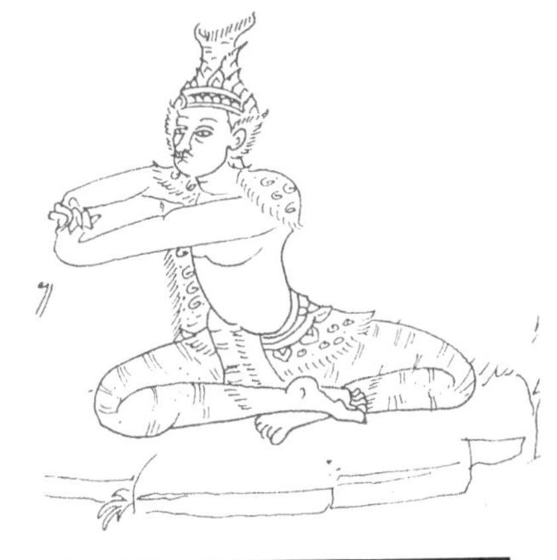

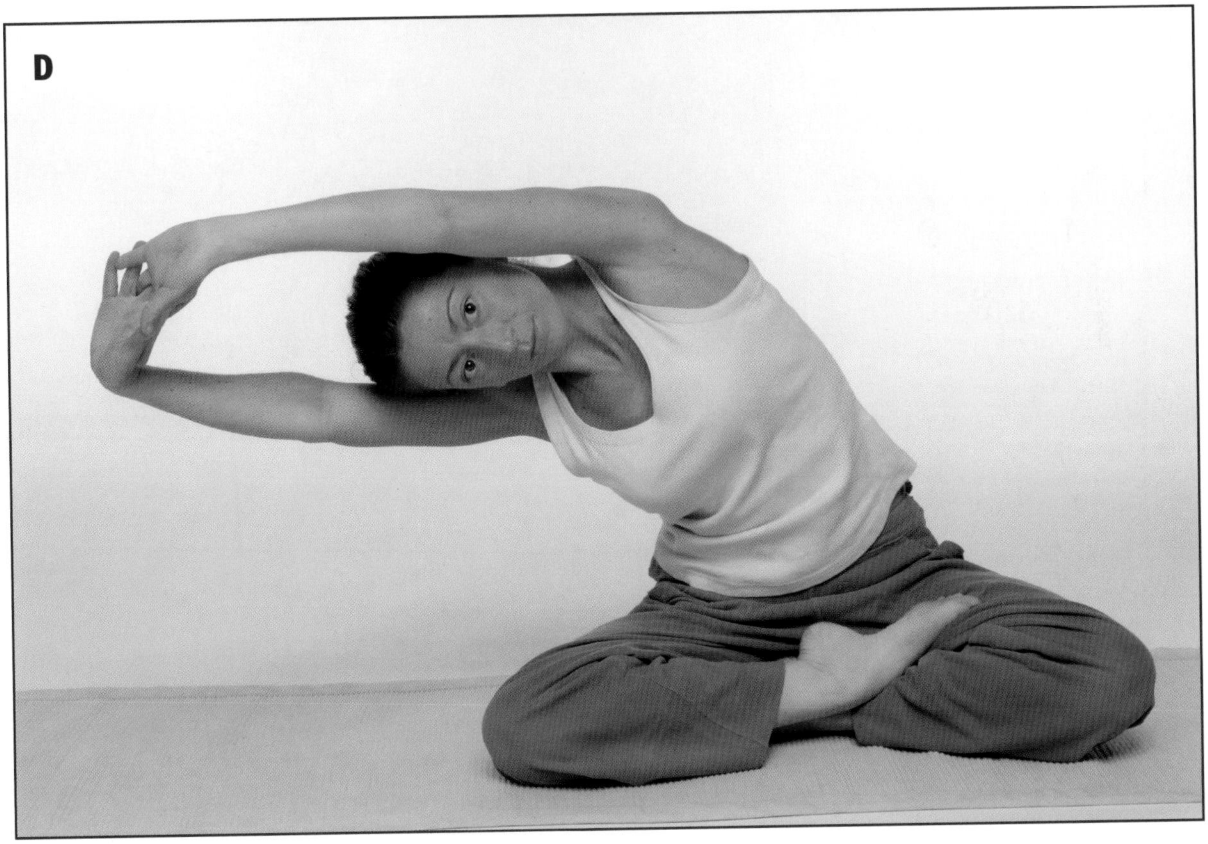

D

While breathing in, bend to the right as far as you can, using your arms to extend the bend (D).

Holding your breath, maintain this position for 3 seconds.

As you breathe out, return slowly to the starting position.

Perform the exercise 3 to 5 times. Then practice the exercise on the other side, now sitting with your left leg over your right and turning and bending to the left.

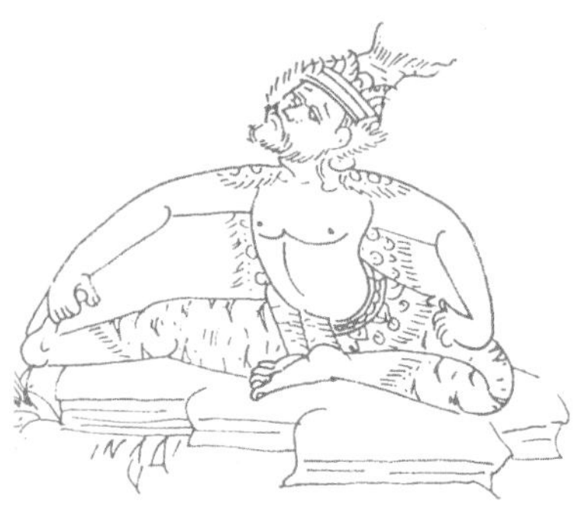

49
Remedy for a State of Drowsiness

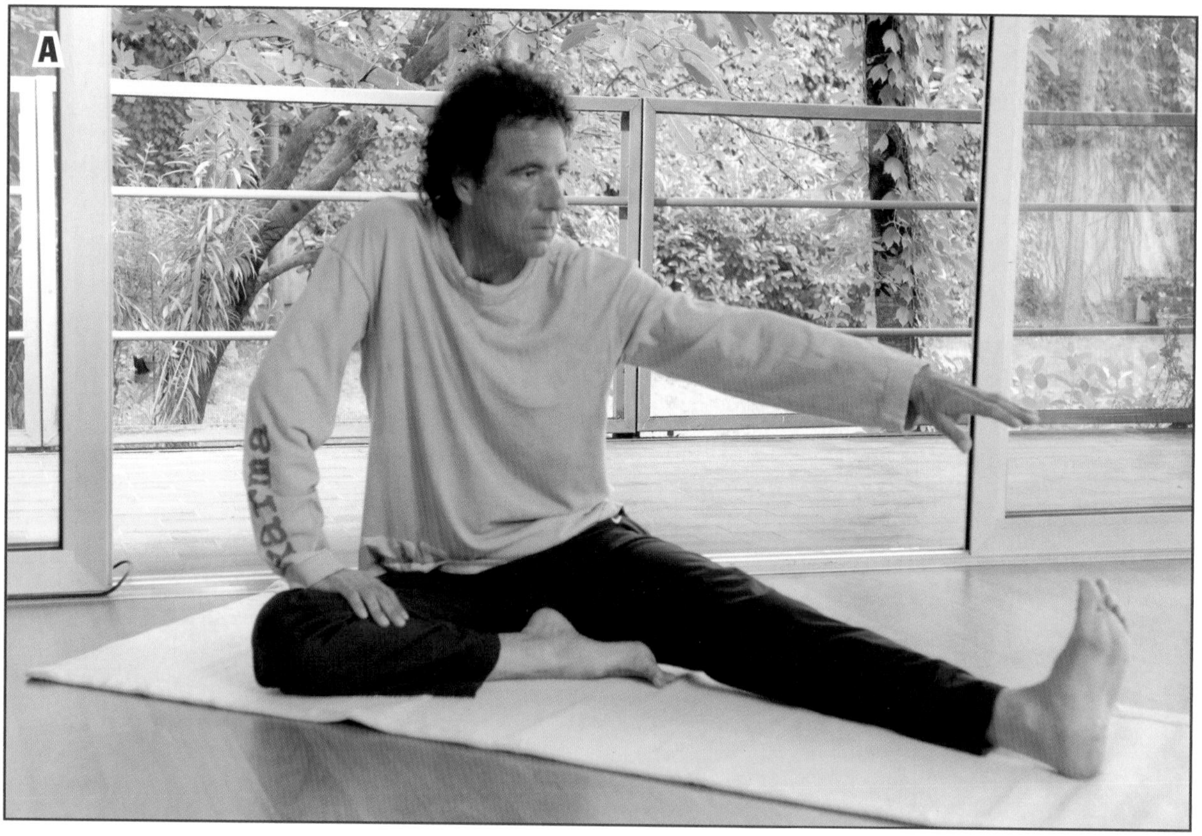

Sit with your left leg extended as much to the side as possible. Fold your right leg in, with its foot against your left thigh. Place your right hand on your right thigh, with your fingers pointing inward, and extend your left arm over your left leg. Turn your head toward your left foot (A).

๑ กมินทร์มือยุดเท้า เหยียดหยัด มือหนึ่งเท้าเข่าขัด สมาธิคู้
เข้าฌานช่วยแรงดัด ทุกค่ำคืนนา ระงับราคหยากจสู้ โรคร้ายพายใน

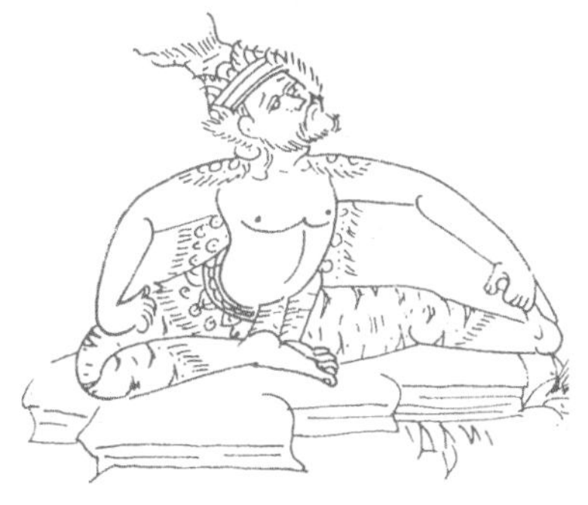

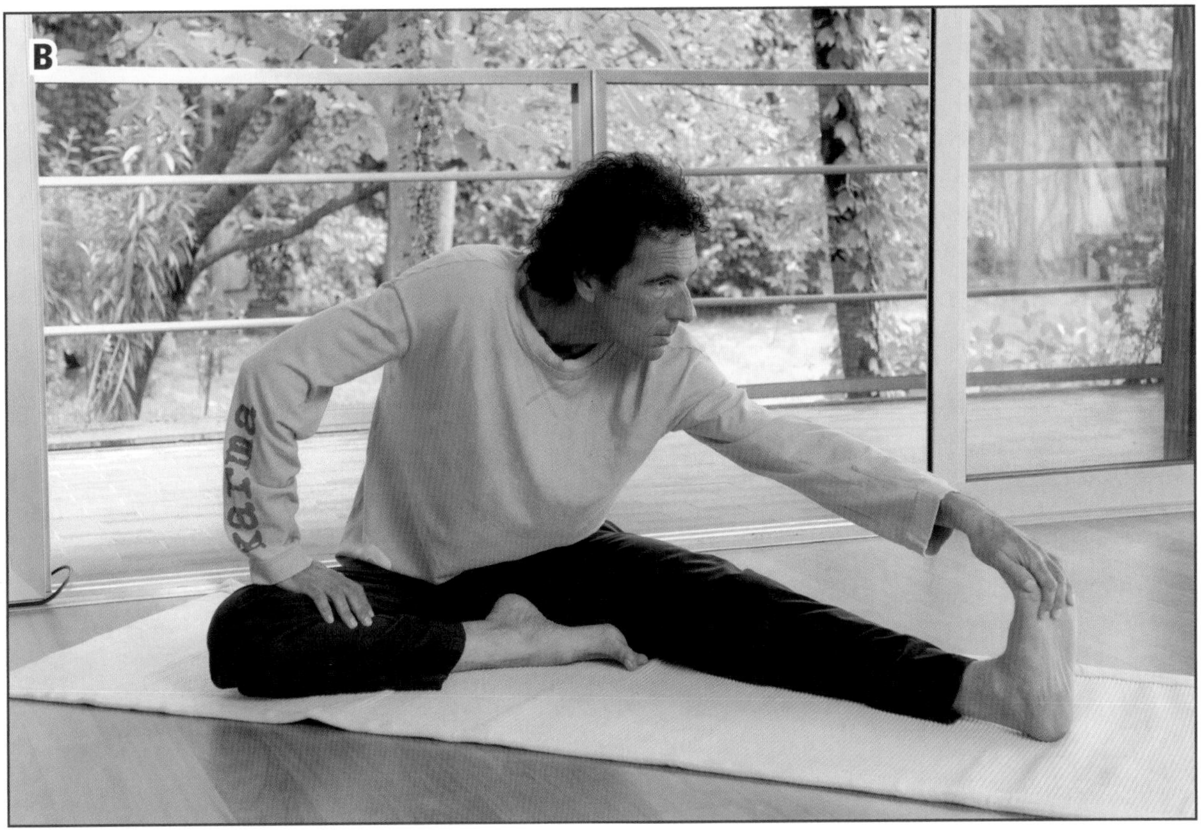

While breathing out, bend forward, pushing yourself with your right arm, and grab your left foot with your left hand (B). If you cannot keep your left leg completely straight, you can bend it slightly.

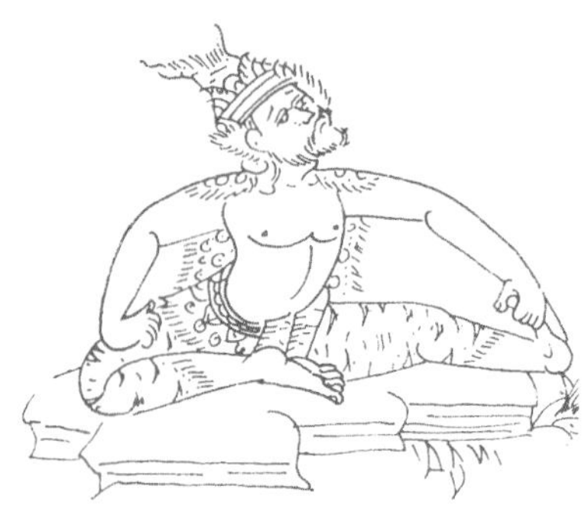

๏ กามินทร์มือยุดเท้า เหยียดหยัด มือหนึ่งเท้าเข่าขัด สมาธิคู้
เข้าฌาณช่วยแมงดัด ทุกค่ำคืนนา รงับภาคหยากจสู้ โรคร้ายพายใน

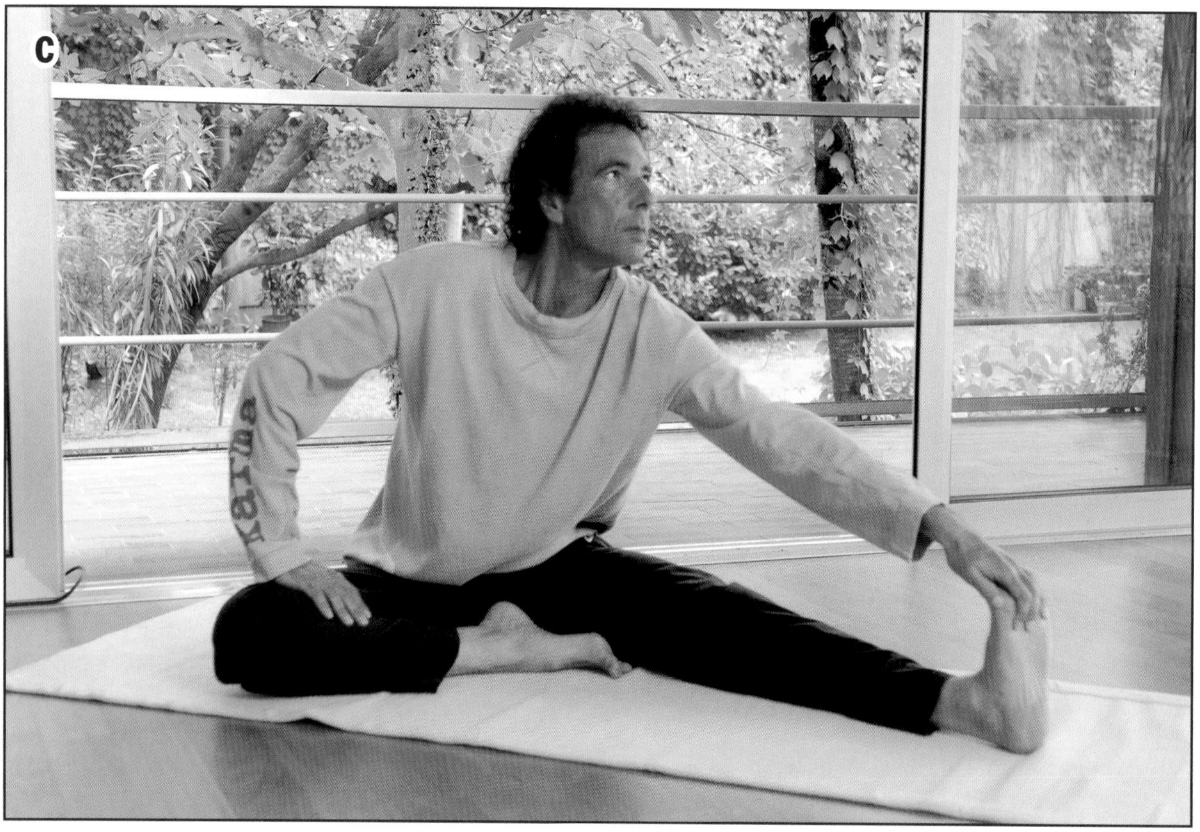

C

As you breathe in, lift your head, straighten your chest, and flex your left foot (C).

Holding your breath, maintain this position for 3 seconds.

As you breathe out, return slowly to the starting position.

Perform the exercise 3 to 5 times. Then practice the exercise on the other side.

50
Remedy for a Feeling of Suffocation

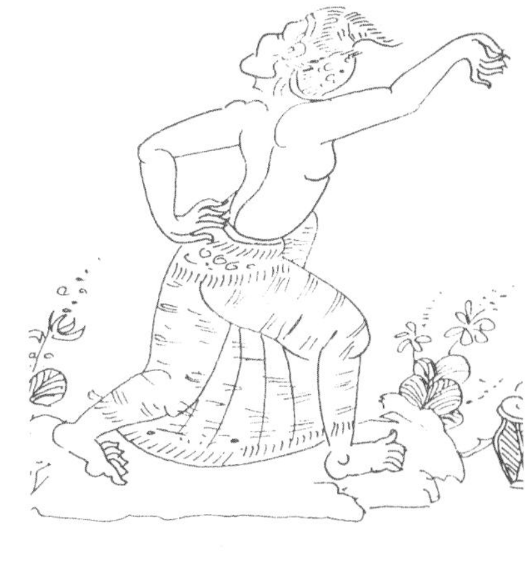

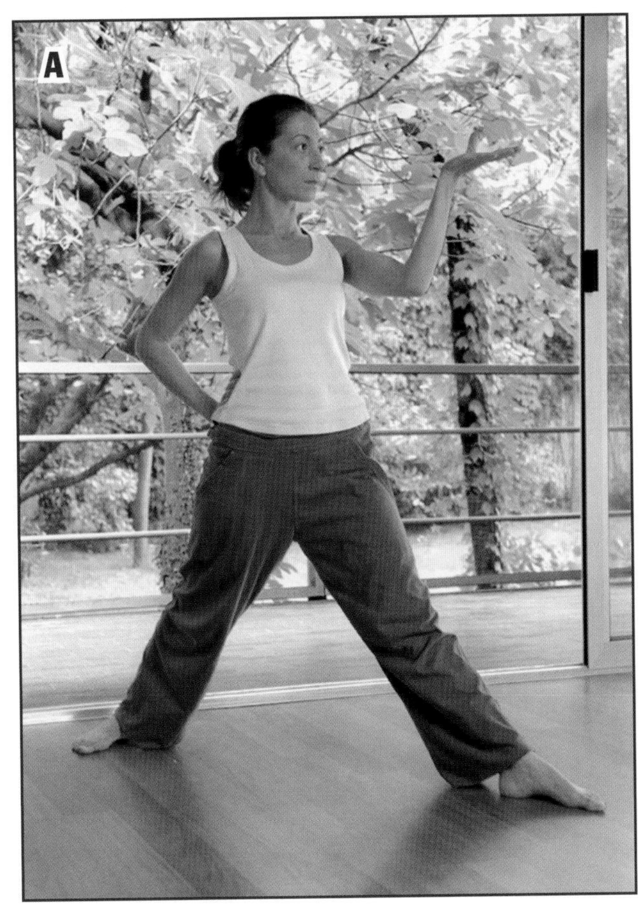

Stand with your legs apart. Pull your right leg back and point your left foot forward, so that your heels are aligned and your feet are perpendicular to each other. Bend your left arm in front of you, keeping the wrist well flexed, and place your right hand on your hip (A).

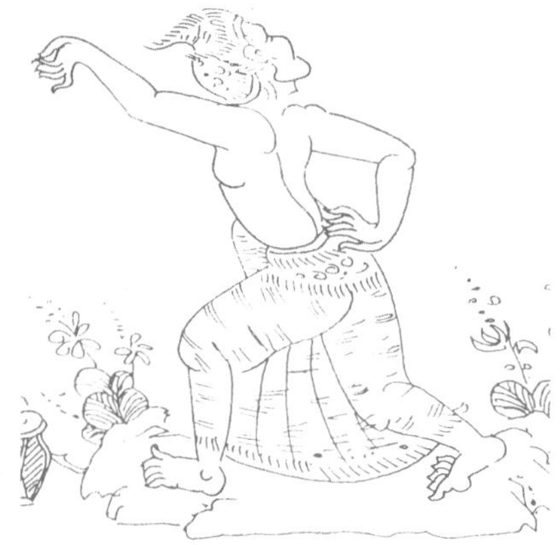

๏ อายันญาณยิ่งผู้ ผนวชเขก เนกพนัศฝ่าแฝก หาบหิ้ว
โรคลมแล่นดูแดก วางหาบ ดัดแฮ แอนอกเอี้ยวสยิ้ว แสยะหน้าเงอหงาย

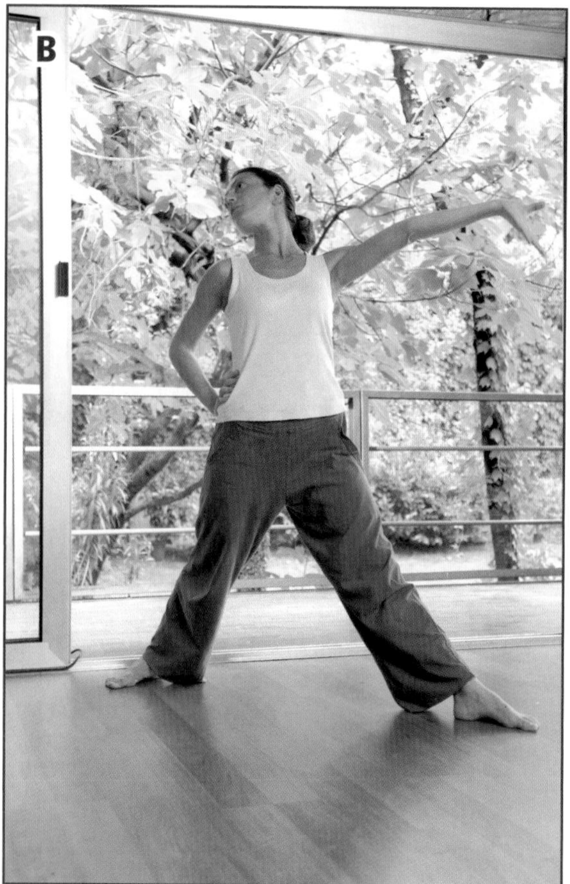

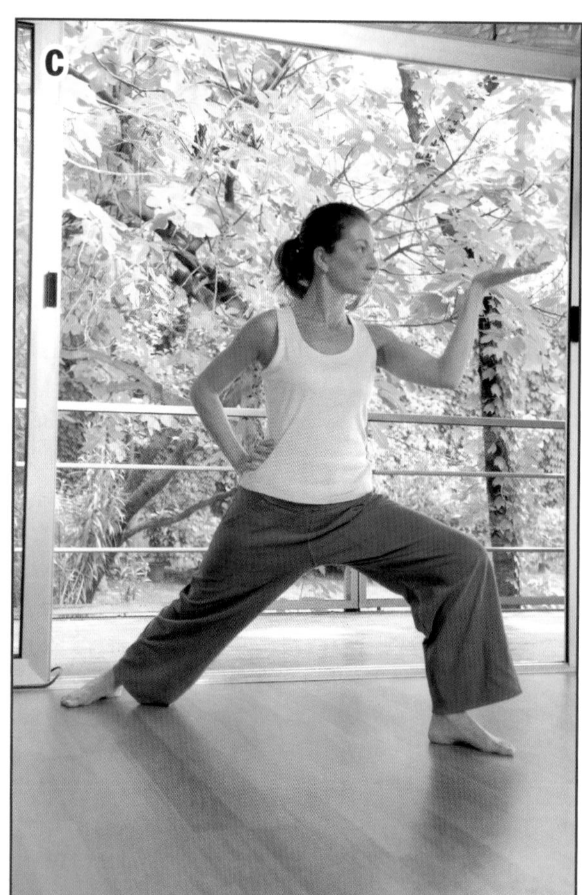

While breathing in, stretch your left arm out straight, and turn your head to the right as far as you can (B).

Holding your breath, maintain this position for 3 seconds.

As you breathe out, return slowly to the starting position.

After taking a breath, breathe out and bend your left leg at a 90-degree angle, stretching your right leg (C).

๏ อายันญาณยิ่งผู้ ผนวชแขก เนกพนัศฝ่าแฝก หาบหิ้ว
โรคลมแล่นดุแดก วางหาบ ดัดแฮ แอ่นอกเอี้ยวสยิ้ว แสยะหน้าเงือหงาย

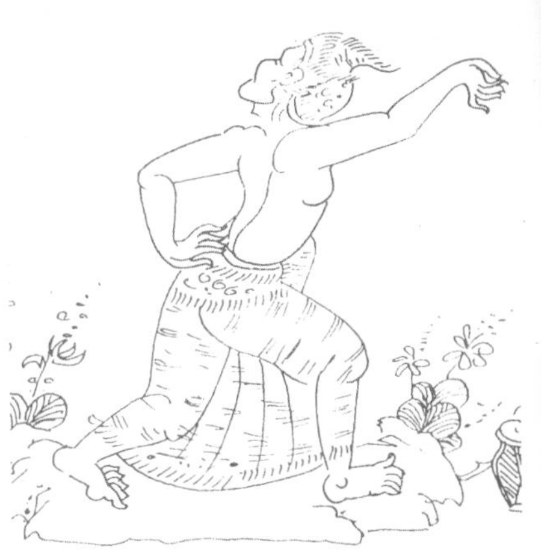

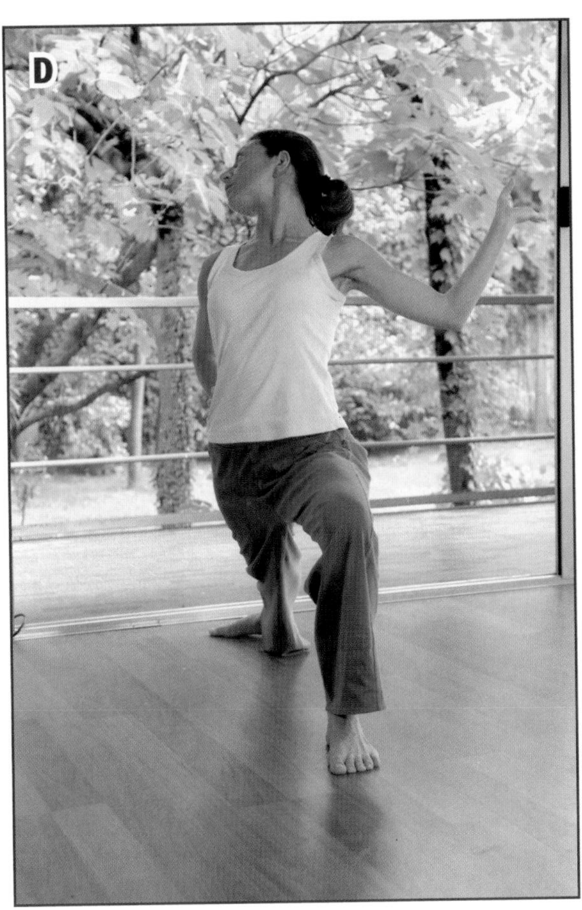

As you breathe in, turn your head to the right as far as you can, and pull your bent left arm to the left, which will cause your chest to open (D).

Holding your breath, maintain this position for 3 seconds.

As you breathe out, return slowly to the starting position.

Perform the exercise 3 to 5 times. Then practice the exercise on the other side.

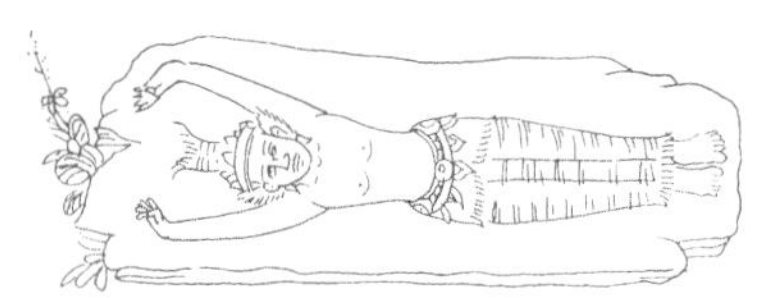

51
Remedy for Shortness of Breath

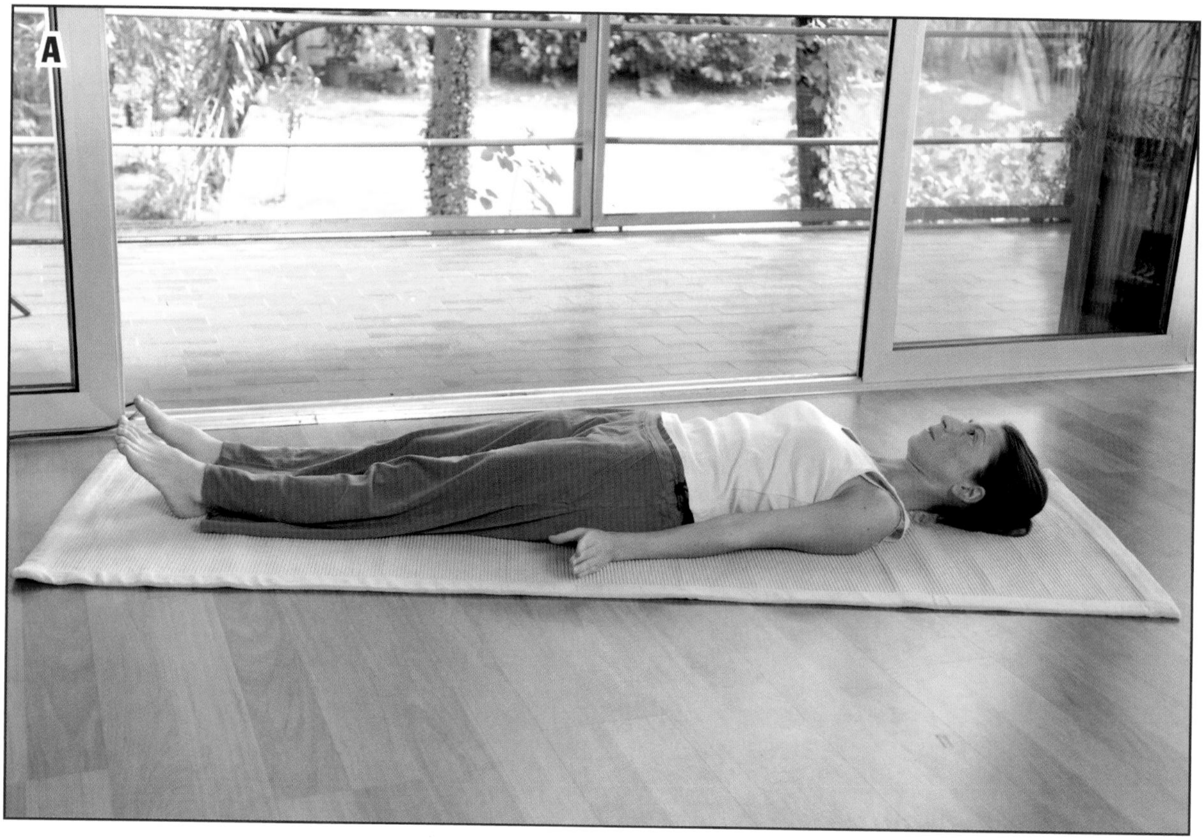

Lie on your back, with your arms at your sides and your wrists well flexed (A).

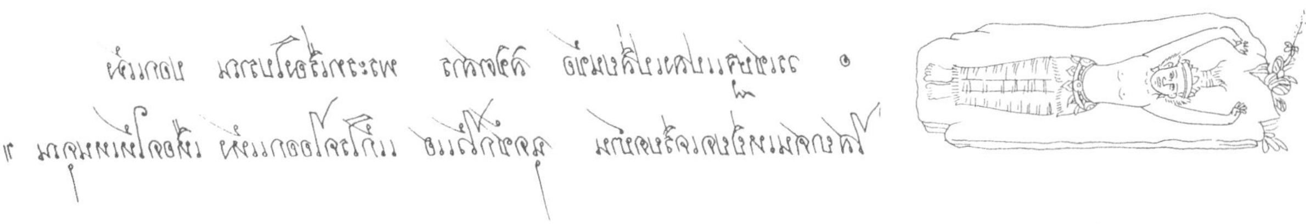

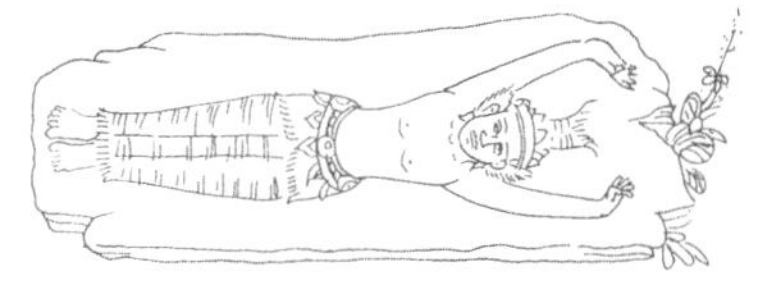

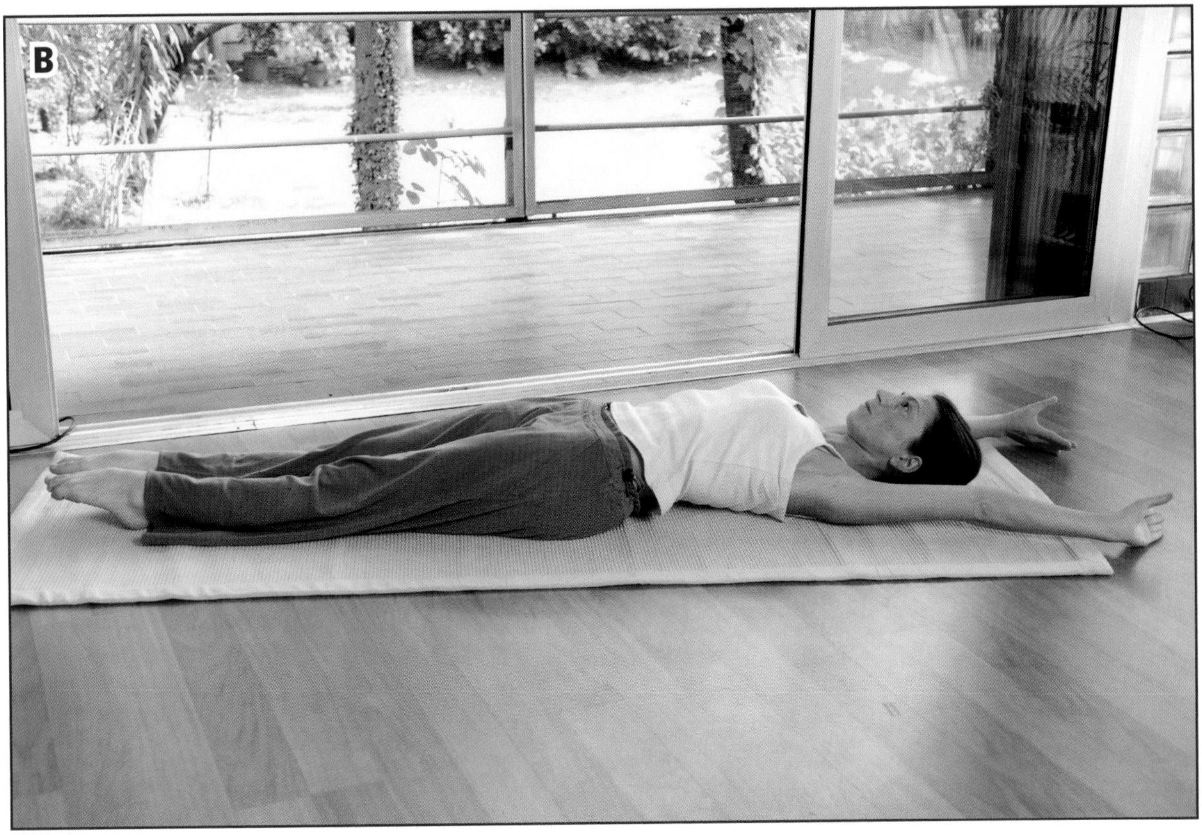

Breathing in, slowly raise your arms over your head, keeping your wrists flexed (B).

Holding your breath, maintain this position for 3 seconds.

As you breathe out, return slowly to the starting position.

Perform the exercise 5 to 7 times.

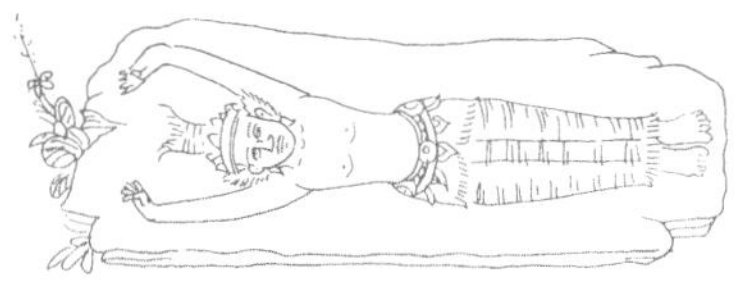

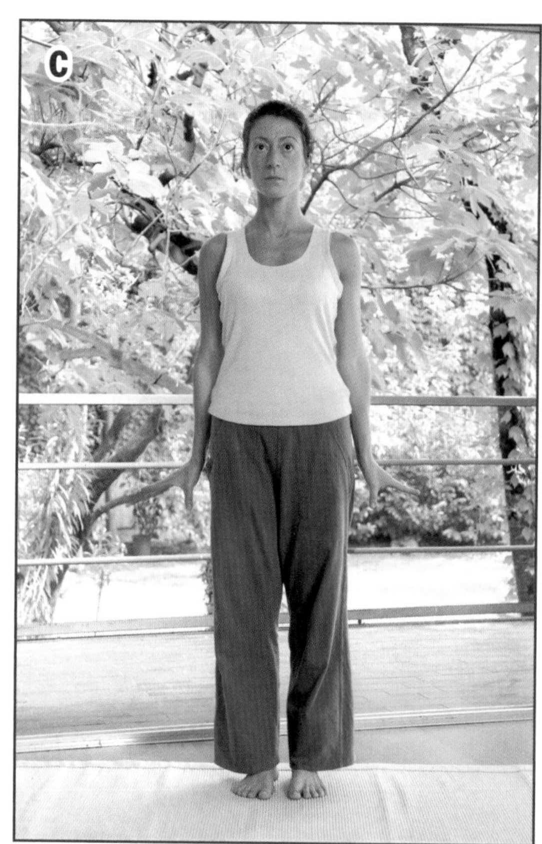

AN ALTERNATIVE FORM OF THE EXERCISE

This exercise can also be performed from a standing position:

Stand with your feet close together and your arms at your sides, with your wrists well flexed (C).

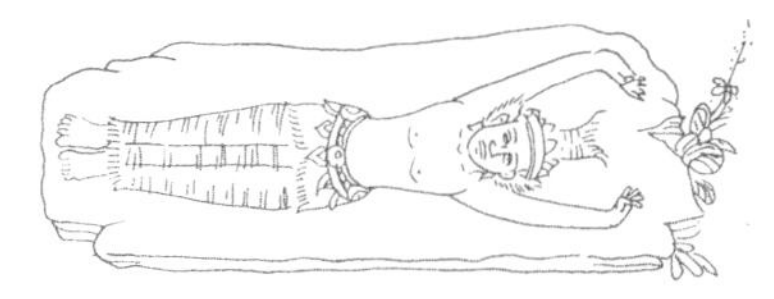

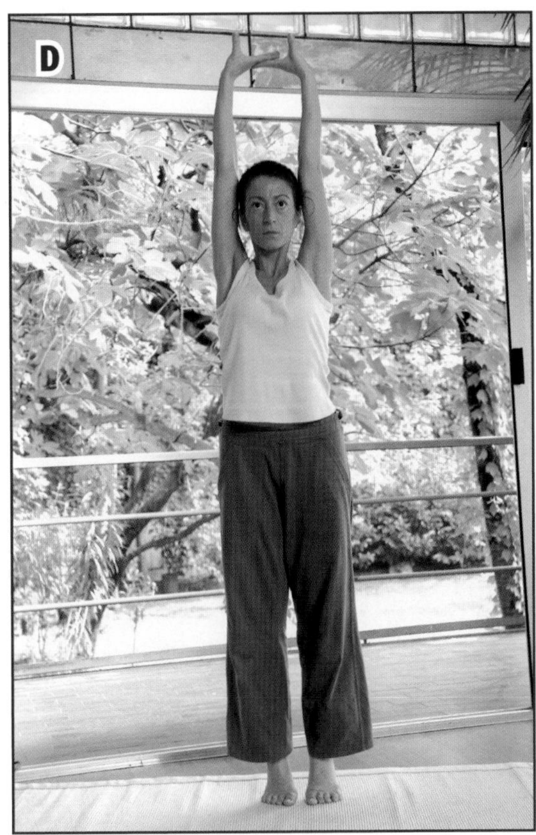

Breathing in, slowly raise your arms over your head, flexing your wrists as much as possible. When your arms are completely stretched, rise up onto the tips of your toes (D).

Holding your breath, maintain this position for 3 seconds.

As you breathe out, slowly return to the starting position, lowering your arms until they are alongside your body and then dropping down from your toes to your feet.

Perform the exercise 5 to 7 times.

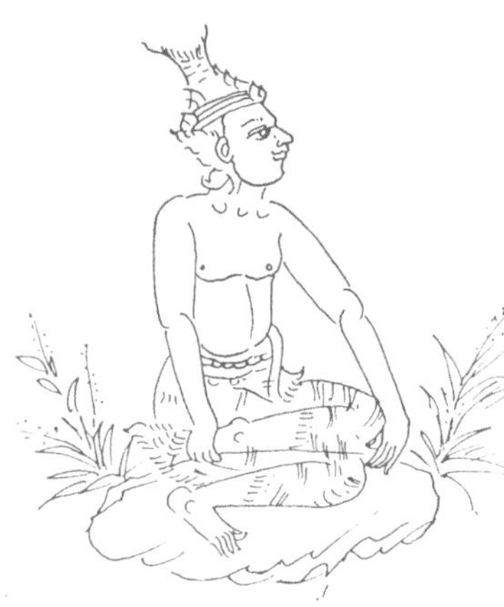

52 Remedy for Feeling Faint

(Additional Symptom—Feet Feel Cold)

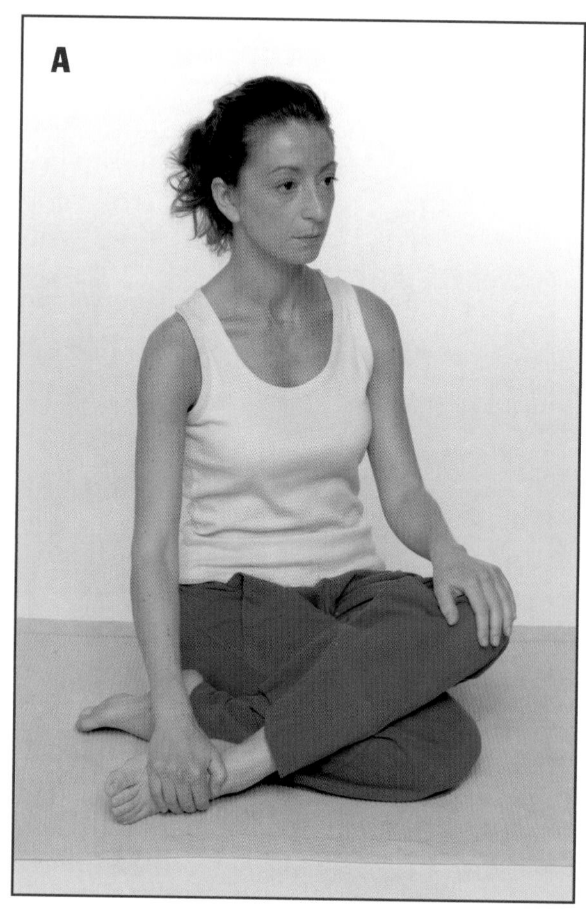

Sit on a cushion with both legs bent to the right, left leg bent over the right. Place your left hand on your left knee, and hold your left foot with your right hand (A).

๑ นักพรตประพฤติสร้าง จรรยา ไชยดชื่อกระปิลดา บทเจ้า
เท้าซ้ายไขว่เพลาขวา มือหน่วงเข่าเอย ลมรงับจับเย็นเท้า อีกทั้งสิ้นสาย

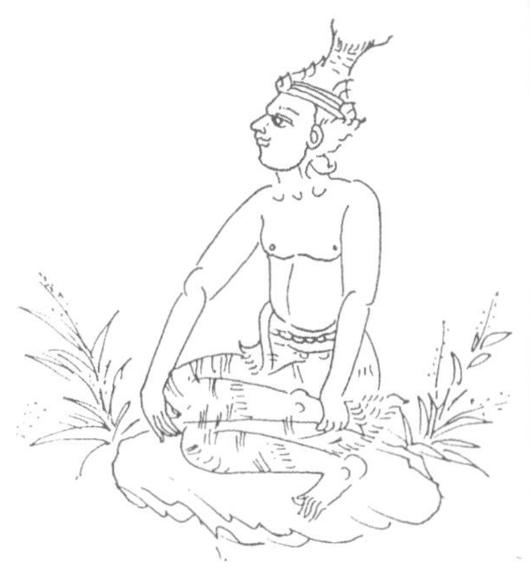

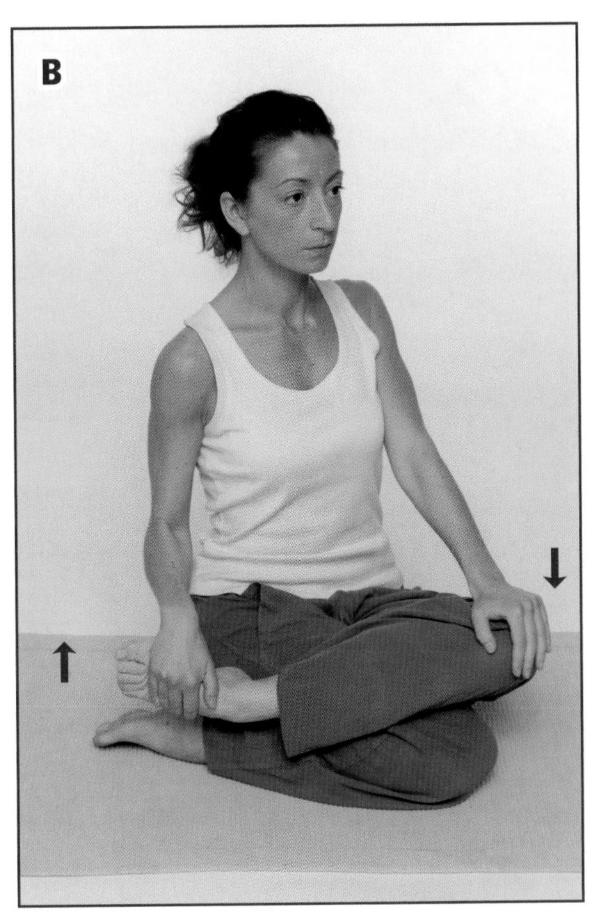

While breathing in, use your right hand to pull your left foot up and toward you, and at the same time use your left hand to push your left knee down (B).

Holding your breath, maintain this position for 3 seconds.

As you breathe out, return slowly to the starting position.

Perform the exercise 3 to 5 times. Then practice the exercise on the other side.

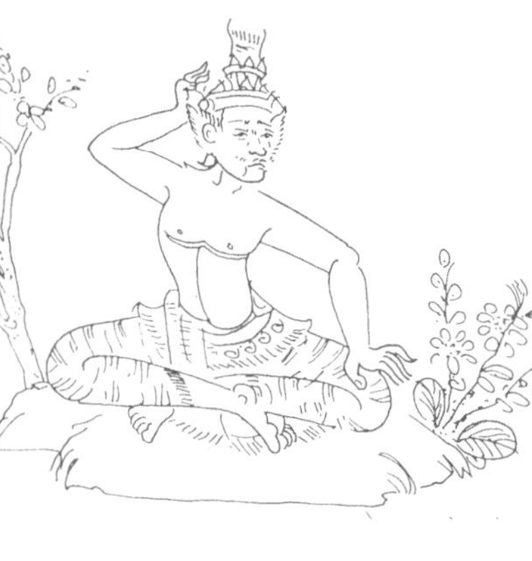

53 Remedy for Nausea and Dizziness

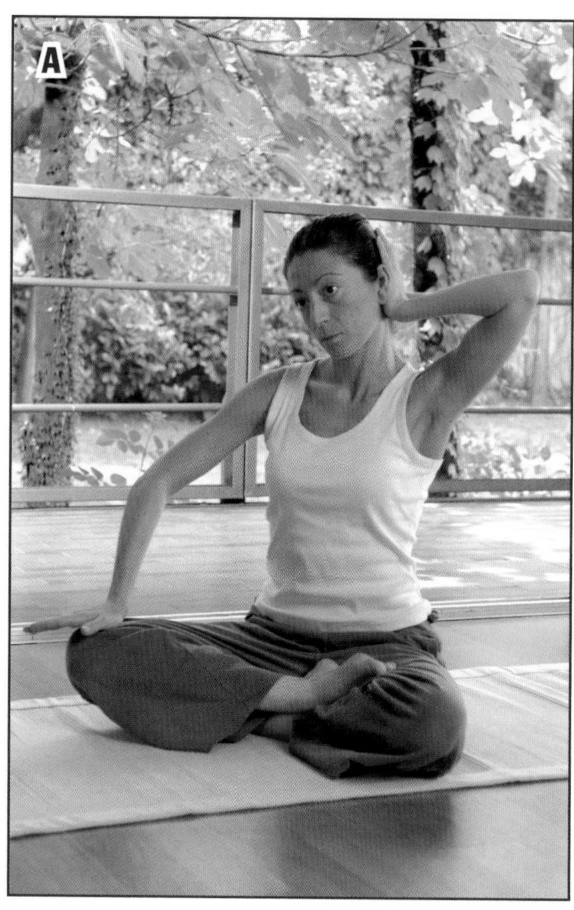

Sit in the half-lotus position. Place the heel of your left hand just below the occipital bone behind your left ear. Place the palm of your right hand on your right knee, with the fingers lifted, the elbow slightly bent, and the shoulder relaxed (A).

๏ สมกิจขัดหัดถ์ยุดทั้ง เพลาเศียร สระสร่างแสลงลมเวียน ศีระเกล้า
นามชะหะพระผู้เพียร ผนวดเน่อนนานแฮ ธะอักษรควบเข้า เพ่อมให้นามกรุง ฯ

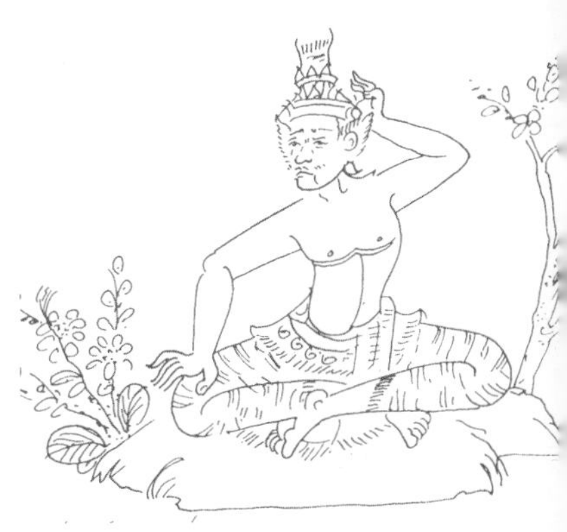

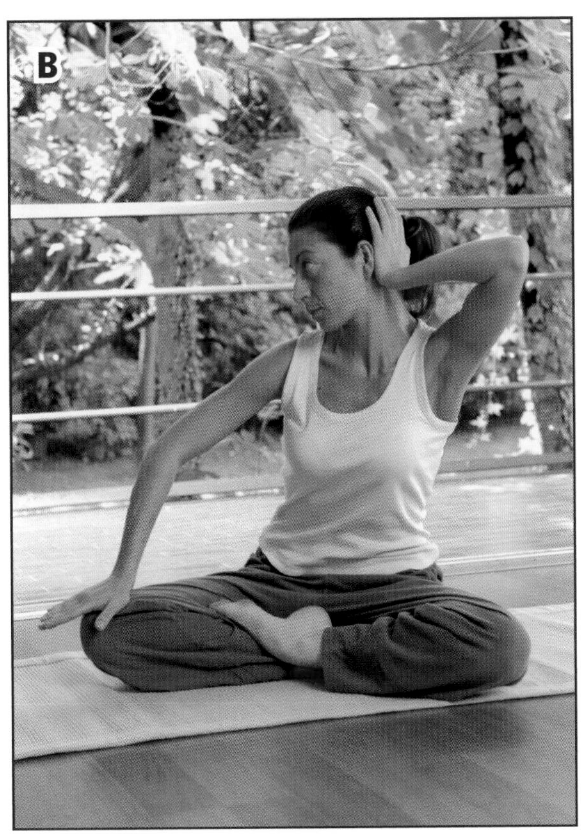

As you breathe in, push against your head with your left hand, turning and bending it to the right as far as you can. At the same time slightly turn your chest toward the left and push against your right leg with your right hand so that your right shoulder remains still (B).

Holding your breath, maintain this position for 3 seconds.

As you breathe out, return slowly to the starting position.

Repeat the exercise on the other side.

Practice the exercise 3 to 5 times.

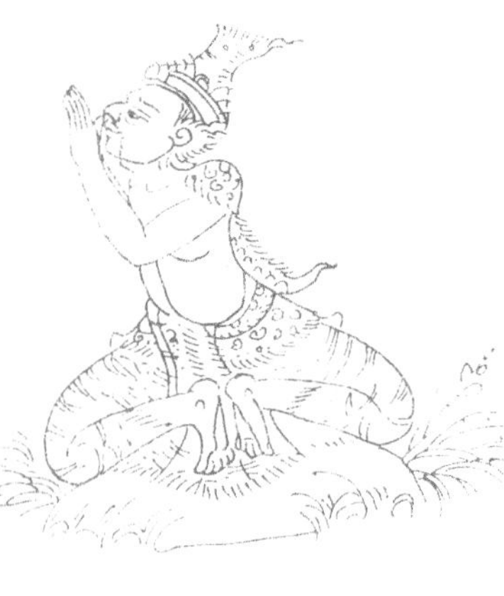

54 Remedy for Vertigo 1

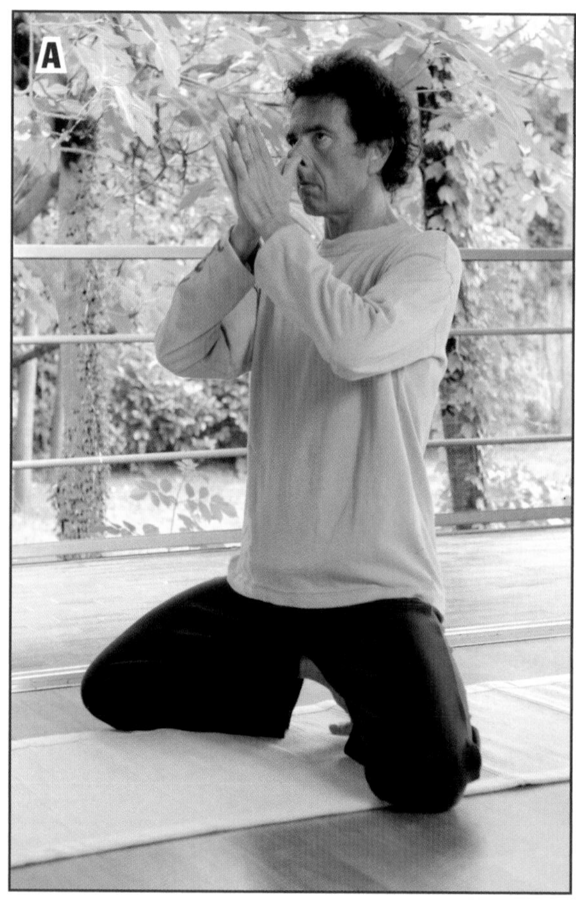

Kneel with your feet flexed, resting your buttocks on your heels and opening your legs as widely as you can. Bring your hands together in front of you, placing the balls of your thumbs over the tops of your nostrils and keeping your palms slightly open (A).

๑ ฤๅษีสุเมธนั่ง ไม่ถนัด กระหย่งเท้าเท่าขัด เหลี่ยมถ้า
เอี้ยวองค์อีกสองหัตถ์ ไห้วเหนี่ยวอยู่เอย แหงนภักตรศีเพ่งฟ้า บอกแก้ลมเวียน ฯ

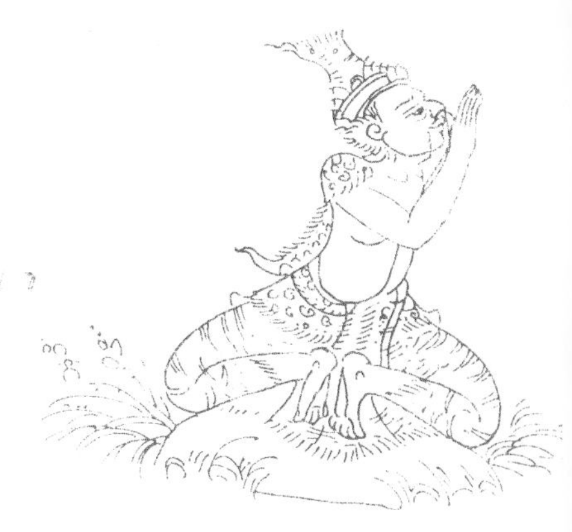

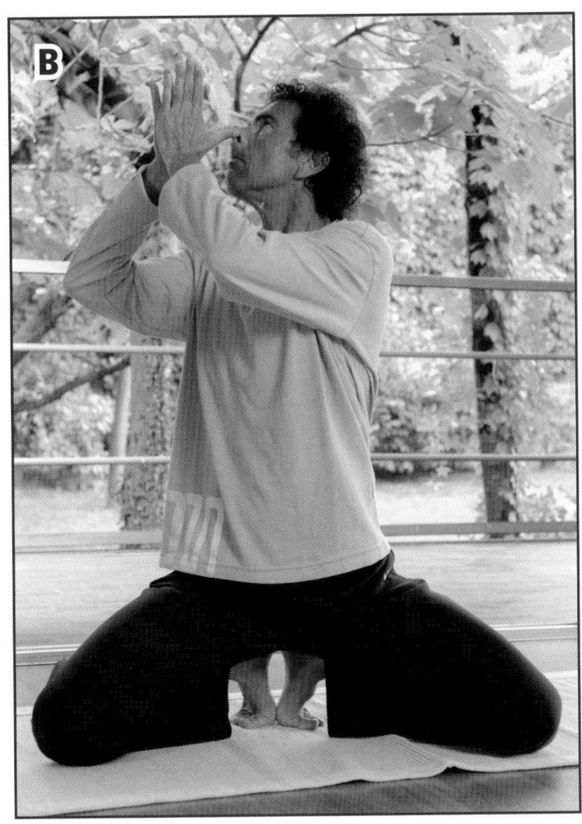

While breathing in, turn your shoulders to the right, and lift your head by pushing up with thumbs against your nostrils (B). This movement will open up the nostrils.

Holding your breath, maintain this position for 3 seconds.

As you breathe out, return slowly to the starting position.

Repeat the exercise, now turning to the left.

Perform the exercise 3 to 5 times, alternating back and forth between sides.

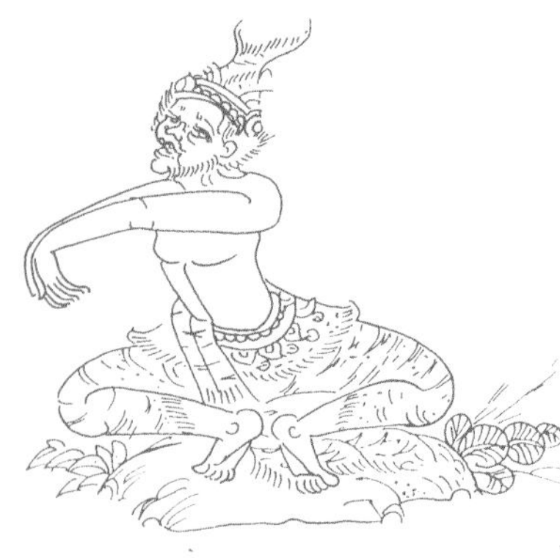

55
Remedy for Vertigo 2

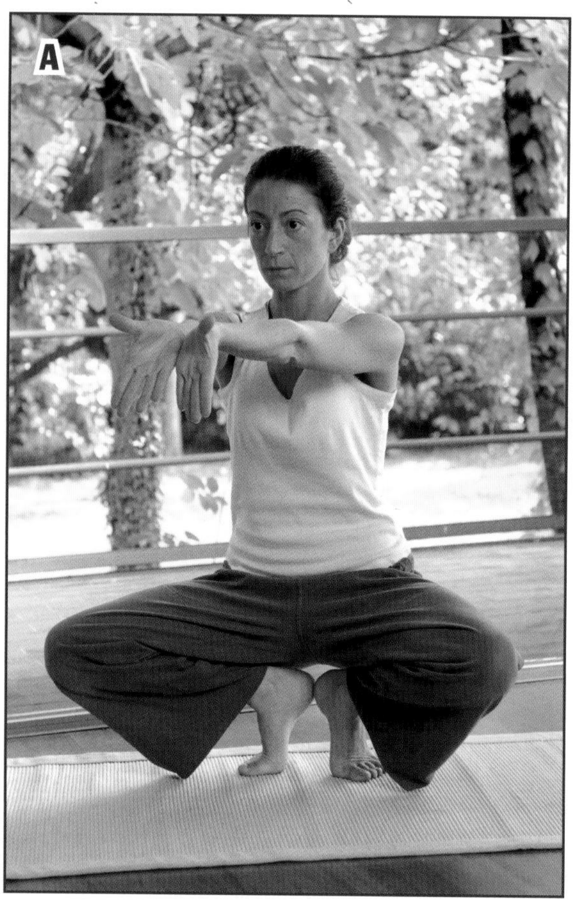

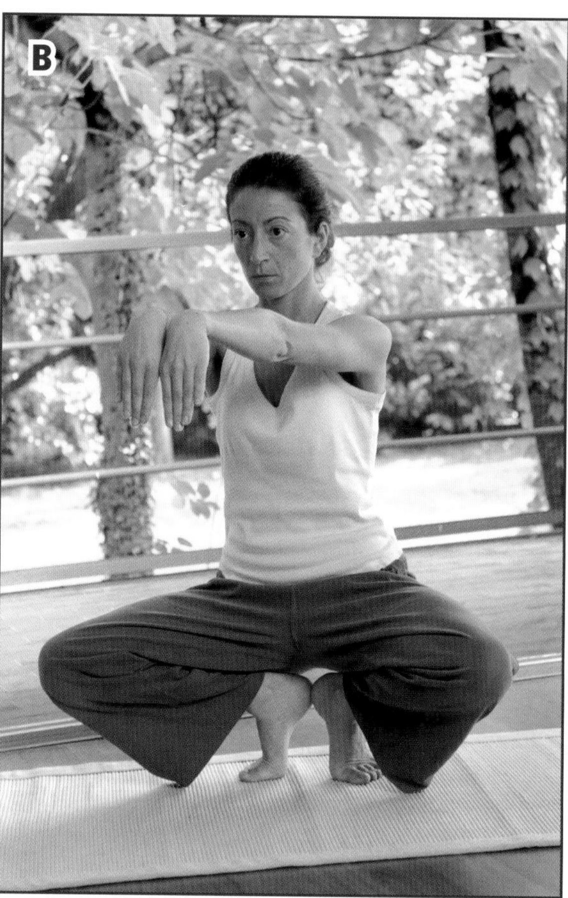

Squat with your heels together and the soles of your feet turned toward each other. Extend your arms in front of you, keeping your wrists flexed, your fingers pointing down, and your palms facing away from you (A).

Turn your wrists over and flex them forward, so that your palms now face you (B).

๏ แบะขคู้เข่าเข้า ชันเสมอ ปิดไหล่หงายเขนเผยอ ยืดไว้
เวียนเศียรจิตรใจเผลอ พลันเสื่อมสั่งนอ พระสุธามันต์ได้ ดัดแล้วอย่าฉงน ฯ

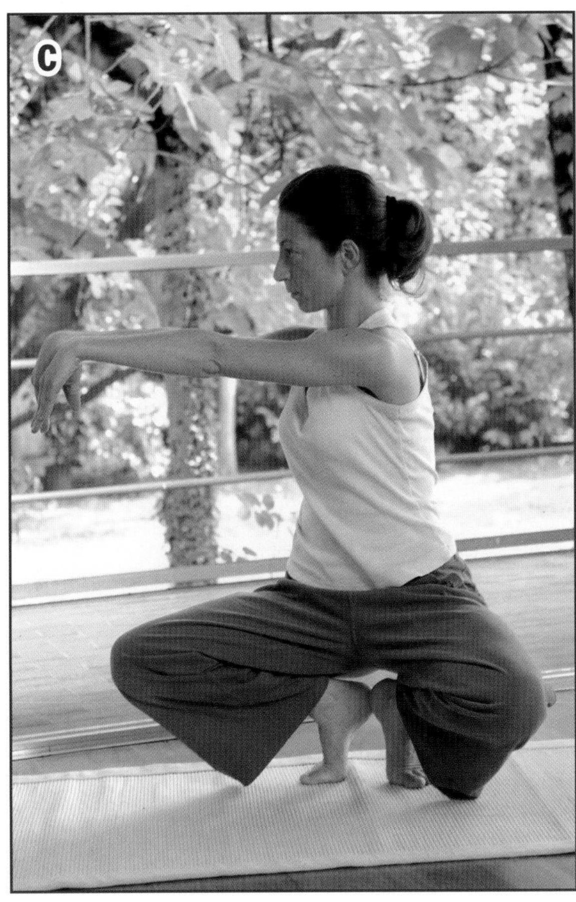

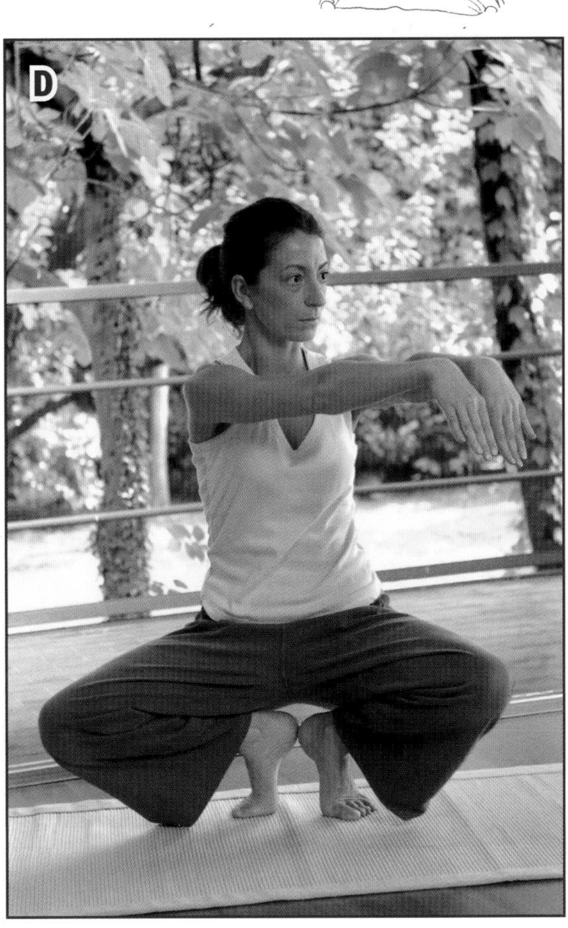

As you breathe in, twist your arms and chest to the right (C).

Holding your breath, maintain this position for 3 seconds.

As you breathe out, slowly return your arms and chest to the front.

Now as you breathe in, twist your arms and chest to the left (D).

Holding your breath, maintain this position for 3 seconds.

As you breathe out, return slowly to the starting position.

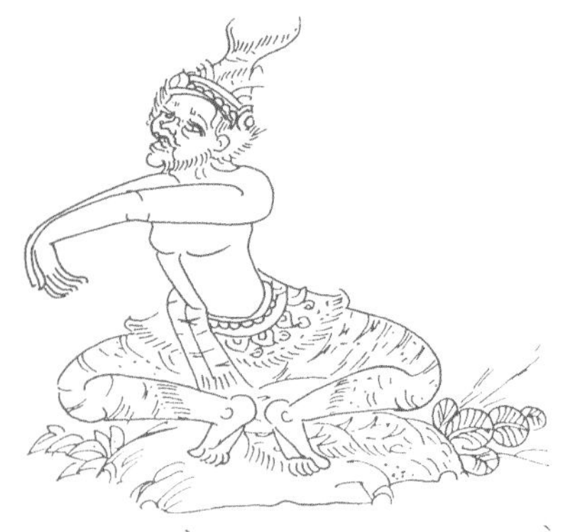

๏ แบะขาคู้เข่าเข้า ชันเสมอ บิดไหล่หงายแขนเผยอ ยืดไว้
เวียนเศียรจิตรใจเผลอ พลันเลื่อมส่างนอ พระสุธามันต์ได้ ดัดแล้วอย่าฉงน ฯ

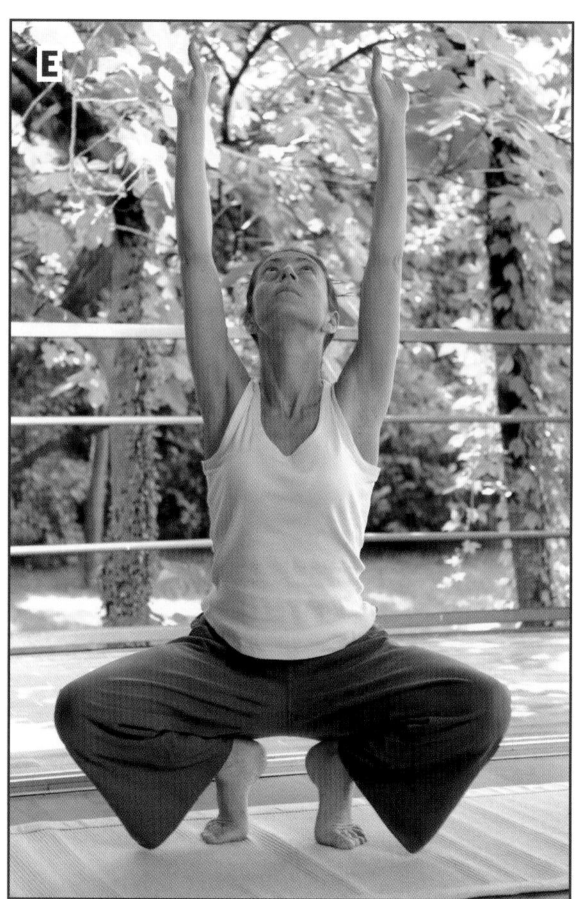

While breathing in, lift your arms over your head. Bend your arms, shoulders, and head backward as far as you can while still maintaining your balance (E).

Holding your breath, maintain this position for 3 seconds.

As you breathe out, return slowly to the starting position.

Repeat entire exercise sequence 3 to 5 times.

56
Remedy for Chronic Muscular Discomfort

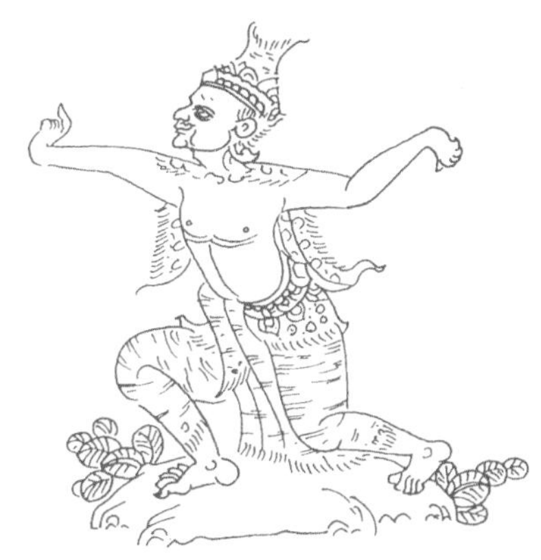

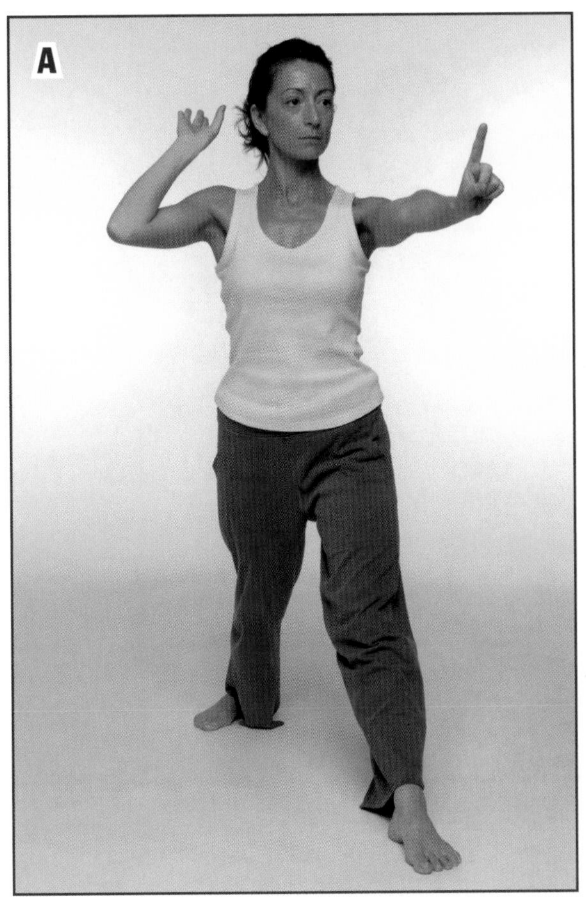

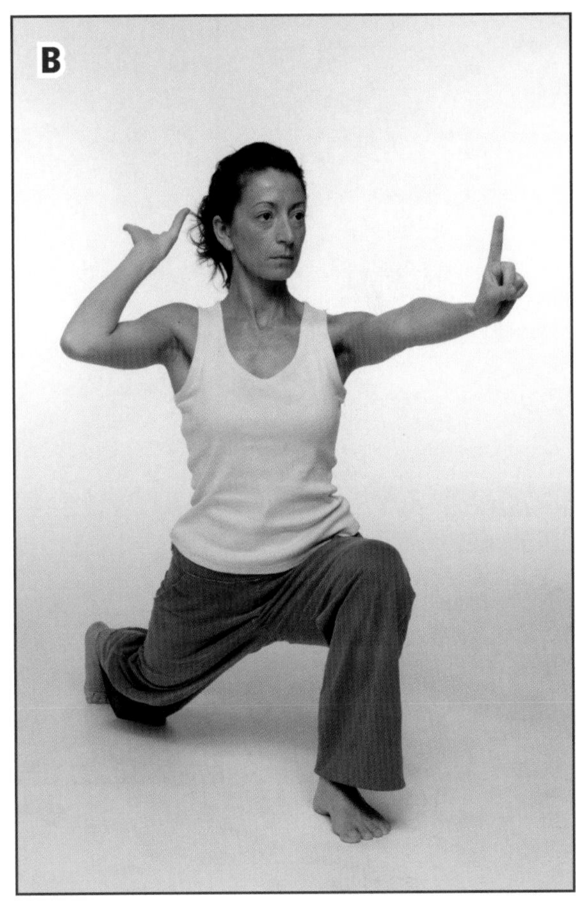

Pull your right leg back to stand with your legs apart and your heels aligned. Turn your right foot out at a 45-degree angle and point your left foot forward. Bend your right arm backward, keeping the wrist well flexed. Stretch your left arm in front of you, closing your hand into a fist with the forefinger pointing upward. Focus your sight on your forefinger (A).

As you breathe out, turn your right foot to align it with the left one, and bend your left leg and flex the right one (B).

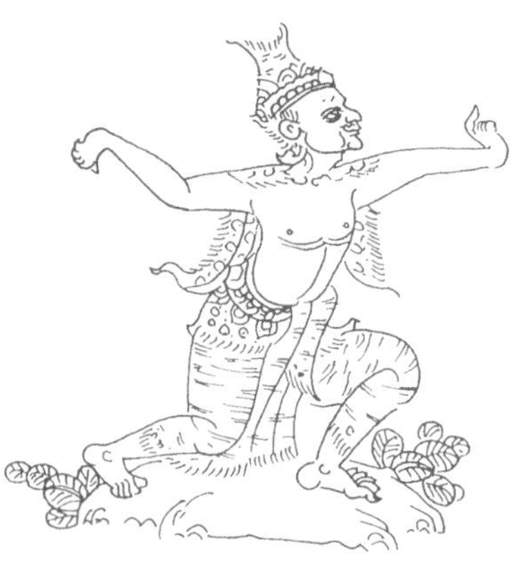

๏ สัขณ์ไลยลี้หลีก ละสงสารแฮ ยืนย่างหยัดเหยียดองค์ อ่อนแล้

สองหัตถ์ท่าทีทม ศรสาตรไปเอย บำบัดปัศฆาฏแก้ กล่อนแห้งหืดหาย ฯ

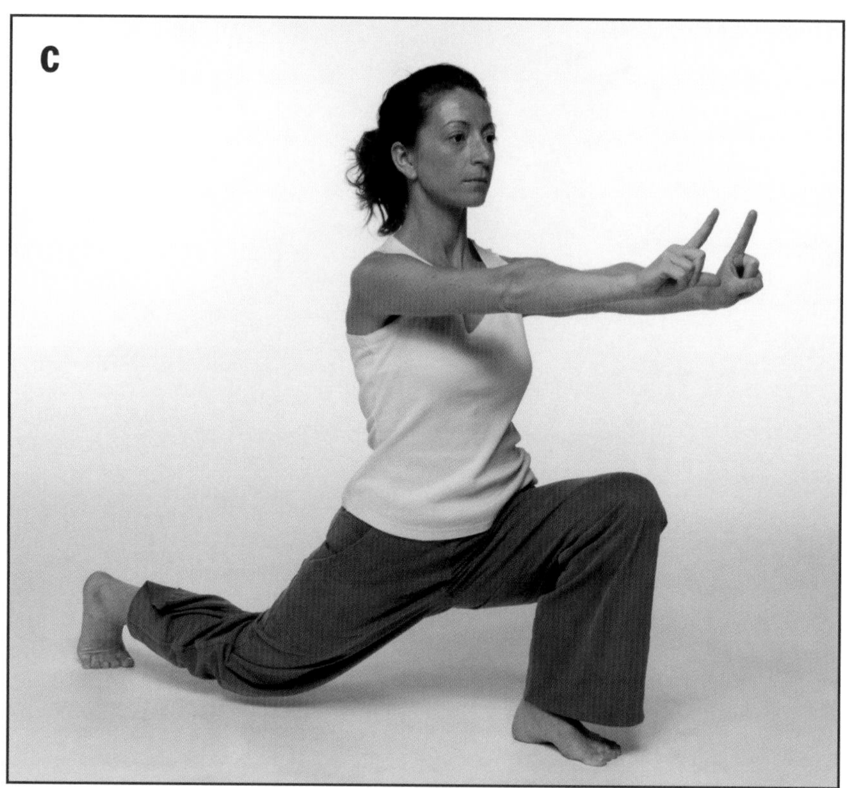

Breathing in, stretch out your right arm to align it with the left one, in the same position. Now focus on both forefingers (C).

Holding your breath, maintain this position for 3 seconds.

As you breathe out, return slowly to the starting position.

Perform the exercise 3 to 5 times. Then practice the exercise on the other side.

57 Remedy for Painful Muscle Cramps

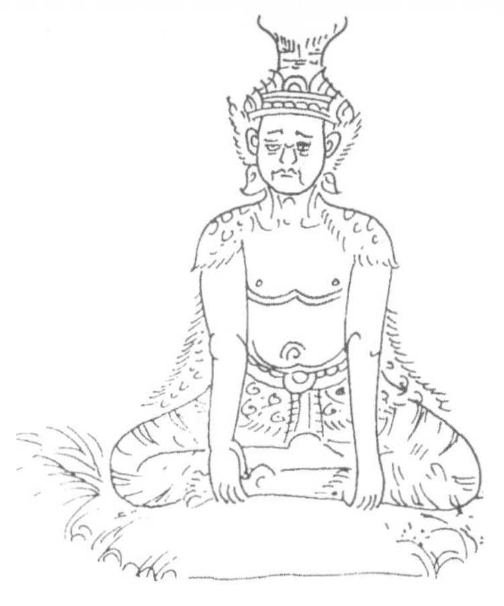

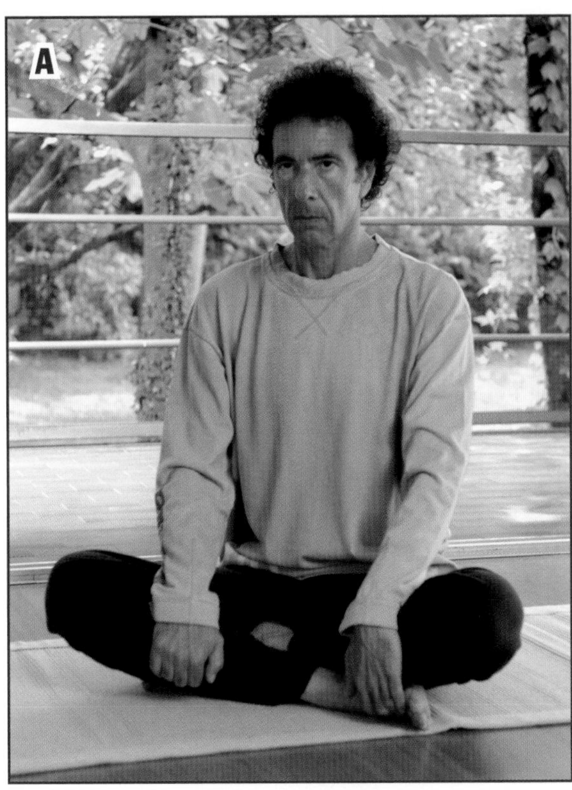

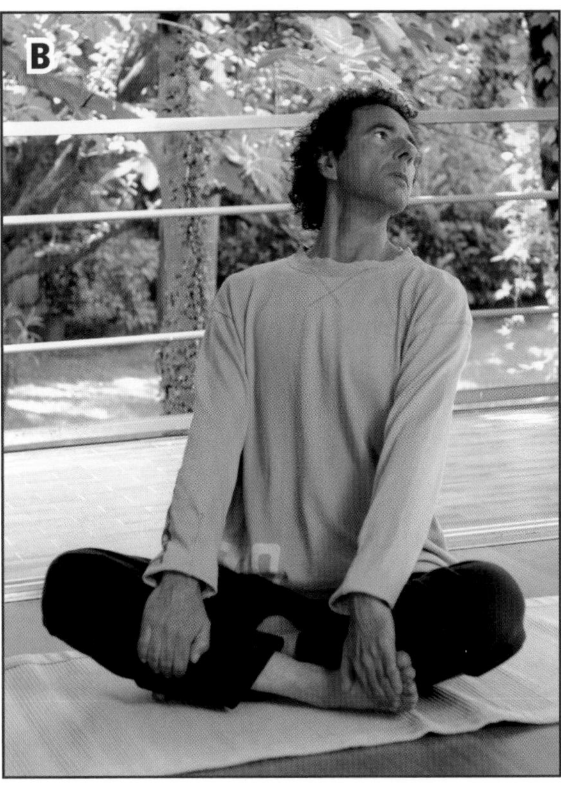

Sit cross-legged. Hold the foot and shin of whichever leg is in front with your hands, keeping your arms shoulder width apart (A).

While breathing in, turn your head to the left as far as you can, lifting it up (B). This movement will stretch your chest. Keep a good grip on your leg to avoid losing your balance.

Holding your breath, maintain this position for 3 seconds.

As you breathe out, return slowly to the starting position.

Alternating back and forth between sides, repeat the exercise 3 to 5 times. (You do not need to change the position of your legs.)

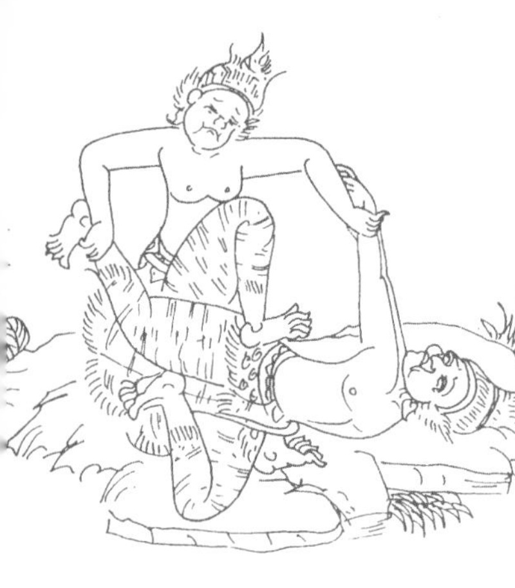

58 Remedy for Muscle Cramps

The original drawing of Jivaka performing this exercise shows another person assisting. The instruction we've prepared allows you to perform the exercise by yourself while remaining as faithful as possible to the original movement.

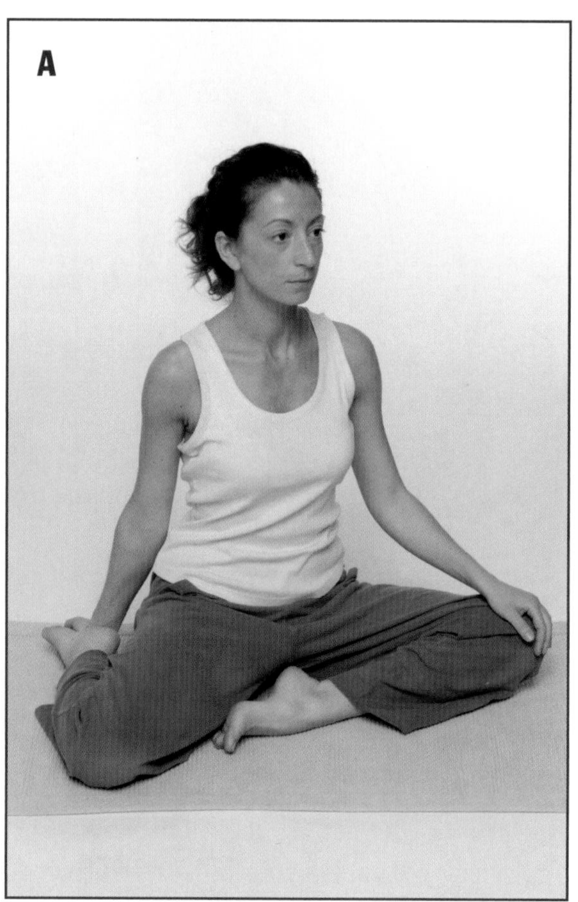
A

Sit in Thai position, with your right leg bent to the outside and your left leg to the inside. Place your left hand on your left knee. Hold your right foot with your right hand (A).

๑ สวามิตคุกเข่าแล้ว เหลี่ยวภักตร์ฝินแฮ วสิทธิเหยียบยันสลัก เพชเคล้น
กรขวาจับบาทชัก เฉวียงฉุดแขนแฮ โรคตะคริวกล่อนเส้น หย่อนได้หลายเดือน ฯ

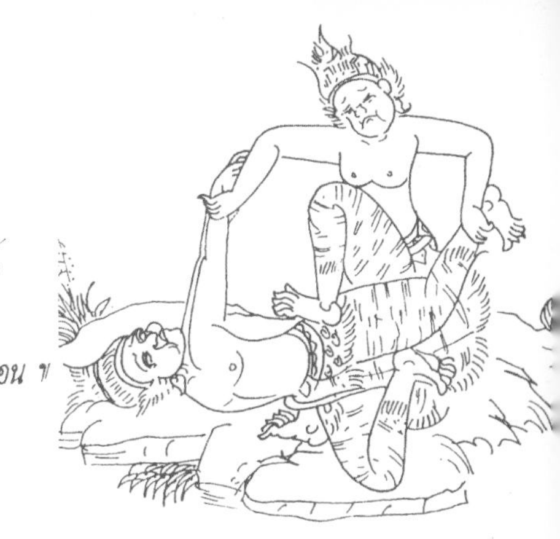

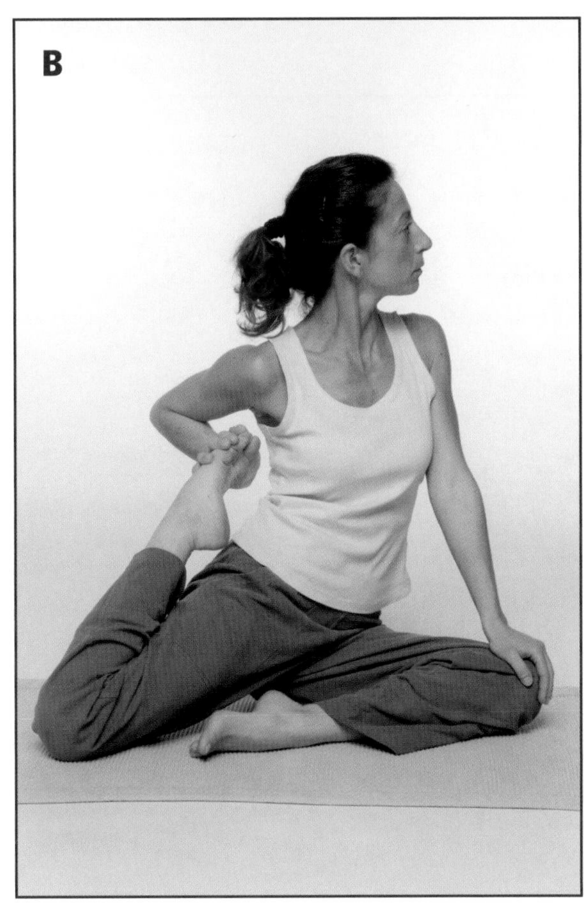

As you breathe in, pull your right leg up and forward, using your outstretched left arm to hold your chest upright (B).

Holding your breath, maintain this position for 3 seconds.

As you breathe out, return slowly to the starting position.

Perform the exercise 3 to 5 times. Then practice the exercise on the other side.

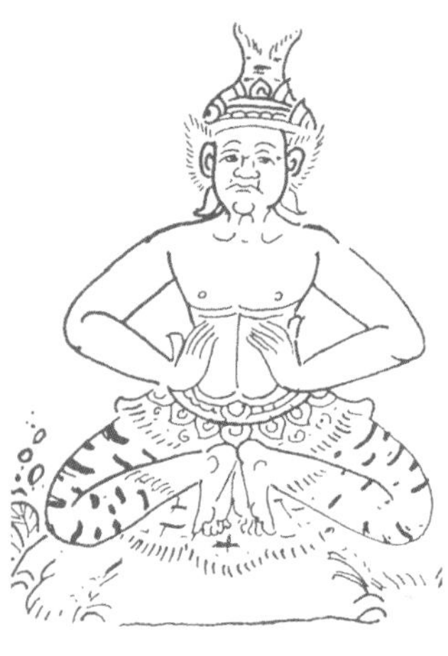

59 Remedy for Hemiplegia

(Paralysis of One Side of the Body)

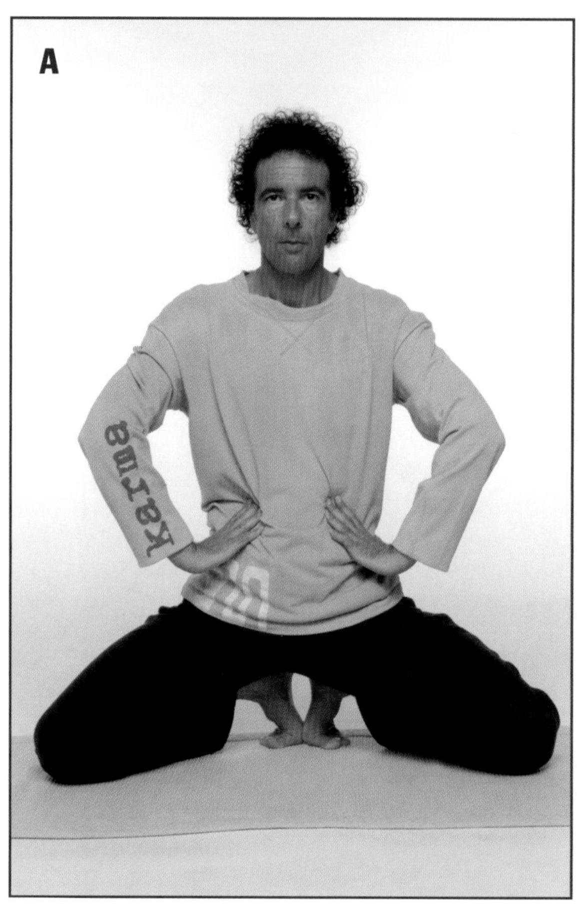

Kneel with your feet flexed, resting your buttocks on your heels and opening your legs as widely as you can. Place your hands on your abdomen just below the rib cage, with your fingers pointing up (A).

๑ โคลินทร์เบะอกให้ รามแผลงอสุรฤๅ สาปไกนนทรีแรง ฤทธิ์เฟ้า
อมพฤกพิบัติแสดง ดัดดับคลายนอ ตั้งชันสองมือเข้า ประทับข้างขีนองค์

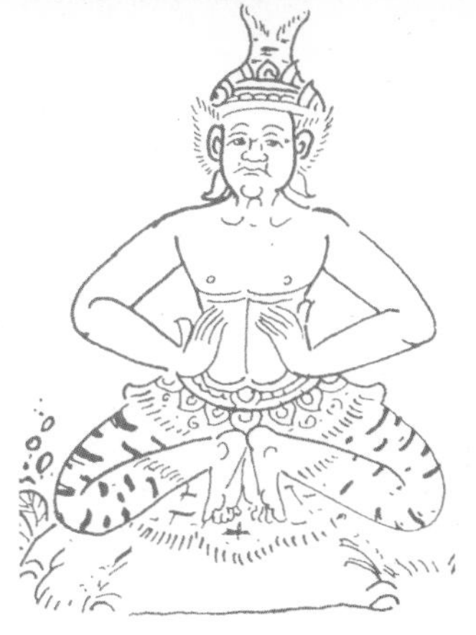

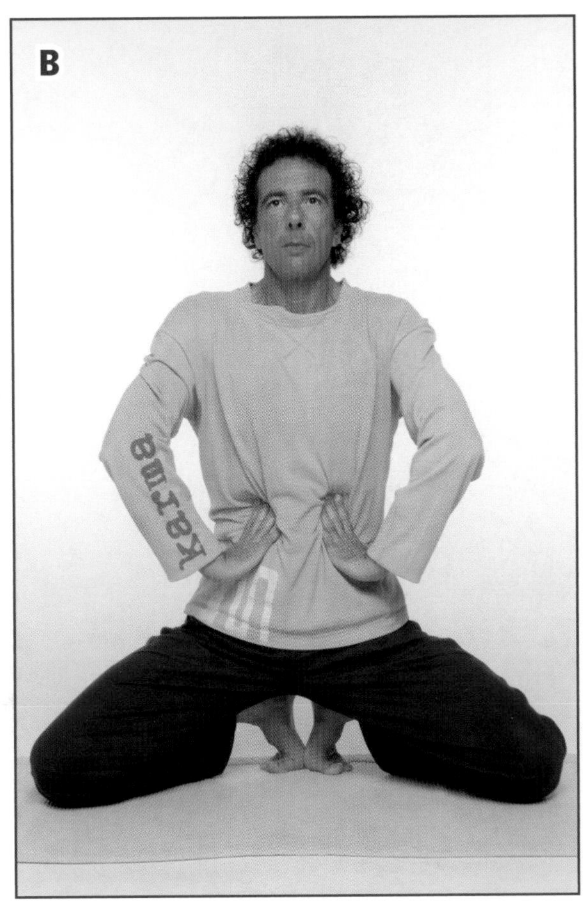

Breathing in, press into your abdomen with your fingers, pushing slightly upward, and at the same time slightly lift your head (B).

Holding your breath, maintain this position for 3 seconds.

As you breathe out, return slowly to the starting position.

Repeat the exercise 3 to 5 times.

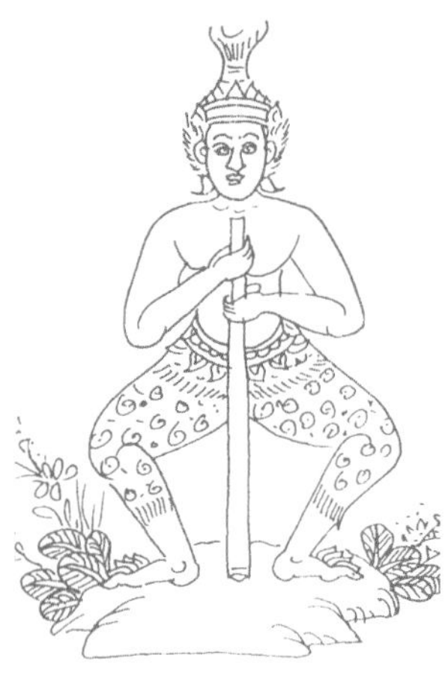

60 Posture for Enhancing Longevity

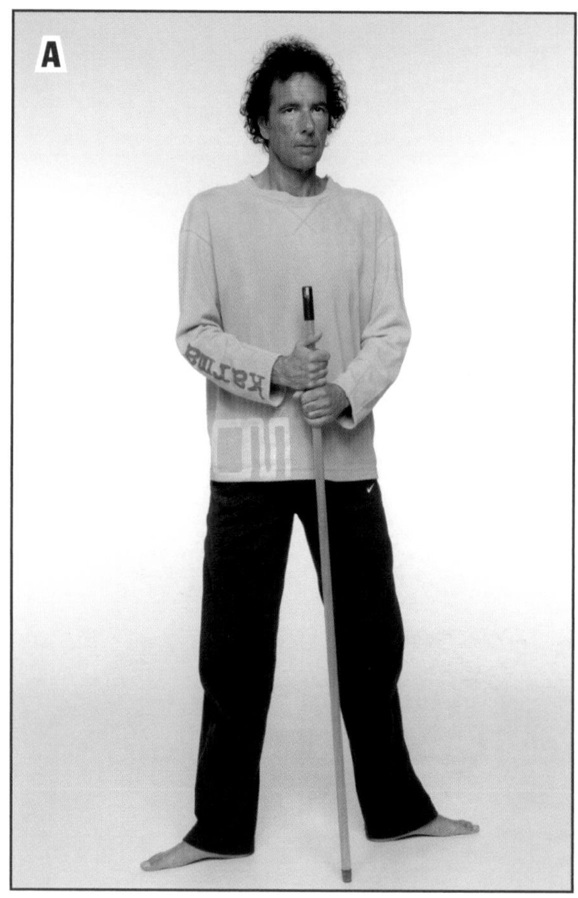

Stand with your feet 10 to 12 inches (25–30 cm) apart. Point your toes outward as much as you can while still maintaining your balance. With both hands, hold a stick upright in front of you (A).

๏ ทิศไภยิโพ้นผนวดช้าง เขาเขอน ทิวพนัศชยเนอน ท่าเถ้า
ประณิบัติคัดองค์เจรอญ ชนม์ชีพพระนา กุมกดธารกรค้ำ พ่างพื้นยืนยัน ฯ

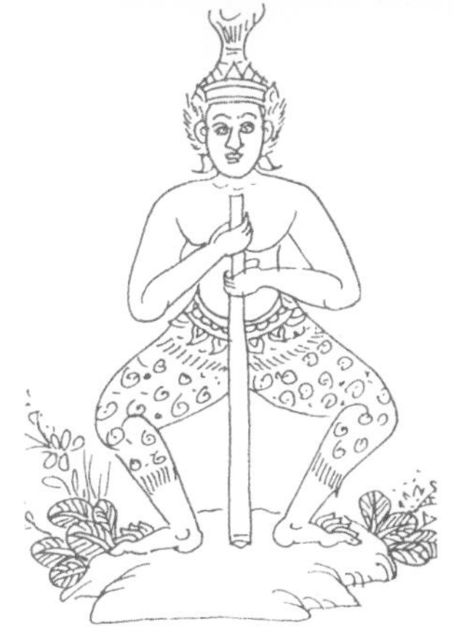

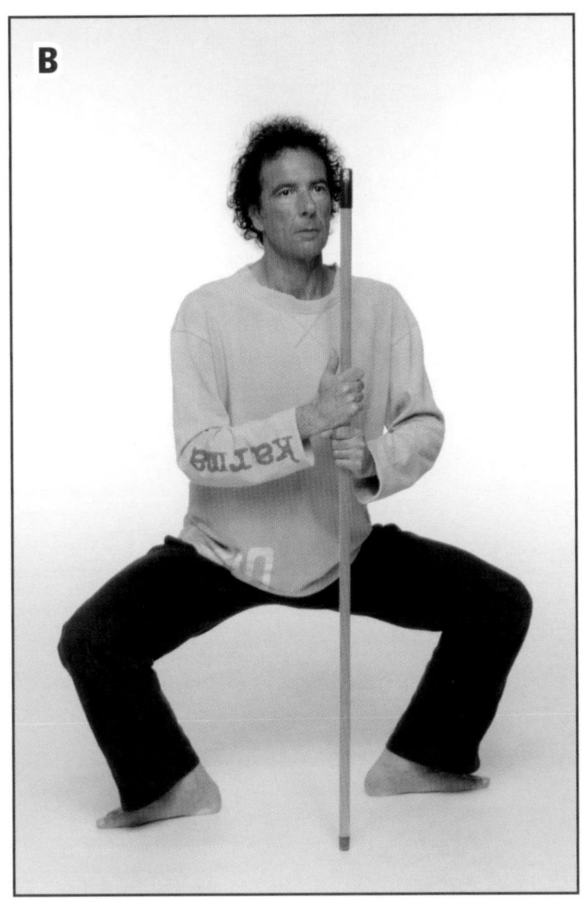

As you breathe in, lower your torso as much as possible by bending your knees outward, using the stick to help you keep your balance. At the same time, contract the muscles in your buttocks and anus (B).

Holding your breath, maintain this position for 3 seconds.

As you breathe out, return slowly to the starting position.

Repeat the exercise 3 to 5 times.

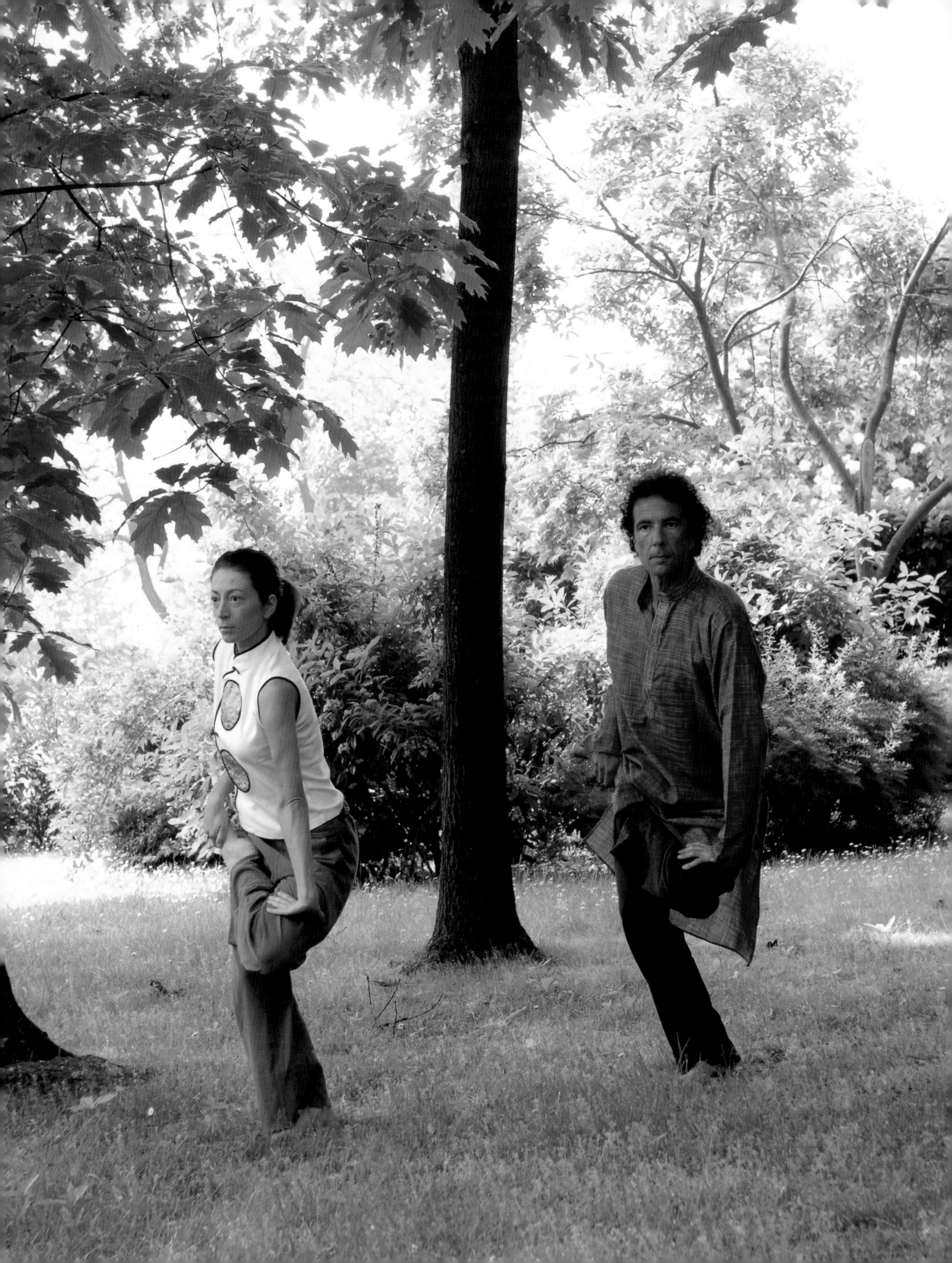

APPENDIX

Ailments from Head to Toe

Although each exercise is named according to its primary therapeutic use, as determined by the creator of this discipline, Jivaka, the exercises have a wider therapeutic value. In fact, most of the exercises provide at least some benefit to all ten of the sen channels. When complementary exercises are practiced as a sequence, Thai yoga can be useful in the treatment of many common ailments, in particular those that limit or cause pain during movement.

Below you'll find exercises grouped according to the ailments they are able to treat or prevent. For best effectiveness, you should practice them regularly, every day if possible, until the symptoms have disappeared or been greatly reduced. If you are not able to practice all the exercises indicated for the treatment of an ailment, try to practice at least some of them daily in order to get good results.

Neck Pain

- Ex 1, Remedy for Tension Headache
- Ex 3, Remedy for Sinus Congestion
- Ex 4, Remedy for Neck Pain
- Ex 5, Remedy for Neck and Shoulder Pain
- Ex 7, Remedy for Shoulder Pain

- Ex 9, Remedy for Shoulder and Shoulder Blade Pain
- Ex 13, Remedy for Chest, Shoulder, and Abdominal Pain
- Ex 24, Remedy for Abdominal Pain and Ankle Pain
- Ex 57, Remedy for Painful Muscle Cramps

Shoulder Pain

- Ex 5, Remedy for Neck and Shoulder Pain
- Ex 6, Remedy for Neck and Shoulder Stiffness
- Ex 7, Remedy for Shoulder Pain
- Ex 8, Remedy for Shoulder Stiffness and Pain
- Ex 10, Remedy for Shoulder and Hip Pain 1
- Ex 11, Remedy for Shoulder and Hip Pain 2
- Ex 13, Remedy for Chest, Shoulder, and Abdominal Pain
- Ex 22, Remedy for Abdominal Pain and Shoulder Blade Pain
- Ex 24, Remedy for Abdominal Pain and Ankle Pain

Arm Pain

- Ex 5, Remedy for Neck and Shoulder Pain
- Ex 32, Remedy for Arm Pain
- Ex 33 Remedy for Arm Stiffness
- Ex 34, Remedy for Joint Pain in the Arms and Hands
- Ex 35, Remedy for Wrist Pain
- Ex 36, Remedy for Arm and Leg Pain
- Ex 47, Remedy for Overall Uneasiness

Middle and Lower Back Pain

- Ex 5, Remedy for Neck and Shoulder Pain
- Ex 16, Remedy for Pressure in the Chest 2
- Ex 21, Remedy for Sharp Pain at the Waist
- Ex 25, Remedy for Lower Back Pain
- Ex 26, Remedy for Lower Back and Hip Pain
- Ex 27, Remedy for Lower Back and Leg Pain
- Ex 28, Remedy for Hemorrhoids

- Ex 36, Remedy for Arm and Leg Pain
- Ex 48, Remedy for a Lack of Motivation
- Ex 50, Remedy for a Feeling of Suffocation

Hip Pain

- Ex 10, Remedy for Shoulder and Hip Pain 1
- Ex 11, Remedy for Shoulder and Hip Pain 2
- Ex 12, Remedy for Shoulder and Leg Stiffness
- Ex 18, Remedy for Intercostal Pain
- Ex 26, Remedy for Lower Back and Hip Pain
- Ex 47, Remedy for Overall Uneasiness

Leg Pain

- Ex 7, Remedy for Shoulder Pain
- Ex 8, Remedy for Shoulder Stiffness and Pain
- Ex 12, Remedy for Shoulder and Leg Stiffness
- Ex 15, Remedy for Pressure in the Chest 1
- Ex 17, Remedy for Heartburn
- Ex 27, Remedy for Lower Back and Leg Pain
- Ex 31, Remedy for Pain in the Testicles and Difficult Urination
- Ex 37, Remedy for Hand and Foot Cramps
- Ex 40, Remedy for Knee Dislocation
- Ex 41, Remedy for Knee and Leg Trouble
- Ex 42, Remedy for Knee, Leg, and Chest Problems
- Ex 43, Remedy for Leg and Neck Pain
- Ex 44, Remedy for Foot Numbness
- Ex 46, Remedy for Heel Pain
- Ex 58, Remedy for Muscle Cramps

Knee Pain

- Ex 38, Remedy for Stiffness in the Knees
- Ex 39, Remedy for Knee Pain
- Ex 40, Remedy for Knee Dislocation

- Ex 41, Remedy for Knee and Leg Trouble
- Ex 42, Remedy for Knee, Leg, and Chest Problems
- Ex 44, Remedy for Foot Numbness

Foot Pain

- Ex 36, Remedy for Arm and Leg Pain
- Ex 37, Remedy for Hand and Foot Cramps
- Ex 44, Remedy for Foot Numbness
- Ex 45, Remedy for Pain in the Sole of the Foot
- Ex 46, Remedy for Heel Pain

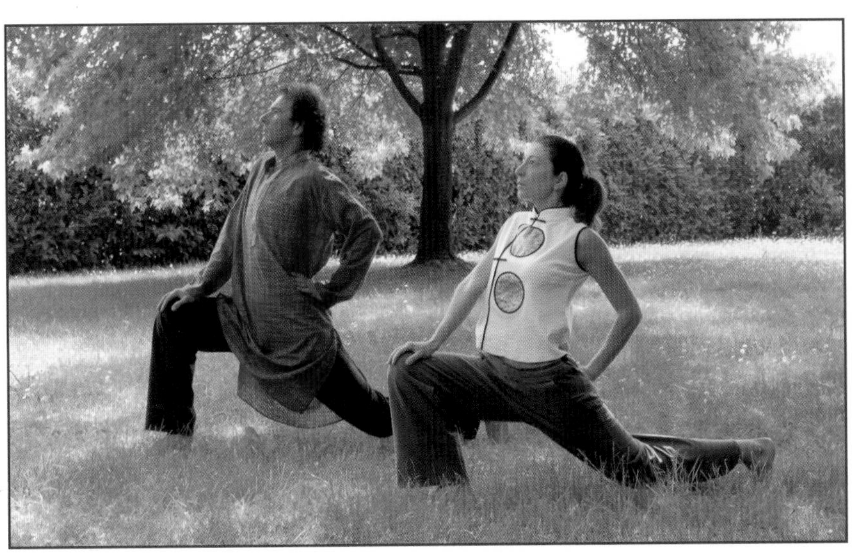

ABOUT THE AUTHORS

Enrico Corsi received his first degree in traditional Thai massage in 1995 from the Wat Pho temple school in Bangkok, Thailand. Since then he has returned to Thailand at least once a year to pursue studies and receive certification in a variety of Thai healing disciplines, including advanced (therapeutic) Thai massage, Thai foot massage, Thai herbal massage, Thai aromatherapy massage, and traditional Thai yoga. At Wat Pho he studied with a number of traditional Thai teachers including Tung and Sonh Pohn. Especially in the discipline of traditional Thai yoga, Enrico has had the opportunity to study with private individuals unaffiliated with any school, including several Thai Buddhist monks. He is the founder of the Accademia di Massaggio Tradizionale Thailandese in Milan, Italy, and lives in Milan.

For more information on Enrico Corsi please visit his websites:

www.thaiacademy.it • www.thaiacademy.org
www.thaiyogahouse.com
E-mail: info@thaiacademy.it

Elena Fanfani received her degree in traditional Thai massage in 2001 from the Wat Pho temple school in Bangkok, Thailand. There she studied with traditional Thai teachers Sunee, Sonh Pohn, Imrak, and Tung. In addition to pursuing studies in traditional Thai yoga and traditional

Thai massage, she has received instruction and certification in a full range of Thai healing techniques at Wat Pho, including Thai foot massage, Thai herbal compress massage (including postnatal applications), Bab massage, Thai aromatherapy and oil massage, and Thai facial massage, with a special emphasis on healing for women and children. To deepen her knowledge, she continues to visit Thailand to meet with her old teachers and to study with new ones, including Kung, at the Bangkok branch of the Khaokho Talaypu Natural Farm. Elena lives in Milan, Italy.

For more information on Elena Fanfani please visit her website:

www.thaiyogastudio.com.
E-mail: info@thaiyogastudio.com

Index

BOOKS OF RELATED INTEREST

Thai Yoga Massage
A Dynamic Therapy for Physical Well-Being and Spiritual Energy
Book & DVD Set
by Kam Thye Chow

Thai Yoga Therapy for Your Body Type
An Ayurvedic Tradition
by Kam Thye Chow and Emily Moody

The Yin Yoga Kit
The Practice of Quiet Power
by Biff Mithoefer

The Heart of Yoga
Developing a Personal Practice
by T. K. V. Desikachar

Self-Awakening Yoga
The Expansion of Consciousness through the Body's Own Wisdom
by Don Stapleton, Ph.D.

Yoga for the Three Stages of Life
Developing Your Practice As an Art Form, a Physical Therapy, and a Guiding Philosophy
by Srivatsa Ramaswami

The Five Tibetans
Five Dynamic Exercises for Health, Energy, and Personal Power
by Christopher S. Kilham

Like a Fish in Water
Yoga for Children
by Isabelle Koch

The New Rules of Posture
How to Sit, Stand, and Move in the Modern World
by Mary Bond

Inner Traditions • Bear & Company
P.O. Box 388
Rochester, VT 05767
1-800-246-8648
www.InnerTraditions.com

Or contact your local bookseller